In *Find Your Peace* Dr. Rodica Malos offers medical recommendations as well as supernatural prescriptions that will never expire to prevent or cure illnesses of a physical or emotional nature or both. The book is not only informative but also an inspiration to those who suffer, those who provide health care, and educators. You will find it a valuable resource.

—Ligia Berci, MD
Child, Adolescent, and Adult Psychiatry
Sacramento, California

As Rodica's daughter, I have seen her journey firsthand, and I can say with confidence that she practices the principles outlined in *Find Your Peace* with excellence. Her passion to promote health through integrating mind, body, and spirit is apparent throughout the entire book. *Find Your Peace* highlights non-pharmacologic solutions to prevent disease and focuses on the Lord's supernatural prescriptions to overcome stress, anxiety, and fear. Rodica's words are practical and profound, supported by in-depth research. This book will strengthen your faith and inspire you to step into the freedom for which God destined you.

—Andreea (Malos) Steward, PharmD
Portland, Oregon

Dr. Rodica Malos miraculously merged the spiritual and scientific worlds in her book *Find Your Peace*. After reading the book, you are confident within the depth of your being that God is a reality of our world and ourselves and that our faith in God has a scientific foundation, which cannot be questioned or doubted any further.

She brings to the surface how much our spiritual health can influence our physical health and how nurturing our souls and minds is as important as nurturing our bodies.

As I navigated through the message of *Find Your Peace*, my faith in our eternal Creator grew stronger and my desire to live and give myself for others was deeper. I value the effort Dr. Malos invested in her work. She is a spiritual giant and a scientist with great capacity to connect the two worlds.

—Emilia Arden, DO, FACC
Cardiologist, GRH Cardiology Clinic
Medford, Oregon

Dr. Rodica Malos treats with realism, warmth, and emotions a topical subject that generates concern. This is a book worth reading by teenagers and older people alike. Man was created with body, soul, and spirit and should be treated as such. Medicine tries to treat the physical and psychological consequences of wrong choices that take place in our hearts. Dr. Rodica is trying to make us aware of the real roots of the problems and to help us take action accordingly.

Find Your Peace is an honest, reasoned pleading for abundant life.

God is truth. There is no contradiction between true science and true religion. Both of them are in the quest of exploring the same truth. Man has departed from his Creator, who gave him clear instructions for living a fulfilled life both physically and spiritually. In *Find Your Peace* we find an accurate description of modern man, quoted from the Bible: lover of self, lover of money, selfish, ungrateful, proud, lover of pleasure, and living a lifestyle that brings stress, anxiety, fear, and worry. The solution is renewing of the mind, a return to God, and trusting completely in Him by knowing His character and His promises.

—Stefan Puscasu, MD, General Surgeon
Founder, Bethesda Hospital and Polyclinic
Suceava, Romania

Dr. Rodica's book *Find Your Peace* brings spiritual food to a starving world. Her book highlights the keys to health as given to us in God's timeless Word. Science is finally catching up with God's plan for humankind, planted deep within our DNA. May this book open our eyes to see, and to know, the truth as we live out our destiny in these end times.

—Kay E. Metsger RN, BSN
Former Nurse Manager, Cardiovascular Operating Room,
Providence St. Vincent Medical Center
Portland, Oregon
Star of Hope International Board Member

Dr. Malos gives an abundance of scientific research that confirms the timeless teachings of the Bible. She shows, through the latest medical discoveries, the clear link between stress, anxiety, negative thinking, and the most common diseases in our society. She also describes clearly the biblical solutions that can prevent and reverse these diseases and lead to optimal health. This brilliant and practical book has the power to transform lives. I highly recommend it to health care professionals, pastors, counselors, and any other person who wants to learn how to live the abundant, healthy life that God desires for all of us.

—Oliver Ghitea, MD
Anesthesiologist
Portland, Oregon

In *Find Your Peace*, Dr. Rodica Malos reveals a remarkable correlation between medical science and biblical principles for our mental and physical health. We are created in the image of God, our heavenly Father, and we have all the potential of His DNA within us. "I am fearfully and wonderfully made" (Ps. 139:14).

My wife and I have had the distinct privilege of knowing Dr. Rodica for more than twenty years, as she worked with us in our local church as well as in missions. Dr. Rodica is a caring, compassionate soul—a visionary person of creativity and impeccable integrity. Her life has been marked by a spirit of excellence and enthusiasm. She is consumed with a passion to enrich and improve the life of everyone she comes in contact with. Hence, *Find Your Peace* is a must-read for invaluable information as well as personal inspiration and transformation.

—Pastors Ed and Cheryl Rebman
New Beginnings Church, Portland Campus

In this groundbreaking new book Dr. Rodica Malos has woven together years of her own personal research to connect spiritual, scientific, and medical facts in a cutting-edge, powerful, and life-changing way. She teaches that the brain, human will, and the ability to choose are incredibly powerful forces. We can break free and overcome negative patterns that have held us captive, perhaps for generations. She lays out a clear, easy-to-understand path to follow to step out of your past and step into your great future.

Dr. Rodica's groundbreaking teachings reveal that medical and scientific truths do not nullify God's biblical spiritual truths. They in fact prove God's biblical spiritual truths. Physical and spiritual realms do not contradict one another. They confirm and complete one another. The teachings in this book are bold, brilliant, and powerful and will change your life, circumstances, and future forever.

—Pastors Larry and Tiz Huch
Senior Pastors, Founders, and Directors, DFW New Beginnings Church, Dallas/Fort Worth; New Beginnings Stream Church, Portland, Oregon; and Global Stream Ministries
Larry Huch Ministries Global TV and Media Outreach Network

Find Your Peace is a fascinating book in which Dr. Rodica masterfully uses the Word of God to explain the science and physiology of our brains. Dr. Rodica weaves together the Bible and biology in a way that brings validity to the Creator and lays out His step-by-step plan for our healing and wholeness.

—Pastors Brad and Lisa Makowski
Lead Pastors, Anthem Church
Portland, Oregon

Find Your Peace is a revolutionary, life-changing book, an essential training manual for the believer, and a must-read for those who wish to walk in victory. Great practical and spiritual applications abound in this book. The extensive research this book brings will impact lives around the world.

I felt gripped throughout as the extraordinary scientific knowledge wrapped alongside the Scriptures came together to highlight the genius of our Creator and the plan He has for us all. It is a book that you can read over and over again—an encyclopedic revelation of the supernatural and a road map for the natural.

—SHANEEN CLARKE
FOUNDER, SHANEEN CLARKE MINISTRIES AND AWC CHARITY; PATRON, RHEMA PARTNERSHIP
SPEAKER, AUTHOR, AND COACH

FIND YOUR PEACE

RODICA MALOS, DNP

SILOAM

Most Charisma House Book Group products are available at special quantity discounts for bulk purchase for sales promotions, premiums, fund-raising, and educational needs. For details, call us at (407) 333-0600 or visit our website at www.charismahouse.com.

Find Your Peace by Rodica Malos, DNP
Published by Siloam
Charisma Media/Charisma House Book Group
600 Rinehart Road, Lake Mary, Florida 32746

This book or parts thereof may not be reproduced in any form, stored in a retrieval system, or transmitted in any form by any means—electronic, mechanical, photocopy, recording, or otherwise—without prior written permission of the publisher, except as provided by United States of America copyright law.

Unless otherwise noted, all Scripture quotations are taken from the Holy Bible, New International Version®, NIV®. Copyright © 1973, 1978, 1984, 2011 by Biblica, Inc.® Used by permission of Zondervan. All rights reserved worldwide. www.zondervan.com. The "NIV" and "New International Version" are trademarks registered in the United States Patent and Trademark Office by Biblica, Inc.®

Scripture quotations marked csb have been taken from the Christian Standard Bible®, Copyright © 2017 by Holman Bible Publishers. Used by permission. Christian Standard Bible® and CSB® are federally registered trademarks of Holman Bible Publishers.

Scripture quotations marked esv are from the Holy Bible, English Standard Version. Copyright © 2001 by Crossway Bibles, a division of Good News Publishers. Used by permission.

Scripture quotations marked kjv are from the King James Version of the Bible.

Scripture quotations marked nasb are from the New American Standard Bible, copyright © 1960, 1962, 1963, 1968, 1971, 1972, 1973, 1975, 1977, 1995 by The Lockman Foundation. Used by permission. www.Lockman.org.

Scripture quotations marked ncv are taken from the New Century Version®. Copyright © 2005 by Thomas Nelson. Used by permission. All rights reserved.

Scripture quotations marked net are from the NET Bible® copyright ©1996–2016 by Biblical Studies Press, L.L.C. http://netbible.com. All rights reserved.

Scripture quotations marked nkjv are taken from the New King James Version®. Copyright © 1982 by Thomas Nelson. Used by permission. All rights reserved.

Scripture quotations marked nlt are from the Holy Bible, New Living Translation, copyright © 1996, 2004, 2007. Used by permission of Tyndale House Publishers, Inc., Wheaton, IL 60189. All rights reserved.

Copyright © 2020 by Rodica Malos, DNP
All rights reserved

Visit the author's website at rodicamalos.com.

Library of Congress Cataloging-in-Publication Data

Names: Malos, Rodica, author.
Title: Find your peace / by Rodica Malos.
Description: Lake Mary, Florida : Siloam, [2020] | Includes bibliographical references and index.
Identifiers: LCCN 2019046199 (print) | LCCN 2019046200 (ebook) | ISBN 9781629996813 (trade paperback) | ISBN 9781629996820 (ebook)
Subjects: LCSH: Peace of mind--Religious aspects--Christianity. | Stress (Psychology)--Religious aspects--Christianity.
Classification: LCC BV4908.5 .M3365 2020 (print) | LCC BV4908.5 (ebook) | DDC 248.8/6--dc23
LC record available at https://lccn.loc.gov/2019046199
LC ebook record available at https://lccn.loc.gov/2019046200

This book contains the opinions and ideas of its author. It is solely for informational and educational purposes and should not be regarded as a substitute for professional medical treatment. The nature of your body's health condition is complex and unique. Therefore, you should consult a health professional before you begin any new lifestyle change, exercise, nutrition, fasting, or supplementation program, or if you have questions about your health. Neither the author nor the publisher shall be liable or responsible for any loss or damage allegedly arising from any information or suggestion in this book.

People and names in this book are composites created by the author from her experiences as a primary care practitioner. Names and details of their stories have been changed, and any similarity between the names and stories of individuals described in this book and individuals known to readers is purely coincidental.

The statements in this book about consumable products or food have not been evaluated by the Food and Drug Administration. The recipes in this book are to be followed exactly as written. The publisher is not responsible for your specific health or allergy needs that may require medical supervision. The publisher is not responsible for any adverse reactions to the consumption of food or products that have been suggested in this book.

While the author has made every effort to provide accurate internet addresses at the time of publication, neither the publisher nor the author assumes any responsibility for errors or for changes that occur after publication. Further, the publisher does not have any control over and does not assume any responsibility for author or third-party websites or their content.

20 21 22 23 24 — 987654321
Printed in the United States of America

I would like to dedicate the book to my faithful husband, Stely (married for more than thirty-five years), and our only daughter, Dr. Andreea Steward (PharmD). I thank God for both of you. With the Lord on our side, we overcame all the obstacles to be where we are today. I appreciate your huge sacrifices. I love you both tremendously.

TABLE OF CONTENTS

Foreword by Irinel Stanciu xiii
Acknowledgments xv
Preface xvii
Disclaimer xxi
Introduction xxiii

PART I: THE SCIENCE OF STRESS AND DISEASE
1 A World Full of Stressors 3
2 Brain Science and Stress 11
3 Your DNA: Body, Mind, and Soul 24

PART II: ROOT CAUSES OF STRESS
4 A World of Problems 31
5 Pain 54

PART III: GOD'S SUPERNATURAL PRESCRIPTIONS
6 Creating Chemical Balance in Your Brain 77
7 Everything Starts in the Brain 89
8 Unexpired, Divine Prescriptions 96
9 Forgiveness Brings Joy 108
10 Identity 124
11 Faith 127
12 Dreams 133
13 Supernatural Healing 143
14 Strategic Choices for a Healthy Lifestyle 149
15 God's Word Reprograms Your Brain 153
16 Favor 162
17 Keep a Biblical Attitude 164
18 Thoughts 174
19 The Will of God 179
20 Gender Differences 185
21 Meditation and Antiaging 194
22 Helping Others 197
23 Prayer Reduces Stress 210
24 Giving Thanks 216
25 Lifestyle Change 223
26 Prayer and Fasting 234
27 Relationships 248
28 Our Hope Is in Heaven 252

Conclusion 271
Notes 273
Index 303

FOREWORD

Rodica has been my best friend and sister-in-Christ for more than thirty years. What stands out to me much more than this is her wisdom, gentleness of spirit, tenacity, perseverance, and hard work. These have been incredibly inspirational examples for me throughout all our years shared together. Her deep love for the Lord and unwavering hope in the midst of numerous difficult circumstances have always been, for me, like a lighthouse in the middle of a raging ocean, proving that trusting the Lord in spite of our doubts, coupled with hard work and perseverance, will get us through, no matter what the circumstances are.

Find Your Peace: Supernatural Solutions Beyond Science for Fear, Anxiety, and Depression is an excellent resource for any person who wants to live a healthy lifestyle and avoid disease. It is not only a fountain of up-to-date, well-researched scientific principles but also a river of life, bringing spiritual renewal of the mind.

From my personal experience of battling breast cancer at a young age, I remember being alarmed and surprised at the diagnosis. I had done, I thought, everything I could to protect myself in advance—I was a doctor, after all. My family and I, like Rodica's, emigrated from Romania years ago in search of a better life, free from communism and religious oppression. But even America's freedom can't solve the root issues that fester in the heart. Even with a better life, a good job, and many blessings, my soul was still dry and worn out from stress that is inescapable anywhere you may be physically located. What I did not realize until after my cancer diagnosis is that my thoughts poisoned my well-being, my anger burned inside me, and the joy of the Lord that is available for all Christians was missing from my life. God used cancer to wake me up and reveal to me what I was missing. I then understood how only He could change me and heal me. I learned the principles to not only control and manage stress but also take each thought captive, changing it from poisoning my soul and body to driving me to the Lord and strengthening my dependence on and trust in Him. Naturally this produced healing in the physical body as well. I was amazed at how interwoven the spiritual and physical realities are, but the Lord has created them both. All of this awakened me to the life-giving facts that Rodica is writing about in this book.

Rodica's book is very easy to read and understand, whether or not you have a medical background. It brings new insights from the most recent scientific discoveries in regard to how stress affects our bodies, and it gives us medication without side effects from the Word of God, the Creator of our entire being, our great physician and healer, Jehovah Rapha. With her extensive medical knowledge obtained during years of studying in the medical field culminating with her PhD thesis, coupled with her experience as a primary care practitioner, filled with the Spirit of God, she reveals the life-giving principles applicable to us all. As an endocrinologist myself, I admire her wisdom and skill in putting together such a masterpiece, useful for every patient in my practice. It uncovers and explains many "hormonal imbalances" that a pill would not be able to completely resolve. Her book is a complementary treatment for anyone with any kind of medical diagnosis and is also the much-sought-after "anti-stress pill" for anyone who wants to maintain a healthy lifestyle or improve his or her lifestyle.

I wholeheartedly recommend Rodica's book to all who want to live a long, healthy life, a life filled with inspirational purpose and meaning! Thank you, Rodica, for being a great example and a blessing to me and my family!

—IRINEL STANCIU, MD, FACE, ECNU, CCD
ENDOCRINOLOGIST
BOISE, IDAHO

ACKNOWLEDGMENTS

THIS BOOK RECEIVED support from the Creator of the universe, who gave the world supernatural prescriptions in His living Word to overcome fear and to manage high levels of stress, anxiety, and depression every day.

I thank Jesus Christ, the Lord and Savior of the world, the Lamb of God, who was slain before the foundation of the world and who delivers those who believe in Him from the stress of sin and from all their fears. Only He gives the joy of salvation, hope, and peace that passes all understanding and guards their minds, spirits, and bodies during stressful situations.

I also acknowledge the Holy Spirit, the great Comforter, who literally transforms and renews our minds and guides every step, giving to those who ask Him inspiration, wisdom, knowledge, revelation, and discernment to cope with high levels of stress, fear, anxiety, and depression.

Also, I give millions of thanks to my beloved husband, Stelica, and my precious daughter, Andreea, for their sacrifices, support, encouragement, and love. You both are a great team, overcoming fear and effectively managing stressful situations to reach your full potential and fulfill your destiny. Millions of thanks to my entire family, all friends, colleagues, and all my patients who were in my sphere of influence who provided support and inspiration throughout my entire life in Romania, in the United States, and everywhere on this planet.

Many thanks to all the writers and scientists cited in this book and all the teachers of truth in churches (the "spiritual clinics"). You sacrifice your time to make the information available, to inspire me and the entire community. We benefit from your spiritual and scientific evidence. You change our thinking and motivate us to have a better lifestyle, to live a quality life here on earth and for eternity.

Special thanks to Kay Metsger "Sora," who was by my side (as the proofreader) during my education at Oregon Health & Science University (OHSU), and special thanks to the editor of this book, Laura Davis, and her husband, Jim, for helping me finish and publish this book.

Finally, many thanks to you for taking the time to read the information in this book. It will strengthen your spirit, renew your mind and thoughts, improve your physical and spiritual health, and prevent physical and spiritual diseases resulting from high levels of stress, fear, anxiety, and depression.

PREFACE

The purpose of this book is to demonstrate the powerful correlation between God's scriptural advice and promises (divine prescriptions) and modern scientific brain research related to stress management.

My goal is to help you learn how to overcome the storms of life by adopting a healthier lifestyle, both physically and spiritually.

High levels of stress, fear, anxiety, and depression can trigger catastrophic health problems—mental, emotional, and physical. The best tools for overcoming the stresses we all face involve a combination of spiritual awareness and faith—beyond science—and a healthier lifestyle.

Building a resiliency to high levels of stress, fear, anxiety, and depression and regulating your emotions are possible through meditation on the promises written in the Word of God. Meditation actually builds new, stronger neurons in your brain. This in turn will help prevent generational curses through the epigenetic mechanism—unaltered gene expression and protein synthesis. *Find Your Peace* will show you how adopting positive lifestyle changes will give you efficient methods for stress management.

When you meditate on God's promises (bringing joy, peace, happiness, and hope to calm your overactive brain), you create new neurons through neurogenesis. New neurons will grow and rebuild your hippocampus and repair your brain, which has been damaged by high levels of stress.[1] Our brains are created by God to regulate themselves and to be rewired for quick responses to high levels of stress and dangerous situations. The brain can actually change its structure based on its neuroplasticity. Your brain structure can shrink or grow based on the quality of your thoughts and attitude.[2]

Our brains are programmed by our super intelligent designer to release the right amount of necessary neurotransmitters and neurochemicals affecting our unconscious and conscious minds, which influence our bodies to function normally. However, due to our human nature we are constantly disturbing the balance in our brains through unhealthy thoughts and unhealthy actions. Emotions from high levels of stress (perceived as threats) activate the sympathetic nervous system (SNS) to release norepinephrine at a high speed in response to stressors, causing rapid heart rate, an increase in blood pressure, sweats, trembling, and other frightening signs and symptoms. The SNS also activates the adrenal gland (medulla and cortex) to release large amounts of adrenaline and cortisol, creating more damage to the body, mind, and spirit.

At normal stress levels cortisol is released for our benefit to increase glucose for energy, to increase the cardiac output, to decrease brain inflammation, and to regulate our emotions through the hypothalamic-pituitary-adrenal (HPA) axis.[3] Our uncontrolled emotion and unhealthy thoughts, however, increase stress levels, causing unhealthy amounts of neurochemicals, including cortisol. These will become toxic for the brain and will kill neurons in the hippocampus area (involved in memory consolidation).[4] Excessive amounts of cortisol will compromise the immune system and circulatory system by damaging the arteries; increasing abdominal fat; and increasing the risk of high glucose, diabetes, hypertension, metabolic syndrome, osteoporosis, and others.[5] High levels of stress cause decreased serotonin levels, making people feel tired, decreasing their attention, and increasing the risk of such ailments as heart attack, depression, and sleep disturbance.[6] A lack of sleep causes depression with all the consequences. Anxiety and depression will decrease the size of the brain.[7] Fearful thoughts will enter through your cortex, but you can change those impulses based on the quality of your thoughts.

Throughout the Bible we find God's supernatural prescriptions and instructions, which will keep our thoughts healthy, thus implicitly regulating all the chemicals and neurotransmitters, releasing them in healthy amounts. Healthy thoughts through meditation and mindful thinking trigger electrical impulses to fire and to release neurotransmitters, causing new neurons to grow and strengthening neuronal connections and communication.[8] That is a miracle growth of the brain size through neuron proliferation called neuroplasticity. Mindful thinking and meditation help you pay attention to your thoughts and enable the release of acetylcholine[9]—important in preventing Alzheimer's. The frontal lobe helps you change your thinking.

For good health it is imperative that we grow healthy neurons by meditating on God's promises, memorizing and quoting Bible verses to consolidate memories in our unconscious minds and growing strong neurons. Healthy thoughts in our conscious minds are controlled by memories and unconscious activities. Our words and actions reflect the activity in our unconscious minds. Put the Word of God inside your heart and mind, and invite the Holy Spirit to help you in any situation. It is the living Word of God, with supernatural power to transform your thinking process, which will enable you to cope with the high levels of stress in your life.

Through joy, peace, happiness, and an active, healthy lifestyle (diet and exercise), our brains have the capacity to release neuroprotective proteins and to grow new neurons.[10] Exercise is a big factor in decreasing anxiety and depression. So keep moving; exercise regularly; be active to stimulate the brain to release the brain-derived neurotrophic factor (BDNF) that is so important for a healthy body, soul, and spirit.[11] Scientists recommend managing stress through intellectual stimulation, enjoying God's creation, physical exercise, recreation, keeping active at work, helping others, and fasting and praying. Be grateful every day, and count your blessings.

Stress management (through healthy habits, meditation, fasting, a healthy diet, and exercise) is truly an antiaging therapy, preventing age-related memory loss. Medically speaking, stress management through exercise, meditation, and healthy thinking are considered antiaging treatments.[12] Conversely, thoughts of fear lead to increased anxiety, shrinkage in the brain, impaired thinking, and neurocognitive disorders and inhibit decision making, thus severely affecting one's quality of life.[13]

With a mind renewed (one of the powerful supernatural prescriptions in the Word of God) through meditation on God's promises—prayer, fasting, compassion, gratitude, worshipping, and rejoicing in the Lord—we embrace this supernatural solution to manage stress from fear, worry, anxiety, and depression.

—Rodica Malos, DNP

DISCLAIMER

Please note: All information written in this book is for informational purposes only. It is not medical advice for any specific individual, nor is it applicable for specific medical problems of any individual. No information presented in this book is written or intended as a substitute for any professional medical intervention for diagnosing or treating, or for medical advice, and the information should not be construed as instruction or medical consultation for a specific person.

You should take no action solely on the basis of this book's contents regarding treatment or diagnosis for your own health condition. Readers must talk to a health professional about any problem regarding their own physical or mental condition. The information found in this book is believed to be accurate, based on the author's best judgment. Readers who fail to seek treatment from appropriate health professionals assume risk of potential ill effects and expenses. Please note that this advice is not specific to any individual. It is generic, and before undertaking any medical or nutritional course of action, you must consult with your doctor. Take your medications as prescribed by your medical providers, schedule follow-up appointments, keep your appointments, and seek and follow medical advice for all your conditions.

—Rodica Malos, DNP

INTRODUCTION

STRESS IS AN inescapable fact of life. An estimated 75–90 percent of doctor visits are related to stress.[1] The Occupational Safety and Health Administration (OSHA) has also declared that stress is a possible workplace hazard.[2] The American Institute of Stress claims that stress costs American industry "over $300 billion annually."[3] All over the world people are suffering from complications of high levels of stress from fear and worry, which cause anxiety and depression. Therefore it is imperative to assess and evaluate the root cause of this pervasive problem. Engrossed in our busy professional lives, we can easily become distracted and even dehumanized, ignoring the emotional and spiritual needs of our patients, friends, neighbors, and coresidents on this planet. Despite all our advanced technology, our lives remain vulnerable to constant tragedies, mass public and school shootings, the 24/7 news cycle that accentuates conflict, and high levels of stress. For this reason more and more health care providers are discussing how to incorporate spiritual care into their medical practice. Let us not allow society to abandon spirituality, which is our best enduring hope for health.

American astronomer Carl Sagan once said, "We live in a society exquisitely dependent on science and technology, in which hardly anyone knows anything about science and technology."[4] Because of this, in our postmodern era we cannot afford to ignore our spirituality. With more and more people living in fear or buried in worry, anxiety, and depression, acute and chronic diseases continue to destroy people's overall well-being.

Scientists, experts, and specialists in health care systems realize that medicine cannot rely only on randomized trials. We make everyday decisions based on our emotions and feelings, as reactions to everyday circumstances. Common sense is necessary when practicing medicine, and that means physicians must address spiritual needs. We are born with an innate need to seek the truth and to call upon God and His eternal presence in our lives. The Book of Ecclesiastes explains, "He has also set eternity in the human heart" (Eccles. 3:11).

Despite health care professionals' constant efforts to educate, entice, advise, convince, indoctrinate, and persuade patients with smooth talk, bribes, guilt, and manipulation to make people understand and follow medical advice, the results are often minimal. People continue to suffer from various diseases and chronic conditions. Many still die prematurely from high levels of stress caused by fear, worry, anxiety, and depression.

Even with people having so much knowledge, the gaps in the way people manage stressors in their daily lives need to be addressed. I hope this book will fill some gaps that we often ignore in our busy health professions and in daily life. The insights you will discover in *Find Your Peace* will transform your way of thinking and give you the tools to change your life and even your eternity. You in turn will change the world around you. When people are transformed, they can better cope with stress and then help transform others. The world can be transformed, one person at a time.

If you experience high levels of stress and are looking for ways beyond science to manage your fear, worry, and anxiety, then keep reading. The following chapters will help you understand the scientific component of stressors and their harmful effects on our spirits, minds, and bodies. Chronic worry produces high levels of stress, affecting our thoughts, emotions, and souls. Our environment is flooded with destructive events and behaviors that trigger unhealthy thoughts, yet we have the power inside us to change our perceptions about life and start thinking healthier thoughts. To protect both the soul and the body from consequences of unmanaged stress, the spirit needs a spiritual prescription. Our spirits and souls need spiritual treatments for spiritual maladies, just as our bodies need treatment or therapy for physical diseases. (See James 2:26.) Despite scholars' many excellent ideas on how to manage stress, people continue to feel stressed out. It is a silent, worldwide pandemic.

Health care professionals who recognize people's need to overcome fear allow their patients to talk about their spiritual needs. According to Dr. Mary Blaszko Helming, who conducted a study of healing through prayer, nurses can help heal patients by allowing them to voice their fears, mystical experiences, and struggles with their own spirituality. Dr. Helming said that many people struggle to verbalize their fears "for fear of ridicule or because no one prompts them to explore these issues."[5] Fears of all kinds must be allowed expression if we hope to conquer stress.

Although stress causes real symptoms, the patient may have no conscious awareness of the connection. Physiological signs and symptoms, and panic attacks from fear and stress, lead to endless ER visits and multiple hospitalizations. Verbal clues of stress can include:

- "I'm too stressed."
- "I'm worn out."
- "I've hit the wall."
- "I can't take it anymore."
- "I can't cope."

- "I'm at the end of my rope."
- "I can't breathe."
- "My world is ending."
- "Life is not worth living."
- "My world is falling apart."

High levels of stress also lead to unhealthy decisions, behaviors, and practices, with their subsequent degenerative diseases. The list of diseases caused by high levels of stress is long and includes heart disease, lung disease, gastrointestinal disease, infections, degenerative and autoimmune diseases, cancer, musculoskeletal diseases, and even neurological deficits, psychological distress, or mental disorders. Researchers have demonstrated that reducing stress levels and bad behaviors can save many lives and trillions of dollars in health care costs.[6] Rising health care costs create economic insecurity, more stress, and more diseases, threatening disaster on every level. It is a vicious cycle. We need to learn how to renew our minds with healthy thinking, resulting in healthy behaviors.

After my own experiences with stress and observing other stressed-out people, I asked myself the question "Who will change the world? Who will fix these problems?" In this book you will find God's supernatural prescriptions to prevent the physical and spiritual diseases caused by worry, fear, anxiety, and depression. Scientists have suggested that chronic stress may lead to long-term changes in brain structure and function that persist after the stressor ends. So for stress, as with many other health issues, an ounce of prevention may be worth a pound of cure—managing and reducing chronic stress may be an effective approach for preventing stress-induced changes in brain structure that may be very difficult to treat after they have emerged.[7]

PART I

THE SCIENCE OF STRESS AND DISEASE

Chapter 1

A WORLD FULL OF STRESSORS

You will hear of wars and rumors of wars.... Nation will rise against nation, and kingdom against kingdom. There will be famines and earthquakes in various places. All these are the beginning of birth pains.
—Matthew 24:6–8

Stress is often defined as physiological and psychological responses to perceived threats. Today's world is rife with threats from chaos, instability, insecurity, violence, news of war, natural disasters, famine, economic crisis, terrorists, occupiers, and political confusion. Sexual immorality, incurable diseases, and unhealthy behaviors are increasing, and societies are in great turmoil. The late Billy Graham, the world-renowned evangelist who preached the gospel on every continent, noted in his 2010 book, *The Journey*, that we live in a world of uncertainty: "The daily headlines don't give us much hope. War, famine, terrorism, racial and ethnic conflict, economic disruption, violence—the list is almost endless. Neither do our everyday experiences give us much hope: family and marital breakdown, sickness, addiction, accidents—again, the list is almost endless. Uncertainty and insecurity seem to be the watchwords of our generation."[1]

Such realities trigger fear, worry, anxiety, depression, bitterness, and increasing stress. Those feelings are like a cancer for the soul—a malignancy that spreads from the soul to the body to entire families, groups of friends, communities, and nations. Listening to the daily news raises our stress levels. Uncertainty grows globally, along with economic and political instability. Even famous and wealthy people are dying from depression, suicide, or overdoses of prescription or illicit drugs. When fears of insecurity, anxiety, depression, and worry grip your heart, they flood your brain with unhealthy levels of neurotransmitters and neurochemicals, causing more damage to the body, mind, and spirit.

Fear is a major factor in increased stress levels. Fear paralyzes people, leading to panic attacks, anger, violence, hate, and murder. All these evils spread darkness and panic, propagating worry, anxiety, panic attacks, and depression. Nations are shaken by terrorism, natural disasters, and other calamities, producing yet more pain and suffering. These are the culprits behind the majority of physical and spiritual diseases.

Despite all our efforts to manage stress from worry and anxiety at the individual and global levels, high levels of stress continue to kill millions. My friend Shaneen Clarke of London, an author and internationally known conference speaker, said in her book, *Dare to Be Great: Forget Your Past! Live Your Dream!*:

> In the words of author Lee Warren, "It should come as no surprise to anyone, especially medical science with all its technological innovations, that if our mind and souls are brimming with negative principles, our health, in general, will deteriorate and disease will be rampant in the world today. The streets, alleys, Skid Row, and mental institutions throughout the earth are crowded with those slain by the Goliath of hopelessness. Man-made philosophies, dogmas and religions stultified with ceremonies, rituals, and traditions have been unable to and have languished in dealing with this problem. They have failed to instill in the minds of the masses, knowledge of the principle of faith in the Creator within them."[2]

In my studies for my master's and doctoral degrees at Oregon Health & Science University in Portland, Oregon, I most enjoyed the courses on health promotion and disease prevention, particularly those on what science says about stress. I became a health care provider and now apply this scientific evidence in my practice, teaching others how to prevent and manage stress. Observing many people struggling with severe stress and its terrible consequences, I concluded there must be more answers than what we learned in school and more than what science teaches us through the best, evidence-based practices.

We share information and knowledge to impact the more vulnerable people in the world through education programs, international leadership conferences, mobile libraries, online discussion forums, and the media, but we must do more. Our view of the world is constantly evolving, especially when we see turmoil in developing countries or the clash of civilizations. I hear at international conferences that the hope of westernization is a mindset project for the entire world, but real hope and transformation come only through a renewed mind through healthy thinking.

THE EFFECTS OF STRESS, FEAR, AND WORRY

> I sought the LORD, and he answered me; he delivered me from all my fears. Those who look to him are radiant; their faces are never covered with shame.
>
> —PSALM 34:4–5

Did you ever experience uncomfortable feelings for no apparent reason? People experiencing high levels of stress from fear and worry—resulting in anxiety and depression—may manifest physical, cognitive, and behavioral symptoms due to an abnormal level of neurochemicals, hormones, and neurotransmitters released in the body.[3] As a biological response to stressors, people at some point in their lives will experience one or more of these signs and symptoms: unexplained pain in the back and jaw, muscle tension, headaches, trembling of lips and hands, light-headedness, dry mouth, difficulty swallowing, heartburn, nausea, stomach cramps, restlessness, increased perspiration, difficulty breathing, chest pain, a heart condition, frequent urination, night sweats, flatulence, diarrhea, and many others.[4]

Mental symptoms of great stress may include such things as anxiety, frustration, anger, depression, confusion, discontentment, loneliness, negativity, defensiveness, low productivity, poor concentration, suspiciousness, or suicidal thoughts. Among other inappropriate behaviors: nervous habits, inattention to grooming, increased alcohol and tobacco use, overspending, gambling, overreacting, fast or mumbled speech, self-pity, social withdrawal, mood swings, crying spells, bad temper, nail biting, and others.[5]

HIGH STRESS AFFECTS ALL OUR SYSTEMS

> Can any one of you by worrying add a single hour to your life?
>
> —MATTHEW 6:27

Let's look at a few examples of how high levels of stress can affect the human body's systems.

Cardiovascular and circulatory system: Increased stress on our cardiovascular systems (due to increased epinephrine and norepinephrine) will increase blood pressure and heart rate,[6] causing palpitations, shortness of breath, fatigue, weakness, dizziness, chest discomfort (felt as pain, numbness, tightness, or pressure), and fainting.[7] People experiencing some of those symptoms may be having a panic attack or anxiety attack[8] and may rush to the emergency room.

Respiratory system: High levels of stress cause vasoconstriction and poor perfusion with oxygen, increased respiratory rate, shortness of breath, and inflammation of the lung tissues, aggravating asthma, the common cold, and flu.[9] Dyspnea (shortness of breath) will further decrease the amount of oxygenated blood in the lungs. All cells will have poor oxygenation, damaging cells throughout the body.

Neurological system: The neurological system under high levels of stress brings on tension headaches, forgetfulness, the inability to concentrate, fatigue, sleep disturbances, anxiety, tremors, weakness, depression, and dizziness.[10] The serotonin-melatonin balance in the brain is disturbed, affecting the quality of sleep.[11] The serotonin level is affected when an overly stressed person ingests carbohydrates in higher amounts, leading to weight gain and obesity.[12] Increased carbohydrate intake due to high levels of stress causes more sleep deprivation.[13] Sleep deprivation and low levels of melatonin increase the risk of breast cancer in women up to 30 percent and prostate cancer in men up to 50 percent.[14] (I will address this later.)

Endocrine system: Stress causes increased levels of cortisol (the "stress hormone"). Cortisol kills neurons and damages regions in the hippocampus,[15] reducing the secretion of acetylcholine, a neurotransmitter that helps us think. The hippocampus is involved in filing information in the brain, but when neurons are destroyed—causing forgetfulness—personality changes can lead to a neurocognitive syndrome. If stress is not managed appropriately, cognition impairment and neurocognitive disorders, such as Alzheimer's and other types of dementia, may result.[16]

Diabetes may develop if cortisol levels remain elevated for long periods of time due to prolonged stress.[17] Bone mass may decrease, leading to osteoporosis.[18] Thyroid function is affected,[19] causing unpleasant symptoms of abnormal thermoregulation. Your thyroid gland regulates the metabolism and temperature in your body. This gland receives messages from the hypothalamus, your "body thermostat," and the pituitary gland, which stimulates the release of the thyroid hormones T3 and T4 (regulating the metabolism rate and production of proteins) and of calcitonin (regulating the calcium used in the bones).[20]

The thyroid gland senses insufficient or excessive amounts of these two hormones and lowers or raises the amount of thyroid-secreting hormone that keeps T3 and T4 balanced. High levels of stress will disrupt the normal functions of the thyroid gland.[21]

Integumentary system under stress: The integumentary system, when affected by stress, increases itching or irritation of the skin and may cause flare-ups of eczema, psoriasis,[22] lupus,[23] and other autoimmune disorders due to decreased effectiveness of the immune system.[24]

Musculoskeletal system: The musculoskeletal system is affected by stress through the inflammation process,[25] which causes degenerative diseases and flare-ups of arthritis,[26] and fibromyalgia with all its complications.[27]

Gastrointestinal system: Stress on the gastrointestinal system causes nausea, vomiting, constipation, diarrhea, irritable bowel syndrome, bladder and bowel accidents, and an electrolyte imbalance.[28]

Lymphatic system: The lymphatic system plays a central role in our defense against different types of infections, microorganisms, viruses, and cancer. It contains lymphatic liquid, a web of lymphatic vessels, specialized cells called lymphocytes, and tissues and organic lymphoid (spleen as an example).[29] The body is vulnerable to interior and exterior attacks, such as traumas, disease, stress, aging, cell destruction, and gene mutations, which develop into cancer.

Immune system: Although extremely vulnerable, the human body has an extraordinary power to protect itself with the immune system. The immune system has the capacity to discern between what belongs to our bodies, and foreign microorganisms and viruses. It attacks any strange particles or molecules to eliminate them. The fascinating part is how the whole defense process stops at the right time to prevent it from self-destructing.

High levels of stress will cause high cortisol levels, leading to higher levels of inflammation, which suppress the immune system and render your body more susceptible to infection and cancer.[30] The immune system secretes natural chemicals to kill foreign microbes; form lymphocytic nodules; promote lymph circulation in the blood; and filter cancer cells, bacteria, and other foreign elements.[31] Cancer cells will alert the key cells from the immune system. New lymphocytes and macrophage can be mobilized within just a few minutes to fight these enemies.[32] It is a miracle. In fact the entire body, mind, and spirit are incomprehensible—an amazing, miraculous creation with visible and invisible functions. We are truly God's masterpieces.

High levels of stress and cortisol will suppress our entire self-defense mechanisms. Stress is the body's enemy—killing, stealing, and destroying—working against our divinely designed immune systems. The body's whole defense mechanism is damaged by high levels of stress from worry, fear, and anxiety.

STRESS IS ENVIRONMENTAL AND DANGEROUS

> But mark this: There will be terrible times in the last days. People will be lovers of themselves, lovers of money, boastful, proud, abusive, disobedient to their parents, ungrateful, unholy, without love, unforgiving, slanderous, without self-control, brutal, not lovers of the good, treacherous, rash, conceited, lovers of pleasure rather than lovers of God—having a form of godliness but denying its power. Have nothing to do with such people.
>
> —2 TIMOTHY 3:1–5

People living in the environment described in 2 Timothy 3:1–5 will develop high levels of stress. This is extremely dangerous for the human body and may cause many diseases. As mentioned before, most visits to a medical office are due to symptoms caused by high levels of stress.

The whole body is affected by stress physically and spiritually, prompting people to seek medical attention and often requiring many unnecessary tests and procedures. Those will increase the costs of medical care and bring on more stress if people do not have adequate health insurance and lack the finances to pay all the bills. Prolonged symptoms lead to acute diagnoses, which, if not treated with the right interventions, will become chronic diseases. More complications and comorbidities may lead to early physical and mental disabilities, putting a burden on oneself, one's family, the community, and society.

All these signs and symptoms can be minimized or avoided if we learn more about what triggers them. We can change our perception about life's problems and learn how to manage stress by following God's supernatural prescriptions. We will benefit by simply taking to heart all the instructions and directions in the Word of God, plus the results of scientific knowledge that God has allowed us to develop in this modern era. I'll have more on this later.

The Brain—Gateway for Stress

There is a strong interdependence among the brain structure, thinking process, and how thoughts are translated into actions in stressful situations. Advanced technology has allowed scientists to discover more insights about the microscopic universe of our neurons. We read increasingly about the results of scientific research about mindfulness and how the brain structures function, connect, grow, heal, restore, renew, and learn.

Your brain is the gate that allows external and internal stressors to stimulate its structures, affecting the whole body. Billions of neurons can release different neurotransmitters in unhealthy, toxic amounts. They flow into the body as a biological response, causing physiological and psychological manifestations through unpleasant signs and symptoms. Sooner or later we all experience high stress levels (rooted in fear, uncertainty, disappointment, insecurity, or unmet expectations), causing emotional distress and pain from multiple chronic conditions. The Book of Ecclesiastes contains a strong prescription—beyond science—to prevent the pain in our bodies that emotional distress causes: "Banish emotional stress from your mind. And put away pain from your body; for youth and the prime of life are fleeting" (Eccles. 11:10, NET). He is able to heal us physically and emotionally of any kind of disease.

Worry, Anxiety, and Depression Hurt

> Why, my soul, are you downcast? Why so disturbed within me? Put your hope in God, for I will yet praise him, my Savior and my God.
> —Psalm 42:5

High levels of stress, anxiety, worry, fear, doubt, and unbelief will cause depression. Depression causes physical pain due to dysfunction of the serotonergic and noradrenergic neurons and pathways. In their article "Understanding Pain in Depression," for *Human Psychopharmacology*, professors Stephen Stahl and Mike Briley wrote:

> A dysfunction of the serotonergic and noradrenergic pathways is commonly accepted as playing a major role in the etiology of depression. Serotonergic cell bodies, located in the raphe nucleus, send projections to various parts of the brain where they are involved in the control of mood, movement, emotions such as anxiety and regulate behaviors such as eating, sexual activity and the feeling of pleasure. Similarly, the noradrenergic neurons, located in the locus ceruleus, project to the same regions where they regulate, in addition, attention and cognition. A further projection to the cerebellum regulates motor control. A dysfunction at the level of the monoamine neurons thus results in the classical symptoms of depression.
>
> In addition to these ascending pathways, however, the neurons in the raphe nucleus and the locus ceruleus also project to the spinal cord. These descending pathways serve to inhibit input from the intestines, the skeletal muscles and other sensory inputs. Under normal conditions, these inhibitory effects are modest, but in times of stress, in the interests of the survival of the individual, they can completely inhibit the input from painful stimuli. A dysfunction at the level of the serotonergic and noradrenergic neurons can thus affect both the ascending and descending pathways resulting in the psychological and somatic symptoms of depression but also in physical painful symptoms.[33]

To prevent dysfunction of the noradrenergic and serotonergic neurons and their pathways (the etiology of depression), we must follow God's powerful prescriptions given thousands of years ago. He admonishes us: do not worry, do not be anxious about anything, do not be afraid, but have faith in the King of the universe and in His promises. He is taking care of our needs so we can avoid depression and physical pain. Throughout the Bible we find spiritual prescriptions full of supernatural potency, which can protect our minds from the disastrous pain of physical, emotional, and spiritual diseases caused by fear and worry. We just need to "banish emotional stress" from our minds, as prescribed in the Book of Ecclesiastes (NET).

Fearful, worried, and anxious thinking causes the brain to release unhealthy levels of neurochemicals from the hypothalamus, which receives messages from the thalamus (the center that processes information and directs it to different brain structures) and from the limbic system (associated with emotions and memories).[34] When we perceive a threat, unhealthy amounts of neurotransmitters are released. Those unhealthy levels of neurochemicals will trigger diseases, as discussed.

The brain was created with its own natural "pharmacy." It produces natural chemicals that can heal and restore when the right amounts of neurochemicals are released.[35] Or it can kill and destroy the body when these are released in unhealthy amounts. Our amazing brains have the ability to produce natural endogenous substances: antidepressants, natural antibiotics, and natural tranquilizers for pain management and healing. For this to work, we need to have the right reactions to circumstances and wise actions to create the right atmosphere in our brains, even when stress is overwhelming.

So many people do not know where to turn for answers and security in tough times. Some will seek refuge in synthetic prescriptions, illicit drugs, alcohol, tobacco, and destructive behaviors. But all those are just bandages for deep emotional infections, which later will result in spiritual septicemia and imminent physical and spiritual death.

Chapter 2

BRAIN SCIENCE AND STRESS

Then God said, "Let us make mankind in our image, in our likeness, so that they may rule over the fish in the sea and the birds in the sky, over the livestock and all the wild animals, and over all the creatures that move along the ground." So God created mankind in his own image, in the image of God he created them; male and female he created them.
—GENESIS 1:26–27

GOD'S FIRST SUPERNATURAL prescription was for human beings to be created in His image—not just to look like God but also to share some of God's creative abilities, enabling man and woman to create visible things from invisible thoughts. Everything created in the beginning originated with God's invisible thoughts, and the visible world was created from invisible things at His command. Human beings were created in His image; thus we also are creative and can participate in the divine nature. (See 2 Peter 1:4.)

He gave mankind the gift of creativity through the power of thoughts. Not only are we God's image bearer; we also carry God's breath in our lungs, and the seed of multiplication. The Holy Spirit is still hovering over the surface of this planet, waiting to get into the inner being of His creation—a population of over seven billion people who are "predestined to be conformed to the image of his Son" (Rom. 8:29.) Through the "seed" planted in our brains we inherit the ability to transform our perceptions of things (thoughts). We have within us the power to create. So often we credit man for inventions and advanced technology, but we forget God's investment in the human brain. He is sharing invisible thoughts, through the power of His Spirit, every moment in every human being. It is written that everything exists not by might, nor by power, but by His Spirit (Zech. 4:6).

God gives revelation, inspiration, discernment, determination, passion, perseverance, and endurance to fulfill His plan for this planet. Thoughts are invisible until we put them into action. God continues to create through our thoughts, in our brains. He drops ideas, inspiration, and revelation into our spirits and brains. Invisible thoughts create things that exist around us. "For by him were all things created, that are in heaven, and that are in earth, visible and invisible, whether they be thrones, or dominions, or principalities, or powers: all things were created by him, and for him" (Col. 1:16, KJV).

Not surprisingly, everything that happens to you begins in your brain. Stress enters your body through your brain (thoughts). It is critical that we learn about physiology and psychology in order to understand the science of stress. We will consider the brain's structure and the body's systems, scratching only the surface of its anatomy, to see how high levels of stress affect the entire body, mind, and spirit—and thus our future. It is well documented in scientific literature that chronic stress leads to excessive damage to the entire body (which is composed of about 37.2 trillion cells, with complex interconnections throughout all the systems).

THE BRAIN: THE CONTROL CENTER

Trillions of highly specialized cells of different sizes are interconnected for different functions, making up our vital organs and all the systems of the human body. Billions of nerve cells with trillions of synapses compute all the information in our brains. The neurons help the body adjust to stimuli in any environment and to inside stimuli when we are physically sick or in emotional pain.

Sensory receptors in our eyes, ears, noses, mouths, skin, muscles, and joints perceive impulses from different stimuli inside or outside the body, then send messages to the nervous system to respond. Neurons communicate among themselves through synapses, dendrites, and axons via neurochemicals and neurotransmitters. Messages are received from outside or inside stimuli through electrical impulses entering the neurons through dendrites. They travel through axons and across the synapses' thresholds as action potential.[1] Connections between neurons are performed through thousands of branches called dendrites and trillions of synapses and axons. Axons facilitate messages from nerve cells to other neurons and can be as long as three feet.[2] Messages are carried through synapses—bridges, as I see them—which are extremely small.

About one hundred neurochemicals are manufactured from amino acids by the neurons throughout the nervous system and are transmitted as a result of perceived external and internal stimuli.[3] They travel across synapses; some are synthesized and stored in neurons. Our thoughts, actions, attitudes, and habits will boost or inhibit many of the neurotransmitters. Neurotransmitters are stored at the ends of axons in vesicles and then are released in the synapses when an electrical impulse (caused by outside or inside stimuli through our five senses) travels to the end of the axon.[4] Those impulses are our perceptions of things, our thoughts, our emotions, and our memories, stored in our brains' structures. They are affected by our good or bad actions in the past or present and by what we see, hear, feel, smell, and taste.

THE LIMBIC SYSTEM

Our feelings, thoughts, and memories take place in our limbic system (situated beneath the cortex). This limbic system consists of the hypothalamus, the amygdala, the hippocampus, the cingulate gyrus, the mammillary bodies, and other brain structures.[5] The hypothalamus controls the autonomic nervous system, with its parasympathetic and sympathetic branches, and the endocrine system.[6] In communication with other areas in the brain and other complex systems, the limbic system contributes to learning, emotions, motivation, and memory.[7]

Just a small example: Dopamine is the neurotransmitter involved in motivation.[8] Our motivation can be affected by drugs. For example, marijuana (now legal in many states) alters the brain's function, leading to amotivational syndrome in marijuana users.[9] On the other hand, stress management (through healthy habits, meditation, fasting, a healthy diet, and exercise) acts as an antiaging therapy, preventing shrinkage of the hippocampus and age-related memory loss.[10]

HOW STRESS BEGINS

The amygdala is associated with emotions, which in turn are attached to thoughts. Emotions from thoughts of fear create memories felt as worry, anxiety, anger, bitterness, irritation, or depression. Each time thoughts of worry and fear bombard our minds, we will experience anxiety.[11] The hippocampus is associated more with conscious memories. The structures in the limbic system bring up good and bad memories in our daily activities in many ways. We are in charge of our limbic system's functions when we decide what kinds of emotions and thoughts to process, store, and memorize. Our response to stress from worry and anxiety begins in our minds and continues in our bodies. Everything the body does begins in the structures of the brain and those billions of neurons and trillions of synapses, axons, receptors, and pathways.

Anatomy and physiology tell us that the brain has three levels: neocortical—for rational thought processing, limbic system—emotional thought processing and memories consolidation, and vegetative—with autonomic responses controlled by two branches (sympathetic and parasympathetic systems).[12]

The autonomic nervous system works automatically at the unconscious and subconscious levels. We are usually not even aware of what we are doing, how we breathe, how our hearts are beating, how we fall asleep and wake up in the morning, and how we function during our daily routines. For example, the parasympathetic branch controls our breathing, blood pressure, peristalsis, sleeping, relaxing, and resting, while the sympathetic branch controls our fight-or-flight response to fear when we are in a dangerous situation.[13] The nervous system contains the central nervous system (brain and spinal cord) and the peripheral nervous system (neural pathways to the extremities).

MYSTERIES OF THE SUBCONSCIOUS AND UNCONSCIOUS

> A good man brings good things out of the good stored up in his heart, and an evil man brings evil things out of the evil stored up in his heart. For the mouth speaks what the heart is full of.
> —LUKE 6:45

We know by now that inside every human being is an invisible world—our thoughts. Let's look briefly at the brain's subconscious functions. The brain receives information from inside and outside the body and computes it all automatically and subconsciously at such a speed, day and night, that you do not even notice what is going on. Dr. Caroline Leaf is a communication pathologist, audiologist, and cognitive neuroscientist—and a biblical and scientific expert of the mind. In her book *Switch On Your Brain: The Key to Peak Happiness, Thinking, and Health*, she mentions that 90–99 percent of the activities in your mind happen at the unconscious level, where thoughts are built. The unconscious thinking process operates at four hundred billion actions per second.[14]

Your thoughts and memories coordinate all the systems unconsciously twenty-four hours a day, seven days a week. For example, the endocrine glands release hormones to regulate body temperature, energy, reproduction, and growth. The nervous system regulates the circulatory, musculoskeletal, gastrointestinal, and genitourinary systems.[15] Think about your musculoskeletal system, with all the bones, joints, and muscle groups connected via tendons, cartilages, sockets, synovial fluids, nerves, fibers, receptors, and pathways for neurotransmitters. All the sockets in each joint assist in mobility—sitting, standing, walking, turning, bending, extending—and all are coordinated by the brain at the unconscious level.

Think about the skin as an amazing organ representing our integumentary system. Its function is to cover and hold together all systems, tissues, and organs lying within the body. Our skin must prevent disconnection and protect us from exposure and unseen environmental factors. It is fascinating how all our internal organs function with precision to keep our bodies alive, even renewing skin cells about every four weeks—something beyond our comprehension. Your body is doing an unimaginable job, continually receiving commands at the subconscious level.

Another small example is how the pancreas reacts within seconds after we eat that yummy ice cream. Blood sugar rises in the bloodstream, ready to release the right amount of insulin to transport the sugar to every cell, providing us with energy to function. Your body is doing an incredible job, digesting and absorbing all the micronutrients and minerals in the gastrointestinal tract.

Then apoptosis (another amazing built-in feature in our DNA, with programmed instructions to constantly clean all cell debris from the body) removes all residuals from our dying cells in order to regenerate our bodies. Our bodies continually fight with residuals from cells, which can cause degenerative diseases, infections, and cancer.[16] We are constantly manufacturing natural chemicals to aid every system in promoting homeostasis for a healthy body.[17] Every cell is working hard every single moment. That is why we need time at night for rest and rejuvenation, another miracle of life.

"God's Glue" Particles Inside Us

The body has such intricate architecture, with orderly interconnections always working at the unconscious level. The anatomy and physiology of the human body is fascinating. Cells are programmed to protect us from invasions of neoplasm and cancer cells. Our cells are held together with laminin, a cell-adhesion protein molecule that is a component of the basement membrane surrounding most tissues of the body.[18] This "God's glue," as I call it, holds the cells and organs together. Laminin molecules are even in the shape of a cross! The Bible tells us that God holds all things together. "For in him all things were created: things in heaven and on earth, visible and invisible, whether thrones or powers or rulers or authorities; all things have been created through him and for him. He is before all things, and in him all things hold together" (Col. 1:16–17). All things are held together at the subconscious and unconscious levels through Jesus Christ, who died on the cross. In Him, through Him, and by Him we have our beings (Acts 17:28).

Another amazing function is that receptors in all systems, including the bladder and intestines, communicate with the brain when to void or when to eliminate waste.[19] This leaves room for new, fresh nutrients to enter the body. Inability to control the bowel and bladder would be a disaster.

Bone mineralization, preventing bone diseases and fractures, is an incredible art. For example, the manufacture of vitamin D in the skin from sunlight exposure is fascinating. Sunlight passes the threshold of the skin, where it is absorbed, manufacturing vitamin D and helping the body to absorb calcium. This strengthens the bones and helps them grow, keeping them healthy and preventing broken bones.[20] If it was not in God's plan for the body to manufacture vitamin D naturally from sunlight, everyone would be in a wheelchair or bedbound from bone fractures. Vitamin D also naturally boosts testosterone levels in men, assisting with reproduction, the immune system, and cognition (helping to regulate outbursts of anger).[21] Thus men need to spend time in the sun, about fifteen minutes a day, for natural testosterone production.[22]

Symmetry in the human body is incredible. In medicine, symmetry is the key to assessing and diagnosing patients who seek medical attention. In fact the existence of the entire universe depends on symmetry. Mathematicians and physicists often discuss the necessity of symmetry. Clearly there is a divine, super intelligent being who designed our bodies as well as the entire universe. Evolution could not produce such mysteries.

SURVIVING STRESSFUL SITUATIONS

> Have I not commanded you? Be strong and courageous. Do not be frightened, and do not be dismayed, for the Lord your God is with you wherever you go.
> —Joshua 1:9, esv

> Do not be afraid of those who kill the body but cannot kill the soul. Rather, be afraid of the One who can destroy both soul and body in hell.
> —Matthew 10:28

Did you ever ask yourself how you've survived so many stressful events? Your brain and body in general are doing amazing work at the subconscious and unconscious levels. The nervous, endocrine, and immune systems are involved in responding to high levels of stress. The job of the autonomic nervous system, with its sympathetic and parasympathetic branches, is to regulate the homeostatic balance in the body for daily normal functions during normal levels of stress as necessary. The autonomic nervous system is responsible for regulating the vital organs and visceral activities, such as "circulation, respiration, digestion, and temperature regulation."[23]

The parasympathetic nervous system will respond to stimuli by releasing acetylcholine to help the thinking process and slow the heart rate. It also assists with digestion to eliminate residual substances from the body, preventing constipation and assisting with bladder function to eliminate unnecessary fluids, maintaining homeostasis in the body. It conserves energy and promotes relaxation.[24]

All these functions can be affected by our decisions to respond to God's prescriptions—or not. When our stress level is high, the sympathetic nervous system will respond to internal or external stimuli by releasing the catecholamines called epinephrine and norepinephrine in large amounts as a fight-or-flight response.[25] God built those features for self-preservation into our bodies to protect us from a dangerous environment. But if they are supra-solicited with no godly thoughts and unhealthy behavior, those features can be destroyed. That is why it is so important to know that too much or too little of these neurotransmitters or neurochemicals released during stressful situations will compromise our entire well-being. I will explain this more in the following chapters.

The endocrine system plays an important role. It is composed of glands, hormones, circulation, and target organs. Hormones released by the glands regulate metabolic functions. The pituitary gland, the master gland of the endocrine system, and the thyroid and adrenal glands are most involved in responding to the stressors mentioned earlier.[26]

The nervous system and endocrine system are connected, forming three metabolic axes: the adrenocorticotropic hormone (ACTH) axis, the vasopressin axis, and the thyroxine axis.[27] The way we respond to stress from fear, worry, and anxiety in our daily lives will influence the functions of the nervous and endocrine systems. We will see in the following chapters how our behavior and attitude can affect the release of neurochemicals, either healing and restoring our bodies, or leading to fatal diseases.

How Stressors Enter the Brain

Let's look at how stressors from the outside world get into our brains. Information from the outside world (your environment) enters your brain as electrical impulses originating from your five senses. These influence your thought formation, decision-making capacity, emotions, and actions. All electrical impulses get through the thalamus, a structure in the brain that connects all other structures of the brain and activates other thoughts that already exist in the neurons in the cerebral cortex. Those thoughts that already exist in the cerebral cortex are brought into our consciousness when triggered by the electrical impulses from our five senses.[28]

Dr. Caroline Leaf, whom I mentioned earlier, states in her book *Who Switched Off My Brain?* that "this wonderfully complex transmission through the cerebral cortex, or the 'breeze through the trees,' alerts and activates attitude. Attitude is a state of mind (all the thoughts on the trees) that influences our choices and what we say and do as a result of our choices."[29]

The Five Senses: Information Gateway

Your five senses are the entryway for outside information, which becomes electrical impulses in your brain. Electrical impulses trigger the thinking process in "the forest" of the neurons (in the cerebral cortex) with a treelike configuration.[30] Dendrites are the branches of those "trees."[31] Thoughts activate other thoughts that already exist with emotions and memories in other brain structures and are sent to the hypothalamus (the fabric of natural chemicals), which sends messages to the pituitary gland, the hormones' master gland.[32] When responding to stress, the pituitary gland in turn sends messages to other glands to release excessive amounts of chemicals such as cortisol, epinephrine, aldosterone, norepinephrine; decreased amounts of serotonin, dopamine, acetylcholine, and melatonin; and other neurochemicals, according to the level of stress perceived.[33] The physical response to the stressors begins, and the whole body will experience the uncomfortable signs and symptoms presented in the beginning of this chapter. When the neurotransmitters or neurochemicals and hormones are released in the central nervous system (CNS) and the endocrine system as a cascade from all the glands in abnormal amounts—in response to unhealthy stressors from fears and worry—the human body experiences the signs, symptoms, and diseases mentioned earlier.

THE STRESS RESPONSE

The stress response consists of "increased neural excitability" and "increased cardiovascular activity" (increased heart rate, stroke volume, cardiac output, and blood pressure). Metabolic activity is increased through gluconeogenesis ("turning glycogen into [higher amounts of] sugar for energy"), mobilizing proteins, decreasing antibody production, and increasing muscle waste. Fats are mobilized to break down into sugar, further elevating sugar to an unhealthy level. Salt is retained, irritating the nerves and producing and increasing neurological sweating, confusion, and salivation. Gastrointestinal system mobility and tonus are changed.[34] The digestive tract responses can result in nausea, vomiting, diarrhea, or constipation.[35] All those symptoms frighten the person experiencing them, causing more stress. The cycle will repeat, damaging the body more and leading to panic attacks, emergency room visits, and unnecessary hospitalization and higher costs. These raise stress levels even more, both for individuals and society as a whole.

Our only hope in stressful circumstances resides in the promises written in the Word of God as supernatural prescriptions—beyond science. These can cause constructive thoughts to form, with healthy restoration and manifestation then taking place.

According to brain research that began in the 1990s, using MRIs and other electromagnetic procedures, scientists see an increase in the brain's aging process when it is repeatedly exposed to high levels of cortisol, "the stress hormone."[36] This damages and shrinks brain tissues irreversibly in the hippocampus area responsible for memory consolidation and increases the size of the amygdala (through the inflammatory process), causing fearful or anxious thoughts and impaired cognition.[37]

NEUROTRANSMITTERS AND YOUR THOUGHTS

> For as he thinketh in his heart, so is he.
> —PROVERBS 23:7, KJV

Scientists have shown interest in researching and investigating how chronic stress and the resulting stress hormones, neurotransmitters, and other neurochemicals induce DNA damage, thus impairing the immune response and often leading to cancer. They have found that the excess amounts of neurotransmitters released in stressful situations will impact cancer progression in the body through a process of transformation at the cellular level. In a scientific paper linking stress to cancer, University of Pittsburgh professors Frank Jenkins, Bennett Van Houten, and Dana Bovbjerg stated:

> Psychological stress, acting through increased levels of catecholamines and/or cortisol, can increase DNA damage and/or reduce repair mechanisms, resulting in increased risk of DNA mutations leading to carcinogenesis. A better understanding of molecular pathways by which psychological stress can increase the risk of cancer initiation would open new avenues of translational research, bringing together psychologists, neuroscientists, and molecular biologists, potentially resulting in the development of novel approaches for cancer risk reduction at the population level.[38]

HOW NERVES SEND MESSAGES

Neurotransmitters play a huge role in our daily functions. Throughout the day and night your brain's structures (such as thalamus, hippocampus, amygdala, and hypothalamus) are communicating with all the other structures at the subconscious and unconscious levels. They store memories, thoughts, and emotions that determine the amount and kind of natural chemicals the brain needs to manufacture, and send messages to different parts of the body to act accordingly. All the cells in our organs are interconnected and are affected by our thoughts, memories, and emotions. This dictates the amounts of neurochemicals circulating in our bodies. About 86.1 billion cells in our brains (neurons) help us think, learn, remember, and reason. We behave accordingly.[39] Neurons help the body adjust to stimuli in any environment. Our eyes, ears, mouths, noses, skin, muscles, and joints have sensory receptors and perceive the impulses from stimuli in our environment. This creates changes at the conscious and unconscious levels every moment, thus preserving our lives so we can exist and function.[40]

Once, when I got home one afternoon, I parked my car in the garage. But before I got the car in the right position, the sensor started sending audible and visual signals that the car was too close to the wall on the right. I ignored all the signals and moved the car a little closer to the right and consequently damaged the right side of the car. The wired equipment in my car had tried insistently to communicate my dangerous position and situation, trying to protect both me and the car from damage.

In a similar way, neurons are communicating messages among themselves through electrical impulses and neurochemicals to alert us and to keep us safe from threatening environments every single moment. Connections between neurons are performed through thousands of branches of dendrites, synapses, and axons. Dendrites facilitate message transmission to the nerve cells, and axons allow messages to travel away from nerve cells to other neurons.[41] The messages are carried through trillions of synapses—one millionth of an inch between the dendrites of one neuron and the axon of the next.[42] It is known that the brain has one quadrillion connections (one million billion) and oversees a transport system that would be one hundred thousand miles long if the blood vessels were laid in one line.[43]

It is also known that about one hundred different neurochemicals made by your body travel across synapses.[44] Neurons synthesize and store neurotransmitters based on our thoughts and actions, which boost or inhibit and influence the amount of these chemicals so necessary for our normal daily routines.

Neurotransmitters are stored at the end of axons in vesicles, and when an impulse or electrical current from our thoughts travels, the neurotransmitters are released from the vesicles in the synapses and travel to the end of the axon.[45] Each thought you allow in your brain will cause impulses that will cause neurochemicals to be released, in the amount according to the quality and kind of thoughts.

The autonomic nervous system and endocrine system are both influenced by the limbic system and the activities taking place in your life, which in communication with other areas in the brain and other complex systems contribute to learning, memory, motivation, and emotions every moment of your life. Your behavior and your thoughts will dictate your ability to learn, to memorize, and to control your emotions and motivation. For example, using marijuana "can cause changes in brain anatomy,"[46] potentially leading to amotivational syndrome.[47] Marijuana users lose interest in studying, learning, or working. Other disturbing consequences are impaired cognition, memory loss, poor coordination, impaired driving skills (increasing fatalities), acute psychosis, paranoia, schizophrenia, dizziness, respiratory insufficiency, sedation, toxicity, and tachycardia.[48] "Getting high" with synthetic cannabinoids can also result in seizures and renal failure.[49] Marijuana opens the door for more dangerous drugs, such as heroin, with all its consequences.[50]

On the other hand, it has been demonstrated that healthy habits prevent shrinkage of the hippocampus and prevent memory loss related to aging. Medically speaking, stress management through exercise, meditation, and healthy thinking are considered antiaging treatments.[51] Conversely, thoughts of fear lead to increased anxiety, cause shrinkage in the brain, lead to impaired thinking and neurocognitive disorders, and inhibit decision-making, thus severely affecting one's quality of life.

HIGH STRESS AND YOUR NEUROTRANSMITTERS

> Be careful what you think, because your thoughts run your life.
> —PROVERBS 4:23, NCV

Your behavior and your life in general are shaped by your values and beliefs because they affect your thinking process. That dictates the kind and number of neurotransmitters released in your body. Let's look at the best-known neurochemicals and their roles and actions in the body in our busy and stressful daily lives. From those one hundred–plus neurochemicals I will mention just a few.

Acetylcholine, norepinephrine, dopamine, GABA, glutamate, serotonin, endorphin, and oxytocin are chemicals produced by neurons and glands, such as the pituitary and adrenal glands. They facilitate the transmission of signals between neurons through synapses. All these neurochemicals are released automatically, either excessively or deficiently, based on the quality of your thoughts and behaviors, subconsciously dictating your signs and symptoms from stress due to fear and worry. Sometimes these can be frightening.

Acetylcholine is the neurotransmitter that stimulates the muscles in the body, assists with the thinking process in neurons, and, in the autonomic nervous system, assists in REM sleep.[52] When acetylcholine is reduced, cognition is impaired; when reduced up to 90 percent due to plaque formation, it leads to Alzheimer's disease.[53] Epinephrine and norepinephrine are also involved in memory formation. During high levels of stress abnormal levels of these neurochemicals will be released, depleting the storage of this neurotransmitter and affecting our cognition negatively.[54] Drugs such as amphetamines will deplete the body's norepinephrine, dopamine, and serotonin.[55]

The neurotransmitter dopamine is a chemical that can have inhibitory action. It has an important role in the brain's reward mechanism. The brain is genetically programmed to search for food, drink, sex, sleep, comfort, and pleasure through thoughts and emotions (automatically generated inside of us) and activates the reward pathway (nucleus accumbens). Anticipation of rewards from eating, drinking, sleeping, sex, comfort, and other pleasures activates neurons that release the dopamine neurotransmitter.[56] Acute or chronic stress overstimulates the dopamine pathways and puts individuals at greater risk of addiction to drugs and other stimulants. In turn chronic drug use alters the brain's stress mechanisms, which can cause excessive dopamine secretion and uncontrollable impulses.[57] Overstressed people can lose self-control, leading to pathological changes and to seeking comfort food, such as carbohydrates, causing excessive weight gain.[58]

The dopamine amount will increase to an abnormal level and will cause very serious addiction if stimulated by the abuse of various drugs or alcohol, gambling, unhealthy sexual activity, or other unhealthy behaviors.[59] This causes lifelong physical and mental disability.[60] High levels of dopamine contribute to the development of schizophrenia, with frightening hallucinations and delusions. Scientists have developed medications to help with this devastating mental condition.[61]

The gamma-aminobutyric acid (GABA) neurotransmitter has an inhibitory action and tells the body when to stop doing bad things and when to calm the brain down, if one is extremely anxious and angry from excessive worrying.[62] Low GABA levels or impaired GABA function causes people to become more anxious and can contribute to disorders such as epilepsy.[63]

Glutamate is an excitatory neurotransmitter, and it is involved in the memory process. In excess amounts it is toxic and kills neurons.[64]

The neurotransmitter serotonin and its receptors exist throughout the body, with many functions.[65] People with low levels of serotonin often become depressed, angry, obsessive, and compulsive[66] and can be suicidal.[67] They also crave carbohydrates and can develop a compulsive eating disorder, gain weight,[68] and develop metabolic syndrome, which involves increased blood pressure and diabetes risk and abnormal cholesterol levels.[69] If left untreated, metabolic syndrome and diabetes can lead to heart disease, stroke, disability, and premature death. Abnormal levels of serotonin will also cause migraines, sleep disorders, mood disorders, and other emotional syndromes.[70] Serotonin is affected also by illicit drugs that trigger high release of serotonin but damage cells that process it, causing hallucinations and impaired cognition.[71]

Endorphins, the endogenous morphine, are naturally manufactured by the human brain. They possess the same functions as synthetic morphine, helping to reduce pain and make people feel well.[72] They slow the heart rate and respiration as needed, when stress from unhealthy thoughts increases. But when people abuse synthetic drugs, such as heroin and opioids that mimic endorphins, the drugs suppress the respiratory center and lower the heart rate to an abnormal level. If carried far enough, the heart and breathing stop.[73] That is why people die from drug overdoses.

The brain is programmed by our super intelligent designer to release the right amount of those necessary neurotransmitters to be able to function normally. However, the human race is constantly disturbing the balance in the brain through unhealthy thoughts and disobedient actions. Throughout the Bible we find God's prescriptions and instructions, which will keep our thoughts healthy, thus implicitly regulating all the chemicals and neurotransmitters, releasing them in healthy amounts—if we follow the divine prescriptions for a healthy physical and spiritual life.

We also have natural, built-in receptors that have calming effects on our brains and with beneficial effects when triggered by our right response to high levels of stress. When people use synthetic, manufactured nicotine and marijuana, they become dependent on those counterfeit stimulants, slowly destroying their bodies and minds.

THE ROLE OF SEROTONIN

We have many receptors throughout our bodies with different functions, built in by our Creator to help our bodies function in a proper, healthy way. These receptors attract neurochemicals or neurotransmitters that either inhibit or stimulate the natural neurochemical release, breaking down molecules to get in and out of cells through different pathways and processes.[74] Neurons make the necessary number of neurotransmitters when receiving the messages and electrical impulses through our five senses and thought processes. We are indeed fearfully and wonderfully made, with all these complex chemicals and their functions to keep us alive and functioning normally. For example, when the serotonin level is low, we can experience depression, anxiety, or irritation. When the serotonin is too high, it can cause restlessness or agitation.[75] In a stressful situation GABA needs to increase to inhibit brain activity in order to decrease anxiety.[76] But if the GABA level is too high, and blocking too many serotonin receptors, it will increase our appetite, then increase our risk of metabolic syndrome, with all its dangers.

While drug companies have developed drugs to increase or decrease serotonin levels, they have many side effects and are very expensive. Scientists have discovered serotonin receptors in the brain, in the gastrointestinal system, and in the blood.[77] Drugs affect not only the brain but many functions of the body. Everything that influences changes in the brain will influence changes in the entire body. For example, increased serotonin through drug ingestion may increase diarrhea and nausea.[78] Due in part to abnormal serotonin levels, people with high levels of stress and worry may develop anxiety, panic attacks, and irritable bowel syndrome (spasms in the intestine).[79] We have many supernatural prescriptions written by divine inspiration in the Word of God for natural serotonin to be released in the body to prevent those unwanted signs and symptoms. God also gave people inspiration to develop synthetic chemicals needed to treat many man-made mental conditions. As a primary care provider I am not against medications. When necessary I prescribe them to treat my patients' acute and chronic conditions. But most of the time they don't experience full relief of the signs and symptoms, and they also report side effects.

We can prescribe many antidepressants and antianxiety medications to keep people happy, but we have a more potent, divine prescription with no side effects. God gave all of us instructions two thousand years ago: rejoice, and socialize with the right people who will encourage us. God wants us to know who we are created to be, and to have confidence and hope, and to feel good about ourselves and our divinely given identity. He tells us to believe the promises in the Word of God—that we are the sons and daughters of the King of the universe, a special people with a heavenly citizenship. We do not need to live under high levels of stress from fears and worries. Those promises make you feel good about yourself and increase your self-esteem, even when you go through tough situations. Your serotonin level will naturally increase to a healthy level and will influence your habits, making you feel fulfilled (even helping you to make the right choices, such as to eat less and lose weight, and influencing the satiety and appetite center in the hypothalamus).

Serotonin helps you sleep and rest better by boosting melatonin, so you can function normally, as you were created to function.[80] Sleeping normal hours will help your entire body rejuvenate, recover, and be restored by boosting your defense mechanisms and immune system to fight diseases caused by high levels of stress. The Word of God gives us instructions to live at peace, to stay still in any situation, and to know that our Creator is our Father and He is God (Ps. 46:10).

Chapter 3

YOUR DNA: BODY, MIND, AND SOUL

You have searched me, Lord, and you know me....For you created my inmost being; you knit me together in my mother's womb. I praise you because I am fearfully and wonderfully made; your works are wonderful, I know that full well. My frame was not hidden from you when I was made in the secret place, when I was woven together in the depths of the earth. Your eyes saw my unformed body; all the days ordained for me were written in your book before one of them came to be. How precious to me are your thoughts, God! How vast is the sum of them!
—Psalm 139:1, 13–17

SCIENCE CLEARLY SHOWS that high levels of stress affect the DNA in every cell.[1] The body contains thousands of incredibly complex systems. Highly specialized in their unique functions and interconnected and programmed to help the whole body grow, they produce energy for motion and reproduction. They also repair, restore, regenerate, refresh, and respond to daily stress. All those commands are embedded within the DNA. Deep within the cells' extreme complexity, stress affects every function. I like what Canadian Bible teacher the late Dr. Grant R. Jeffrey explained in his book *Creation: Remarkable Evidence of God's Design*. Jeffrey described the cell as functioning like a "modern city," possessing defense systems, chemical factories, energy-producing facilities, a heating system, a transportation system, a communication system, an administration office, an information warehouse, a library, and a waste-disposal system.[2]

TRILLIONS OF "MODERN CITIES" INSIDE YOU

Let's take a look inside the cell to discover how its functional complexity can be affected by high levels of stress when you allow fearful, worried thoughts to run out of control. You do not need to memorize the cell description that follows. In

Fundamentals of Anatomy and Physiology, professors Frederic Martini, Judi Nath, and Edwin Bartholomew talk about how each cell has a complex structure, including a cell membrane, cytosol, a nucleus, non-membranous organelles, and membranous organelles. They go on to say: "Nonmembranous organelles include the cytoskeleton, centrosome with centrioles, ribosomes, and proteasomes.... Membranous organelles include the endoplasmic reticulum, the Golgi apparatus, lysosomes, peroxisomes and mitochondria." The cell membrane is composed of a "lipid bilayer containing phospholipids, steroids, proteins, and carbohydrates"; its functions are "isolation; protection; sensitivity; support, [and controlling] entry and exit of materials" from the cell. "The cytosol is the fluid component of the cytoplasm" that "distributes material by diffusion." The cytoskeleton is composed of "proteins organized in fine filaments" used for "strength and support; movement of cellular structures and materials." Microvilli are membrane extensions "containing microfilaments"; they help to "increase surface area to facilitate absorption of extracellular materials." The centrosome is part of the cytoplasm and contains two centrioles, each made of 9 microtubule triplets; the centrosome and centrioles are "essential for movement of chromosomes during cell division" and "organization of microtubules in [the] cytoskeleton." Ribosomes are RNA+ proteins that can be "fixed ribosomes bound to endoplasmic reticulum" or "free ribosomes scattered in cytoplasm" for protein synthesis. Mitochondria have a "double membrane, with inner membrane folds...enclosing important metabolic enzymes"; they "produce 95% of the ATP required by the cell." The endoplastic reticulum (ER) is a "network of membranous channels extending throughout the cytoplasm" that is necessary for "synthesis of secretory products; intracellular storage and transport.... Rough ER has ribosomes, and it modifies and packages newly synthesized proteins. Smooth ER does not have ribosomes and synthesizes lipids and carbohydrates." The Golgi apparatus comprises "stacks of flattened membranes (cisternae) containing chambers" used for "storage, alteration, and packaging of secretory products and lysosomal enzymes." Lysosomes are vesicles that contain powerful digestive enzymes and are used for "intracellular removal of damaged organelles or pathogens." Peroxisomes are "vesicles containing degradative enzymes" and are used for "neutralization of toxic compounds." The nucleus is composed of "nucleoplasm containing nucleotides, enzymes, nucleoproteins, and chromatin"; it is "surrounded by a double membrane, the nuclear envelope." The nucleus controls metabolism, stores and processes genetic information, and controls protein synthesis. Part of the nucleus structure, the nucleolus contains DNA and RNA and is the "site of rRNA synthesis and assembly of ribosomal subunit(s)."[3]

High levels of stress, thoughts of fear, anxiety, and worry of all kinds are an outside insult, like "a tsunami" affecting every cell—this "modern city" in your body—bringing devastating, irreversible damages. It is extremely important to follow God's prescriptions (presented later in this book) to obtain His promises in our lives so that we can reduce our anxiety and stress levels.

Stress "Tsunamis" Affect Your DNA

> My soul is overwhelmed with sorrow to the point of death.
> —Mark 14:34

Our DNA tells our cells (where the DNA resides) what they need to produce in order to maintain life. The genetic code, life's blueprint, is packed into the DNA. I believe this is God's language built into our human chromosomes, designing and developing every organ in our extremely complex bodies. To quote Dr. Grant Jeffrey again:

> To record the genetic instructions encoded in human DNA we would need more than five billion letters that would require up to three thousand volumes to print out. This enormous amount of information would fill a library shelf over one hundred yards long. Yet it is intricately encoded in a tiny double helix curled up in a microscopic cell. This degree of microengineering is so far beyond the ability of humans that it fills the mind with wonder at the work of the Creator.[4]

If your stress level is very high and lasts for a long period of time, it can even modify your marvelous DNA through gene mutation.[5] Genetic mutation can lead to abnormal, uncontrollable cell division—what we call cancer.[6] DNA, the genetic blueprint, has encoded instructions for growing, reproducing, repairing, restoring, and building life.[7] You were created in such an orderly, disciplined way that your DNA synthesizes proteins and enables your organism to produce energy to regenerate, repair, restore, heal, reorganize, and reproduce.[8] All these functions of every cell, with help from the DNA, are affected by the high levels of stress, worry, and anxiety you experience, along with the actions and behaviors you exhibit as a result.[9]

The Unconscious Brain

> For God does speak—now one way, now another—though no one perceives it. In a dream, in a vision of the night, when deep sleep falls on people as they slumber in their beds, he may speak in their ears and terrify them with warnings, to turn them from wrongdoing and keep them from pride, to preserve them from the pit, their lives from perishing by the sword.
> —Job 33:14–18

Studies have shown that past emotional memories from stressful events affect our future at the unconscious level, as well as the way we react to future situations.

In a research paper on the effects of stress on cognitive versus emotional function, professors Aparna Suvrathan, Rajnish Rao, and Sumantra Chattarji affirmed:

> Explicit memories of facts or events, encoded by a brain structure called the hippocampus, tend to fade away with time. In contrast, unconscious emotional memories of stressful experiences, formed in a brain structure called the amygdala, appear to leave an indelible mark that may last for a lifetime. The rapid and efficient encoding of fearful memories by the amygdala help us cope with threatening stimuli in the future, but it also comes at a high price. These emotional memories etched into the amygdalar circuitry can also become maladaptive. For example, high anxiety and mood lability are cardinal symptoms of many stress disorders. Here we review recent findings that provide insights into the cellular and synaptic mechanisms underlying the cognitive and emotional effects of stress.[10]

The brain has built-in features of incredible computational power at the unconscious and conscious levels. The unconscious mind (in areas such as the amygdala and nucleus accumbens) assesses threats and sends signals to the body through the neurochemicals and neurotransmitters, released in the body automatically as a response to your thoughts of fear, worry, and anxiety. Just a quick calculation of the power of your brain, based on what is known at this time, shows that many neurons can fire fifty times per second when the electrical impulse arrives to pass the synapses' threshold.[11] Some estimate that neurons may have up to ten thousand synapses, meaning that our brains have as many as one thousand trillion synaptic connections to process our thoughts, communications, and actions.[12]

It is beyond our comprehension how the body has been created by the super intelligent designer, the Creator of the universe. Indeed we are amazing, complex creatures and wonderfully made, as the king and psalmist David stated thousands of years ago—before modern, scientific evidence flooded our libraries. He wrote: "I will praise You, for I am fearfully and wonderfully made; marvelous are Your works, and that my soul knows very well" (Ps. 139:14, NKJV). Deep in his inner being David knew (approximately three thousand years ago) about these complex functions of the human body, mind, soul, and spirit, having been shown this by the Spirit of God. It is extremely important to select quality thoughts that trigger healthy neurotransmitters and not to destroy neurons and synapses, with their great impact on our cognition.

STRESS AFFECTS YOUR NEUROCHEMICAL BALANCE

> The human spirit can endure in sickness, but a crushed spirit who can bear?
>
> —PROVERBS 18:14

> You will keep in perfect peace those whose minds are steadfast, because they trust in you. Trust in the LORD forever, for the LORD, the LORD himself, is the Rock eternal.
> —Isaiah 26:3–4

Studies show that those who have suffered from chronic depression can develop metabolic syndrome (glucose intolerance, diabetes, hypertension, dyslipidemia, and obesity) and vice versa.[13] Those who suffer from metabolic syndrome can likewise develop depression, with its complications. The cycle repeats itself. Diabetes is increasing so much that in America researchers predicted that between 2015 and 2030 we would see a 54 percent increase in the number of Americans suffering from this disease, with the medical and societal costs of the disease projected to reach $622 billion.[14] This can be reduced if people learn they can help prevent depression and diabetes by changing their lifestyle, way of thinking, and attitude when fear, worry, and anxiety hit. We need to react appropriately to avoid bad habits. Diseases and high costs will cause stress levels to go up even more. This becomes a problem affecting everyone in the world, now and for future generations.

Stress and unwise behaviors cause more damage, making people more dependent on others. If the world ignores God's prescriptions for managing stress, there will be larger numbers of dependent people and fewer able to provide care to all those affected by the diseases and consequences of bad behavior and unhealthy thinking. Changing the world's thinking is urgent if we want to prevent the disaster of a stress pandemic. God's prescriptions, which function beyond the scope of science, will lead us in the right direction. They can heal emotionally broken people for all eternity. With God's healing, people are stronger at that place of brokenness, just as in a human body a broken bone is stronger after it heals. As Psalm 147:3 says: "He heals the brokenhearted and binds up their wounds." When God heals us, we are stronger in the place of brokenness and able to comfort the world around us with the same comfort. We can help heal people's brokenness with a godly approach. We can grow healthier and stronger by knowing God and His prescriptions for stress management.

PART II

ROOT CAUSES OF STRESS

Chapter 4

A WORLD OF PROBLEMS

Therefore, I urge you, brothers and sisters, in view of God's mercy, to offer your bodies as a living sacrifice, holy and pleasing to God—this is your true and proper worship. Do not conform to the pattern of this world, but be transformed by the renewing of your mind. Then you will be able to test and approve what God's will is—his good, pleasing and perfect will.
—Romans 12:1–2

A SCAN OF DAILY news headlines is all we need to know the entire world is suffering from unsolved problems. Fear, worry, and anxiety are everywhere, and stress is rising exponentially. Many people fear the future. They worry about being rejected, or not forgiven, or unable to forgive. They worry about their lack of finances, poor health, or lack of friends. Loneliness further affects their thinking process. People fear losing their jobs, losing a loved one, facing rejection or failure, or chronic health conditions—it can seem as if the situation is getting worse despite their efforts to overcome.

You may have the same question I often had: Who will fix the world's problems? Who will change conditions? Many think advanced technology, or armies, or corporations, or talented people, or new scientific discoveries will save us. Even in this postmodern era so many problems remain unsolved, leaving people under constant pressure. When we are under constant stress, dangerous levels of neurochemicals and neurotransmitters are released as cortisol, the "stress hormone." High levels of cortisol released in the hippocampus area kill neurons.[1] Unfortunately most people do not understand these disease processes and how high levels of stress, fear, worry, and anxiety can damage their brains—indeed their entire bodies.

Since the dawn of creation, mankind has made great progress in many directions, yet in many areas humanity is experiencing drastic deterioration. When people experience fear and worry from uncertainty, financial insecurity, separation, divorce, drug abuse, abortion, guilt, discouragement, bitterness, and other problems, stress levels keep going up, further damaging the whole body. The supernatural prescription for preventing physical and spiritual damage resonates in my mind: "Do not conform to the pattern of this world, but be transformed by the renewing of your mind" (Rom. 12:2).

Unhealthy Individuals, Unhealthy Society

The world's culture is deteriorating, marred by widespread drug use, alcoholism, violence, anger, immorality, pornography, prostitution, and human trafficking—all leading to fear, worry, and anxiety. The result: multiple chronic diseases and death. If not properly addressed, all the unhealthy behavior displayed in this generation will lead to physical and spiritual diseases—and physical and spiritual death. You have likely heard the cliché that it takes a village to raise a child. But in order to have a healthy child, that village must itself be healthy.

We must change our thinking about family life, the foundation of any society. A society cannot remain healthy if individuals, families, and the educational system are unhealthy and political leaders untrustworthy. Schoolteachers know that nothing can be fixed at school before the family is fixed at home. Too many children do not have their biological fathers in their lives as role models. As a result, they often become rebellious at home, at school, and in their communities. They may have a stepfather who is trying hard to provide care, but this is not the same thing. Children can become bitter, feeling rejected by their biological fathers. Accumulating bitterness in their souls can express itself in outbursts and angry episodes. All too often we see teens committing murder or dying because of suicide.

When the biological father is not in a child's life—not available to share feelings, needs, joys, and sorrows—then bad feelings accumulate in the area of the brain associated with memories and emotions (the limbic system's hippocampus and amygdala), causing anger and leading to violent, destructive behaviors.[2] They do not know what it means to honor their fathers, to be encouraged, to show respect, and to feel their fathers' love. Divorced and dysfunctional families are epidemic. All the distress, depression, anxiety, dissatisfaction, and other unhealthy emotions are transmitted from a single mother to her children. Children without both parents suffer and cannot concentrate to perform well at school, leading to low self-esteem. On the other hand, passive, permissive, inconsistent, and poor parenting creates more problems in society. We live in a painful world, and we need to have clear expectations for children in order to avoid chronic problems in the future.

Stress Starts in Childhood

> Jesus said, "Let the little children come to me, and do not hinder them, for the kingdom of heaven belongs to such as these."
> —Matthew 19:14

> He took a little child whom he placed among them. Taking the child in his arms, he said to them, "Whoever welcomes one of these little children in my name welcomes me; and whoever welcomes me does not welcome me but the one who sent me."
> —Mark 9:36–37

A wealth of scientific literature has documented that the brain structure is altered in children facing family adversity during their childhood. One 2014 article on the role of a particular protein in processing emotions said:

> Accumulating evidence suggests a role of FKBP5, a co-chaperone regulating the glucocorticoid receptor sensitivity, in the etiology of depression and anxiety disorders. Based on recent findings of altered amygdala activity following childhood adversity, the present study aimed at clarifying the impact of genetic variation in FKBP5 on threat-related neural activity and coupling as well as morphometric alterations in stress-sensitive brain systems.
>
> Functional magnetic resonance imaging during an emotional face-matching task was performed in 153 healthy young adults (66 males) from a high-risk community sample followed since birth. Voxel-based morphometry was applied to study structural alterations and DNA was genotyped for FKBP5 rs1360780. Childhood adversity was measured using retrospective self-report (Childhood Trauma Questionnaire) and by a standardized parent interview assessing childhood family adversity. Depression was assessed by the Beck Depression Inventory. There was a main effect of FKBP5 on the left amygdala, with T homozygotes showing the highest activity, largest volume and increased coupling with the left hippocampus and the orbitofrontal cortex (OFC). Moreover, amygdala-OFC coupling proved to be associated with depression in this genotype. In addition, our results support previous evidence of a gene-environment interaction on right amygdala activity with respect to retrospective assessment of childhood adversity, but clarify that this does not generalize to the prospective assessment. These findings indicated that activity in T homozygotes increased with the level of adversity, whereas the opposite pattern emerged in C homozygotes, with CT individuals being intermediate. The present results point to a functional involvement of FKBP5 in intermediate phenotypes associated with emotional processing, suggesting a possible

mechanism for this gene in conferring susceptibility to stress-related disorders.[3]

We now know that stressors in childhood form memories of traumatic events, which can affect us as adults and our offspring, from generation to generation.[4] Everything parents go through reflects on their children due to the mirror neurons in the brain.[5] As a child I lived in a big family of eight children, and my father worked prolonged hours to provide for our needs. One day my mother fell ill, and my father came home and rushed her to the hospital; there wasn't a telephone to call for an ambulance. My mother had been falling on the floor because she had weak legs from acute thrombophlebitis and other complications.

When I saw her falling, something broke in my heart and mind. Distressed, I started to cry—almost paralyzed by thoughts of discouragement. I was only eleven years old when I experienced those feelings of hopelessness and helplessness. But those painful memories are still fresh in my mind, stirring emotions each time I visit the storage of old memories (even after more than forty-five years).

Even now when I see disabled people who are suffering, those memories stored long ago are activated. They produce emotional pain if I do not suppress them with the promises of God, that He is our constant healer and great physician. Children feel the stress of their parents' problems, which remains with them for a long time if not addressed properly. The mirror neurons built into our brain structures are involved in this process. But for children it is more intense because their brains are not completely developed until their twenties.[6]

Children will generally mirror their parents' behavior. What children learn at home on a daily basis remains with them when they grow up. If they see parents loving each other, they will imitate them later in their lives. If they see parents fighting, hating, divorcing, committing adultery, drinking, consuming drugs and alcohol, and smoking, the children will likely do the same. Thus the cliché "Like father, like son." Children mirror their parents' behavior by consolidating those memories, which influence their behavior in the future.[7]

Once, looking through some drawers, seeking information for the business demands of the day, my eyes fell on a folder with pictures of my best friend, Mary, who died of cancer long before. All the memories were so fresh in my mind, as if it had just happened. Divorced, Mary had three small children who were emotionally devastated by seeing their mother die at such a young age. I already knew their struggles and understood why they did not have a father like a normal family. Their mother needed to fill that gap left by her husband, who had abandoned his family for another woman. Even now those children continue to struggle emotionally—even though their parents were intellectuals with advanced educational degrees, and even though their mother provided a home for the children to live in and money for food, clothing, and other expenses.

Despite good advice and committed help from good friends who were available for those children after their mother passed away, they used up all their personal resources and have had a difficult time succeeding. You could easily read the distress in their hearts on their faces. Children with no family structure struggle to make it in life.

Mirror neurons enable children to actively mirror those around them, helping with mental development and growth. Children are forming a mirror image of the behavior they see repeatedly and will behave later in the same way.[8] For example, children living with depressed parents or siblings, or with divorced parents, or drug addicts, or alcoholics, will suffer later because of these mirror neurons. Science has discovered that mirror neurons are active in a child's brain when health care professionals are doing play therapy.[9] Our Creator built mirror neurons into our bodies for nurturing, empathy, healthy growth, self-actualization, and great achievements.[10] To build a healthy society, we must create a healthy environment for children so they will do the same for their future families.

In today's society stress levels are high, and children feel it too. We know that such levels of stress will reduce the serotonin level in the brain, causing more depression. Statistics tell us that millions of people are on antidepressants. Demands in this postmodern era stress out millions, which is why the use of antidepressants is on the rise.[11] When stress is high, our brains register stimuli that influence our thinking process in unhealthy ways. The atmosphere is created for more cortisol to be released in the brain, killing neurons responsible for producing serotonin, and then more depression is seen in the children. Families often put stress on children, expecting high performance and perfection in everything at a young age. Children also experience high levels of stress and anxiety from dysfunctional families—no love, rejection, low self-esteem—and in a short time they can become depressed. But here is hope in the supernatural prescription: "Jesus said, 'Let the little children come to me, and do not hinder them, for the kingdom of heaven belongs to such as these'" (Matt. 19:14).

STRESS IN ADOLESCENCE

Start children off on the way they should go, and even when they are old they will not turn from it.
—PROVERBS 22:6

From infancy you have known the Holy Scriptures, which are able to make you wise for salvation through faith in Christ Jesus. All Scripture is God-breathed and is useful for teaching, rebuking, correcting and training in righteousness, so that the servant of God may be thoroughly equipped for every good work.
—2 TIMOTHY 3:15–17

Now let us look into what is happening in the brain of a child or an adolescent who becomes addicted to illicit or prescription drugs, which will invariably lead to unhealthy behaviors. The prefrontal cortex, the conscious part of the brain used to evaluate situations and to make decisions, is the last area to finish developing in children.[12] Young children, then, cannot be expected to make good decisions consistently. Adolescents are impacted by memories of their childhood and also by peer pressure, activities, school attendance and performance, friends, sleep disturbances, medical issues, and family dynamics—any of which can cause physical and psychological pain.

Poor parental modeling as well as psychological stress (fear, anxiety, and depression) will cause abnormal nervous system activities.[13] This will lead to withdrawal from society, missing school, and poor socialization.[14] Pain will cause more stress and emotional thoughts. Fear itself can cause a child to avoid healthy behavior. It can also cause more pain, leading the young person to be overly worried and sensitive to pain, which then can bring on further anxiety and depression. Chronic illness is a potentially sad result.[15]

Parents usually restrict children from some otherwise healthy activities when they are ill but allow them to stay home and play games on the internet—an immediate reward system for illness through the dopamine neurotransmitter. I already mentioned that high dopamine levels can lead to substance abuse, such as alcohol, stimulants, opioids, sedatives, marijuana, and tobacco.[16] A healthy family life and wise parental decisions play a major part in a child's recovery. The more attention you pay to the pain, the more the pain will grow, causing the sufferer to seek painkillers, with an increased risk of addiction. Positive confrontation is needed to recover from pain. Parents must interact with children positively and provide a healthy home environment. In a family under constant stress the children will develop psychological pain. Culture, beliefs, behavior during illness, social interaction, and emotional support play a huge role in an adolescent's recovery from pain.

Some will seek narcotics when they're experiencing stress, anxiety, or worry. Fear and anxiety increase the adolescent's risk of substance abuse, including alcohol, cigarettes, and/or medication. The adolescent craves something to relieve the pressure and tension built up from psychological distress.[17] The results can be low self-esteem, trouble with peers, poor grades in school, poor socialization, weak coping mechanisms, or feelings of rejection.[18]

Parents' behavior directly affects their children's behavior. Parents need to know that pain "loves" an audience. Over-coddling children to reinforce bad behavior is never good, but reasonable expectations are vital. Do not allow children to avoid healthy activities. Escaping activities shouldn't be the solution to avoid consequences from pain. Good relaxation techniques, such as deep breathing, will decrease anxiety and loosen tight muscles—a mindfulness approach to relieving stress.

Increased pain will increase stress. So we need to teach children to use positive coping strategies that provide a distraction. Reducing the focus on pain will reduce physiological arousal, which produces physiological changes that will reduce pain.[19]

We can suppress an existing habit by understanding the source of that habit and redirecting it to a better source. Rewards for participation in activities are contingent reinforcement to pain-control strategies. If a child fails to meet specific goals, it helps to ensure there will be consequences. For example, let the child know that he or she has normal privileges when attending school and no privileges if the child misses school.

Parents need to help their children learn how to deal with pain. It takes good, family-based, problem-solving management to guide children toward success and prevent school failure, addictions, and other tragedies. Help children manage the associated stress if they have a medical condition. Help them reengage in life and manage their pain when they face a crisis. Allowing children to withdraw from physical activities will only increase their anxiety. "Start children off on the way they should go, and even when they are old they will not turn from it" (Prov. 22:6).

Volunteering in the community is a wonderful, positive activity. Our brains like to be active all the time. Neurons require constant stimulation to stay alive. An inactive cell is a dying cell.[20] My daughter was in middle school when she started volunteering with the elderly in foster homes. Later she volunteered at Portland Adventist Community Services Health Clinic, where I volunteered as a primary care provider, and then at a hospital, working with children suffering from cancer. She also volunteered in the church, working with small children. Volunteer experience gave her the drive to study more and helped her choose a profession with a great future. She never touched drugs or engaged in other unhealthy behavior, and she enjoyed a healthy adolescence.

Constructive thoughts, facing our fears, and moderating our pain language will improve our mood, help us be more active, decrease our anxiety, and increase our whole quality of life.

Too many young people live with feelings of anxiety and depression, a lack of self-esteem, and rejection. They start looking for affection, love, and acceptance in the wrong groups, leading to unhealthy behaviors and bad habits—drugs, gangs, or adultery, which can result in AIDS or contracting a sexually transmitted disease (STD). They become emotionally disabled at a very young age as a consequence of behaviors that were triggered by an unstable environment, creating psychosocial distress in their lives. Some become so overwhelmed that they resort to violence or suicide.

When young adolescents consume high doses of marijuana, they develop delusions and cannot think clearly. With distorted thoughts, they develop amotivational syndrome, which will eventually ruin their future.[21] They are not motivated to study to finish high school, not able to get and keep a job, and often not able to get married and have a family. Their future is destroyed. As we learned earlier, marijuana damages the brain, with long-term consequences. As the gateway to more dangerous drugs such as heroin, it is the road to disaster for individuals and for society as a whole.

It is obvious to most of us that the world is going in the wrong direction. To change the world, we must fix things that are not right. We must influence our communities, including political leaders, to identify the root causes of problems that adversely affect our society, and start from there to correct the defects.

Frequently young patients come into the clinic asking for a prescription for a medical marijuana card for different kinds of "pain." When I check their health records and ask about their disease history, there is nothing indicating they need that drug! We need to change our approach in the health care system and educate our adolescents to think productive, healthy thoughts by bringing spirituality back into medicine because "all Scripture is God-breathed and is useful for teaching, rebuking, correcting and training in righteousness, so that the servant of God may be thoroughly equipped for every good work" (2 Tim. 3:16–17).

The Burden of Hidden Stress

> Come unto me, all ye that labour and are heavy laden, and I will give you rest. Take my yoke upon you, and learn of me; for I am meek and lowly in heart: and ye shall find rest unto your souls. For my yoke is easy, and my burden is light.
>
> —Matthew 11:28–30, kjv

People suffering from hidden stress often have unexplained signs and symptoms, making a doctor's heart "sink." In my practice I see patients presenting with the same symptoms repeatedly but with no physiological causes. Patients become more worried about their sickness and are restless if their provider cannot find a diagnosis for their symptoms. Physiological diseases get much more attention than psychological problems. Yet doctors need a psychological framework to achieve better outcomes when dealing with hidden stress. People with hidden stress may experience many of the signs and symptoms listed in the first chapters. They visit emergency rooms (ERs) frequently and consult with specialists for tests, with no physiological explanation. Even psychiatrists cannot diagnose them. It is costly and frustrating due to all the workups and false positive results. Though doctors rule out serious illnesses, the patients remain ill. People are reluctant to accept "hidden stress" as a cause of illness. It may not be mental illness, or delusional, but they have hit the wall and are deficient in self-care skills.

Childhood stress can carry over into adult life.[22] From long-term stress the intestines develop permeability, and nutrients "leak out" and are not absorbed into the bloodstream. Then the cell can't get the right nutrients for health, resulting in unpleasant physical symptoms.[23] From childhood emotions stuffed in the back of their minds (physical, psychological, sexual, or substance abuse, or domestic violence), chronic stress diminishes self-esteem.[24] Later those children may be involved in drug use, suicidal attempts, alcohol abuse, anxiety, panic attacks, and depression.[25]

Often specialists have those patients journal their feelings and address them directly toward the people who abused them in their childhood. It has been shown that writing down feelings, addressing them to the people who caused trauma to their souls, and forgiveness will bring much-needed relief and healing. Writing about stress and worry is more helpful than people realize. We need to reflect, think of solutions, and learn self-care skills. Finding activities we enjoy and finding time to focus on our spiritual needs are important. Become aware of bad habits, and reinforce positive habits. Patients with massive stress are not always consciously aware of it.

Anger is transferable. Mothers with displaced anger will transfer that to their children. For example, if after a divorce the mother needs to overwork to take care of everything and then uses words that are verbally and emotionally abusive, her children will suffer emotional damage.[26] Stress from childhood can be hidden for a long time—even a lifetime—whether we are consciously aware of it or not. But similar thoughts will trigger memories and emotions later, with unpleasant feelings and disastrous illnesses if not properly addressed. You can find rest for the burden of hidden stress when you follow Jesus' instruction: "Come unto me, all ye that labour and are heavy laden, and I will give you rest" (Matt. 11:28, KJV).

STRESS LEADS TO UNHEALTHY LIFESTYLES

> Be very careful, then, how you live—not as unwise but as wise, making the most of every opportunity, because the days are evil. Therefore do not be foolish, but understand what the Lord's will is.
> —EPHESIANS 5:15–17

Due to thoughts of hopelessness and disorientation in life, many people are prone to unhealthy lifestyles. Overeating, a lack of exercise, and inactivity will develop into metabolic syndrome—a cluster of diseases (hypertension, diabetes, dyslipidemia, obesity) that damage the body, mind, and spirit. It is a vicious cycle with no hope. Hope is complete when we are connected with God, as we read in Romans: "Since we have been justified through faith, we have peace with God through our Lord Jesus Christ, through whom we have gained access by faith into this grace in which we now stand. And we boast in the hope of the glory of God" (Rom. 5:1–2).

Hope in the Word of God does not disappoint. God is speaking to people through dreams, visions, and signs but most of the time through His Word. We have access to His grace by faith in Christ, and faith in His Word helps to prevent unhealthy lifestyles. The brain, through communication between the prefrontal cortex and basal ganglia, has the ability to learn new habits and modify bad habits.[27] Meditation on the promises of God will help the brain focus on positive thoughts and healthy coping mechanisms to deal with stress and overcome it to prevent an unhealthy lifestyle.

Risky Technology Addiction

Addiction in the body is triggered by a high level of dopamine (through the immediate reward mechanism), a neurochemical that, when released, produces "feel good" emotions. Scientists have found that in order to overcome addiction, people need to strengthen their anterior cingulate circuits, found in the frontal lobe, in order to control the neurochemical dopamine involved in addiction.[28] Dopamine in unhealthy levels clouds the brain and reduces one's judgment capacity[29]—which can be lethal. To strengthen the neurochemical fabric in our brains, we must control our thought process and change our thinking. Only the Word of God has the power to transform our minds and thinking.

People often get addicted to video games, gambling, internet pornography, web-based shopping, overeating (junk food causes you to gain weight, leading to metabolic syndrome and all its signs and symptoms), drinking, drugs, and internet dating—anticipating the immediate gratification of feeling good. These bad habits will boost the dopamine level in the brain. High levels of dopamine can cause immediate gratification, but in the long run the storage runs out,[30] creating emptiness in people's hearts and terrible, lifelong consequences.

Preserve your ability to store dopamine by staying away from compulsive, unhealthy behaviors so you can preserve good judgment and enjoy a better quality of life. You are in control of your life and your thinking process. You have the ability to reconstruct your neurons, brain, and judgment. When you feel euphoria, it comes from a high dopamine level, which is responsible for motivation and rewards. We want more and more of those feelings, described thousands of years ago in Proverbs: "There are three things that are never satisfied, four that never say, 'Enough!': the grave, the barren womb, land, which is never satisfied with water, and fire, which never says, 'Enough!'" (Prov. 30:15–16). When people develop compulsive, unhealthy behaviors that cause addiction, there will never be *enough*.

All addictive activities activate the neurons in the prefrontal cortex, which controls short-term memories and decisions. This releases more dopamine (responsible for pleasure) and leads to dependency with bad consequences.[31]

Worry Increases Stress

> Therefore do not worry about tomorrow, for tomorrow will worry about itself. Each day has enough trouble of its own.
> —Matthew 6:34

The root causes of stress are many, but the biggest one is worrying about tomorrow, which causes increased anxiety and depression. But the Bible gives us the prescription for this ailment. Matthew 6:34 tells us not to worry about it! Every single day, God gives strength to those who are burdened by worry. I was worried and anxious many times in my life, and yet I couldn't seem to do anything to get out of my hopeless situations.

I had to trust in God every day and believe in His divine intervention to bring supernatural solutions for my problems. I had to meditate on the promises of God and repeat them constantly, through the worst and best times of my life. Many Bible verses are written for our benefit, to prevent us from worrying about tomorrow. The Word of God teaches us how to cope and manage stress to prevent the brain from responding to high levels of stress by releasing toxic chemicals and neurotransmitters that would destroy our health. The threats of worry about tomorrow—the stressors—will send signals through the pathways that the Creator wired inside the body to fight threats. But if we ignore God's instructions and allow our minds to engage with worry and anxiety, our brains will be flooded with many neurochemicals in abnormal quantities—toxins poisoning and affecting the whole body.

Excessive Worry

Acute stress syndrome (ACS) can result from excessive worries about anything when people experience traumatic, catastrophic life events, such as a natural disaster, an assault, or a car accident. ACS brings uncomfortable signs and symptoms and toxic amounts of neurotransmitters. People endure endless tests, with negative results, and yet their uncomfortable and unexplained medical signs and symptoms remain. Normal life includes a normal amount of anxiety for success, but excessive amounts cause unhealthy amounts of neurochemicals to be released, which will cloud your mind.[32] If you feel irritation building inside, or tension, sleep disturbance, and fatigue, or if your cognition is affected, or you have other signs and symptoms discussed in this book, then your anxiety is growing and your mind is clouded from too many neurochemicals.

I remember the nuclear accident in Chernobyl, USSR, in the spring of 1986. The resulting nuclear cloud reached all over northwestern Europe.[33] Millions of people were affected; even today many diseases and disabilities, especially of the thyroid gland, remain in adults who were children at that time.[34] Using that analogy, the "clouds" of neurochemicals released in your brain and body from unhealthy thoughts can modify your DNA through epigenetics. The gene's expression is altered, increasing the risk of diseases in future generations.[35] Just remember that meditating on the promises of God in His powerful Word pushes away the "clouds" of unhealthy neurochemicals and neurotransmitters from your mind and builds new neurons through neurogenesis, divinely strengthening your mind and body.

No matter your age, you can still benefit from making changes. All stress-related mental and physical conditions start with anxiety, cognition impairment, increased short-term memory loss, or depression. MRI tests have shown that mild cognitive impairment can precede Alzheimer's disease.[36] People with excessive worry, known as generalized anxiety disorder, and those who do not sleep enough develop early signs of neurocognitive disorders.[37] The best way to prevent cognitive impairment is to start today to reduce excessive worry, anxiety, and depression and focus on positive attitudes and faith in God's prescriptions.

Use relaxation techniques and deep breathing whenever you feel stressed. Take your mind off those things that cause you anxiety and emotional distress, and redirect your thoughts to past positive experiences that brought you success and victory. Take a quick walk (even if just five or ten minutes) when you feel overwhelmed with worry and fear. Physical exercise, even walking, is equivalent to pharmacotherapy; just one and a half miles a day will be a benefit. More is even better. The faster you can walk, the longer you are expected to live; speed correlates with longevity.[38] Evaluate the increased level of stress in your life by verifying your feelings at the end of the day. Are you emotionally drained? Do you feel tired when you get up to face another day of work? How is your relationship with those around you? Do you feel burned out, frustrated, hardened emotionally, uncaring, or victimized?

FEAR AND WORRY

> My life is consumed by anguish and my years by groaning; my strength fails because of my affliction, and my bones grow weak.
> —PSALM 31:10

Fear comes from doubt and unbelief. Healthy faith comes from meditating and hearing positive promises for your life from God's Word and verses such as "The one who is in you is greater than the one who is in the world" (1 John 4:4) and "If God is for us, who can be against us?" (Rom. 8:31). Neuroscientists have discovered that meditation affects the alpha brain waves, enabling the brain to filter unnecessary information and focus on the most important information to improve cognition for basic operations in our daily lives.[39] Meditate on this promise, and do not let people speak fear into your life, causing doubt and unbelief. Doubts and unbelief are unhealthy faith, which is called fear.

Both faith and unbelief come by hearing. If you hear discouraging words, your faith decreases and fear increases. That produces stress, with all its physiological and psychological manifestations. The brain perceives fearful thoughts as a threat. When you speak encouraging words, your faith will be increased and your fear will disappear. Faith brings hope, peace, and joy. Our words hold the power of life and death.

Nearly two thousand years ago James wrote about our tongue: "The tongue also is a fire, a world of evil among the parts of the body. It corrupts the whole body, sets the whole course of one's life on fire, and is itself set on fire by hell" (Jas. 3:6). That statement is still true. We see all over the world today that the tongue is like a deadly poison. It causes damage when one speaks words against the promises of God, and then the spoken words enter someone else's brain, and the spoken words are transformed into electrical signals that travel through synapses and axons to neurons, forming fearful or threatening thoughts. These trigger poisonous amounts of neurochemicals to be released from those neurons that affect the emotions, mind, spirit, and body.[40]

Use your tongue to declare encouraging words from the life-giving promises of God. It is very important to pray God's promises over your life. Your prayer will be full of healthy words, and hearing those words will build your faith. God loves people with great faith, who believe the promises written in His Word. Faith is essential: "Without faith it is impossible to please God, because anyone who comes to him must believe that he exists and that he rewards those who earnestly seek him" (Heb. 11:6). The reward for your faith will be a healthy, happy life—here on earth and in eternity.

People live with fear every day, refusing to believe God's promises. Growing up in Romania, for many years I feared losing everything. The communists threatened us because of our values and beliefs. Christians had to live on the margins during Nicolae Ceaușescu's communist regime—a harsh dictatorship—or take the exile route. We suffered brutality, ruthless repression, harassment, and death threats. Communists in Romania suffocated our individual freedom and human rights with Marxist-Leninist atheistic doctrine. Ordinary Christians were arrested, brainwashed, and threatened with losing their privileges, education, and jobs. But for me the fear of God was stronger than the fear of men.

FEAR OF FAILURE BRINGS STRESS

> Being confident of this, that he who began a good work in you will carry it on to completion until the day of Christ Jesus.
> —PHILIPPIANS 1:6

Insecurity and fear of failure bring anxiety and depression. Fear of failure is not uncommon. We are afraid of not being excellent or not being perfect. I often experienced anxiety from the fear of failure, especially in Romania's communist regime. I needed to avoid the persecution of the communists, whose mocking attitude never ended until they were overthrown. Then, when I moved to the United States, I grew even more anxious. I did not speak English and was unable to express myself and make my needs known. To illustrate, one time somebody told me to bring something from an area from the right side of the building. I said, "OK," and then to that person's amazement I turned to the left and started to walk away. I did not have a clue what she wanted me to do. I was so embarrassed; it felt as if the earth were sinking under my feet.

In college all the exams were very difficult, and I had an inordinate fear of failure. I had to work harder, spending prolonged hours to meet all my school requirements while at the same time operating my business responsibly. I learned many times from my own mistakes, even though I was afraid. I worried that I would fail to manage the business and I might lose it. You must give yourself permission to learn from mistakes. While this quote has been attributed to a number of people and is of uncertain origin, I like the wisdom it expresses: "I learned that good judgment comes from experience and that experience grows out of mistakes."

Fear and Anxiety Paralyze

> A thousand may fall at your side, ten thousand at your right hand, but it will not come near you. You will only observe with your eyes and see the punishment of the wicked.
> —Psalm 91:7–8

The devil wants to mutilate us and reduce us to silence. The power to do what is right is built into us. Maybe that is why the Creator designed our systems with neurotransmitters to inhibit abnormal actions and calm our brains down when we are overwhelmed by anxiety or agitated by fear and worry. GABA, the inhibitory neurotransmitter, brings calmness but must be activated through the power of the Holy Spirit with the promises of God and His primary instruction for life that appears dozens of times in Scripture: "Do not be afraid."

The Holy Spirit is our helper and brings the Word to our memory. According to Genesis 1:2, the Holy Spirit created order in the universe when it was just chaos. The same Spirit is hovering over us, ready to intervene, according to God's promises in the Word of God. The Comforter will bring order into our brains when we are under excessive pressure from worry and stress—but only when we give Him permission. Through prayer we enter into the spiritual realm, activating the promises of God. Many times fear has gripped my heart about uncertain things, but whenever I was afraid, I prayed.

Nothing will harm you when you pray and do the right thing, "for the eyes of the Lord are on the righteous and his ears are attentive to their prayer, but the face of the Lord is against those who do evil" (1 Pet. 3:12). God fights for you. He reduces the wicked to silence. "He will guard the feet of his faithful servants, but the wicked will be silenced in the place of darkness" (1 Sam. 2:9). I believed the promises of God, which said that man could do nothing to me when I trusted in the promises of God despite my fears and struggles.

Thanks to Psalm 91:7, I believed nothing would touch me. I experimented with this truth in my life as a youth in Bucharest without parents or any support nearby. I had no one to protect me at that early age. In my early teens I arrived in Romania's capital of Bucharest, where I didn't know anybody. Growing up in my small village, where I knew each family, and then going to a completely strange environment was a shocking experience. No family and no friends! It was dangerous to live in a big, corrupt city ruled by communists who had no fear of God. But I put my trust in Him, and He protected me always and watched my steps. He will keep you from evil when you trust Him. As 2 Thessalonians 3:3 promises: "But the Lord is faithful, and he will strengthen you and protect you from the evil one."

Fear will disappear when you focus on God's promises. He will keep you from falling when things go wrong and there appears to be no hope. "To him who is able to keep you from stumbling and to present you before his glorious presence without fault and with great joy—to the only God our Savior be glory, majesty, power and authority, through Jesus Christ our Lord, before all ages, now and forevermore! Amen" (Jude 24–25). The enemy will be blocked by the Spirit of the Lord when you shift your focus from the things that bring worry and fear to the fear of the Lord. God is faithful to His people who obey Him. He will punish your enemy that causes fear in your life. "According to what they have done, so will he repay wrath to his enemies and retribution to his foes; he will repay the islands their due" (Isa. 59:18). You are in the Father's hands. (See John 10:27–29.)

Do not let your thoughts be controlled by your enemies: worry, fear, and anxiety. God is in control of your life.

Low Self-Esteem and Distress

> But the Lord said unto Samuel, Look not on his countenance, or on the height of his stature; because I have refused him: for the Lord seeth not as man seeth; for man looketh on the outward appearance, but the Lord looketh on the heart.
> —1 Samuel 16:7, kjv

Low self-esteem makes people anxious. It can even cause depression. Stop everything you are doing and look at yourself in a mirror. See how perfectly everything has been made and programmed by a super intelligent designer. Think about all your vital organs and your extremities that keep you moving all day. You are "fearfully and wonderfully made" (Ps. 139:14).

Many men and women pay a lot of money for their beauty, fashion, makeup, and jewelry, but your beauty comes from the Lord. I always saw myself as less physically attractive, but I was confident that what I had inside me was more precious than my looks. Many times since my childhood people have told me, "I'd like to have your brain." I am glad they did not ask for my nose, because I have a big one and could feel offended by that! But in my brain I had the beauty of the Lord, which meant God's Word in it came out through my thoughts, vocabulary, and behavior. No one could miss that.

I didn't hear anybody say, "I'd like to have your face, either." When I was two years old, my older sisters were cooking corn at the farm, and reaching for the pot with boiling water, I burned my face. I got a severe burn on the right side of my chin that has stayed with me all my life. So you can see why a lack of self-esteem could have destroyed my future, if I had not held on to the promises of God. Instead I value how He created me and what He poured into me through the baptism of the Holy Spirit at a very young age. All my beauty was internal, from the power of God's Word at work in my mind through the Holy Spirit.

Rejection Leads to Destruction

> As you come to him, a living stone rejected by men but in the sight of God chosen and precious.
> —1 Peter 2:4, esv

> In him we have redemption through his blood, the forgiveness of our trespasses, according to the riches of his grace, which he lavished upon us, in all wisdom and insight.
> —Ephesians 1:7–8, esv

Some people have a strong fear of rejection, even from childhood. They work hard to be accepted, but when they feel as if everything is falling apart, they make bad decisions and end up in the wrong crowd. As a result, there are many teens committing suicide, many families going through separation and divorce, and many children with one or no parents, who also experience feelings of rejection or abandonment. They keep looking for a group that will accept them. This leaves them vulnerable to the wrong groups, which, while accepting them, draw them into destructive addictions.

The Bible teaches that we are accepted through Jesus Christ, as Ephesians 1:7–8 assures us. People everywhere are hungry for love, affection, acceptance, and a sense of belonging. God is love. Run into His arms, and you will feel the love of our eternal Father in heaven, who saved us through the blood of His own Son, Jesus. In Him you will find divine acceptance and protection.

Avoiding Responsibilities

People often choose to disregard the Word of God and run from their responsibilities. In every city I visit I look for homeless people because I think they are the most vulnerable population. This group just moves my heart. I asked a security person one time how we can help the homeless besides giving them money for food and clothes. The security person said there are shelters and housing available for them, but they refuse them because they do not like to follow rules or take responsibility for their own behavior. They choose to live in misery, even with unmet basic needs. The same thing happens with people who run away from the Word of God. Their spiritual needs remain unmet and their spiritual lives are miserable. But spiritual irresponsibility and unbelief do not change who God is or the truth of His Word.

BITTERNESS, DISCOURAGEMENT, AND YOUR LIMBIC SYSTEM

> The LORD is close to the brokenhearted and saves those who are crushed in spirit.
> —PSALM 34:18

> He heals the brokenhearted and binds up their wounds.
> —PSALM 147:3

What goes on in your brain affects your whole body and your well-being. That is why it is essential to feed your brain with healthy thoughts that bring joy and peace. The devil's goal is to steal, kill, and destroy, and he knows that if you feed your brain with healthy thoughts, he cannot destroy your body. Satan tries to bring bitter and unhealthy thoughts to destroy you emotionally and physically. As I mentioned in chapter 2, harmful emotions such as fear, anger, and bitterness are processed in the limbic system. This causes a cascade of unhealthy amounts of neurochemicals to be released, poisoning every cell in your body—enough to alter your gene expression, damage your DNA, and change your personality.

All those negative feelings and their consequences can be prevented by healthy thoughts and healthy emotions, through prayer and meditating on the Word of God. Prayer and meditation prevent fear and worry, increase peace, calm your brain, keep you healthy, increase your mental function, help you solve conflicts, improve your relationships, and help with forgiveness so you can be more optimistic and live a happier, healthier, longer life. Prayer and meditation alleviate anxiety and bitterness, dissipate anger, dissolve feelings of depression, reduce blood pressure and blood sugar, reduce pain, improve your immunity, and increase your positive outlook on life.[41]

Discouragement and bitterness will go away if you pray. Our Lord Jesus Christ, in the Garden of Gethsemane, was brokenhearted and filled with sorrow. He prayed to the Father, and after He prayed, He accepted the will of God in His life to die on the cross for the sins of the world to save humanity from eternal punishment. His inner fleshly man was bitter and discouraged that He had to endure the cross, but His spiritual man wanted to die for the sins of the world to save us as His heritage for eternity. The Father strengthened Him to accomplish that.

Run to God when you are discouraged. Find rest in Him. God is involved in your life when you are discouraged. His love for you is the same everywhere, in every situation. Tell Him about your fear and worry, talk to Him, and stay in His presence. He is the only One who can help you when you are in distress. I am writing from experience. I felt the healing power of God during my brokenness, bitterness, and discouragement in the most difficult time of my life.

Wrong Conclusions Bring Discouragement

> My clan is the weakest in Manasseh, and I am the least in my family.
> —Judges 6:15

> I am the only one left, and now they are trying to kill me too.
> —1 Kings 19:10

The devil brings wrong thinking, wrong accusations, wrong conclusions, and wrong comparisons, which are activated when you are discouraged. Inactivity brings even more discouragement and destruction. Brain cells die from inactivity.[42] When you are discouraged and worried, get busy and involved in constructive activities. That will build you up. You need to go to work and be active. Distract yourself from thoughts of bitterness and discouragement with healthy activities, and God will give you new ways to overcome your difficulties. You are in the center of His attention. God is interested in each one of us.

In the Old Testament, when Gideon was approached by an angel of the Lord with a divine plan, he complained, "My clan is the weakest in Manasseh, and I am the least in my family" (Judg. 6:15). Gideon was the least in his own eyes, and discouraged and bitter in his soul, but the angel of the Lord came to reveal to Gideon who he was in God's eyes and what God could do through Him. God lifted Gideon from insignificance and gave him courage and hope for his future. He can do that with you too. You have more value in God's eyes than your own. Gideon was comparing himself with people around him. He thought, "I am not better than my parents." Well, do not compare yourself with others. Competition has consequences. Be who God made you to be, with purpose in life. The one true God is calling us to leave behind discouragement and bitterness and move forward to a life of prayer, repentance, and the desire to know Him and reach new spiritual dimensions.

Another example is Elijah, who was very discouraged. After fleeing Jezebel, he lamented, "I am the only one left, and now they are trying to kill me too" (1 Kings 19:10). He was wrong. He felt so lonely, afraid, anxious, and depressed, but God told Elijah that He had seven thousand faithful followers in Israel and that Elisha would take his place. God does not want you to isolate yourself. Loneliness can lead to bitterness and destruction. You must pray as Jesus did when He was left alone in Gethsemane and all His disciples had left Him in the hands of the enemy. The Bible tells us that God sends His angels to keep company with lonely people and strengthen them. He sends His angels for you too.

When you feel alone, remember that an angel is beside you at all times to strengthen you. One of my friends said, "God is always with me, and He keeps me company every moment to comfort me when I am discouraged." Find rest in God, like Elijah under the juniper, and talk to God when you are alone. When you do, your faith will increase, creating a shift from discouragement to hope. Healthy thinking will release the right neurotransmitters, preventing illness in your body. We were created to talk. Talk with God, and the right people around you, who will know how to encourage you. God will send an angel to strengthen you, as He did for Jesus after His forty days of fasting. He will encourage you, just as He sent angels for Gideon and Elijah when they were at their lowest moments.

After a few years of struggles I was extremely discouraged and at a low point in my life while waiting for my daughter and my husband to get visas and come to the United States. The Lord knew my brokenness and sent an angel in a dream, showing me that my family would come soon. My discouragement and bitter thoughts scattered immediately. A few months later my husband and my daughter received their visas. God knows the details and feelings of brokenness deep in your heart, and He will replace them when you stay firm in your faith and trust in His promises.

Sin Creates Stress

> For our struggle is not against flesh and blood, but against the rulers, against the authorities, against the powers of this dark world and against the spiritual forces of evil in the heavenly realms.
> —Ephesians 6:12

Sin destroys your soul, your emotions, your life, and those around you. It will bring fruits of its own kind; as the prophet Hosea said, "They sow the wind and reap the whirlwind" (Hos. 8:7). Yes, sin activates a destructive cascade of unhealthy neurochemicals in the brain, ultimately weakening us. But repentance cleans our brains' structures from bad memories,[43] which result from the emotional distress of all the garbage from years of unbelief and sin.

Sin Brings Discouragement

> The heart is deceitful above all things and beyond cure. Who can understand it?
> —Jeremiah 17:9

When we focus on harmful thoughts rather than the power of God, we end up discouraged and depressed. You can read discouragement on people's faces. They know deep in their hearts when they have done something wrong. The voice in our spirits will whisper to our minds. It is the Spirit of God's role in our brains to make us vigilant when an evil thought crosses our minds and to help us inhibit bad actions. If we have sinned, we can cry out in prayer and ask for forgiveness, and

God will answer and provide a pathway to our restoration. His forgiveness brings us joy, peace, and hope and welcomes us back to God's kingdom.

Sin originates in the hearts of people, as Jeremiah 17:9 says. We can see proof all around us that the heart is deceitful. Only through the love of Jesus can the heart be changed.

Follow God's prescriptions and maintain a good relationship with God Almighty, who is love. Love always makes a difference and is a key ingredient in our relationship with Jesus. Being born again, you love the Lord and you cannot get enough of Him. Spend time in His presence, and He will saturate your soul. Be ready to answer God's call in your life, cheerfully obey Him, and have faith that you are created to do good work, activated and multiplied by the Spirit of God. You are saved by grace.

Guilt and Shame

The wages of sin is death.

—Romans 6:23

Sin makes people feel ashamed, withdraw from social activities, and become lonely and depressed. It's a vicious cycle. The designer of the universe did not create us to bear emotional distress from guilt and shame (originating from sin in our souls and/or our bodies). Identify the sin in your life, confess it in your prayers to God, and let your requests be known to Him. Run from sin, which will kill—eternally.

People always ask why bad things happen to good people. It is a cause-and-effect relationship. The cause is sin, and the effect is that bad things happen. The effect of sin continues from generation to generation. Our Father God's desire is that all people will come to repentance so none will perish, but all will have eternal life (John 3:16). Sin is forgiven, but the consequences of original sin still remain. Humans must die because of the sin committed in the Garden of Eden by the first human beings, Adam and Eve. They disobeyed God's prescriptions and did what was specifically forbidden. Through the sin of disobedience, death entered into God's creation. Sin results in death, but the antidote for sin is the blood of Jesus. It is important for every human being to confess sin and be cleansed by the blood of Jesus. Search your heart, turn from evil, and let your spirit, soul, and body be healed.

The sin virus enters the spirit just as viruses enter computers, or our human bodies, causing signs and symptoms in the spirit that can be recognized in our lives as bad emotions, unhappiness, depression, bitterness, ungratefulness, ignorance, negligence, loneliness, anxiety, agitation, anger, resentment, chronic fatigue, and weakness. Strengthen your spiritual immunity, and prevent the sin virus from contaminating your soul. Do not allow anything from the world to contaminate you or keep you from reaching your full potential. God gave you a glorious destiny. When you follow His prescription for repentance and live in obedience to His Word, He pours out "so much blessing that there will not be room enough to store it" (Mal. 3:10). By knowing the Word of God and living accordingly, you become a new person with a changed mind and a new way of thinking (Rom. 12:2). When you meditate on His Word, you will discover God's will and His perfect plan for your life.

When you sin against God, you sin against people too. Be careful—your gestures and words can hurt. Distance between us and the Word of God also creates distance in families, between spouses, and between parents and children. When you get closer to the Word of God, you get closer to your family and your loved ones. We must turn away from sin through repentance: "Repent and be baptized, every one of you, in the name of Jesus Christ for the forgiveness of your sins" (Acts 2:38).

Desire for the Supernatural

> Then Manoah intreated the LORD, and said, O my Lord, let the man of God which thou didst send come again unto us, and teach us what we shall do unto the child that shall be born. And God hearkened to the voice of Manoah; and the angel of God came again unto the woman as she sat in the field: but Manoah her husband was not with her.
>
> —Judges 13:8–9, kjv

God put the desire for the supernatural in humans at creation. For that reason we are not satisfied with who we are, what we are, and what we have. Our desire for the supernatural was hijacked in the Garden of Eden by Satan, who put evil thoughts in the mind of man to pervert that desire for a supernatural God into a desire for worldly satisfactions. That is why God gave us His Word, to teach us, direct us, and keep us focused on Him. Only God can fulfill our hearts' desires.

A physician friend I will call Lea started to see this after she was diagnosed with cancer.

She was a scientist, but when the news came about her deadly disease, she needed an answer from God, and she was comforted by His supernatural prescriptions, beyond science. She knew she could not lean on her own understanding, but the Bible answers the mysteries of life. Her spiritual eyes were opened.

After deciding to acknowledge that Jesus is the Son of God and make Him her Lord and Savior, she was born again. The Word of God began to work in her heart, giving her eternal hope on her deathbed. The Word spoke to her soul, giving her confidence, reassurance, and hope for eternal life.

Lea started to see the world around her in a totally different way. She felt so sorry for people who didn't know Christ and the Word of God, and she regretted wasting so many years ignoring God and living an atheistic, worldly life with no meaning. The Word of God had the power to change her story and her spiritual résumé after she accepted Jesus as her Savior. Her passing was peaceful, with new hope in God, who saved her soul. She passed away with confidence in her eternity.

Spiritual Needs

In my profession I care for dying people and often witness their last desire to hear the Word of God. It speaks to the soul even during the dying process. My friend Dr. Lea wanted to have a Bible study in her home every day before her death. I saw people coming night after night to her house, which I thought would be too tiring for her. I intended to stop them to protect her from being overly tired in her last days. When I asked her how she felt about canceling the meetings, to my surprise she said, "This Bible study is the only thing that sustains me every day."

She had been an atheist and didn't believe in God or own a Bible until she was forty-three years old. When she was diagnosed with an incurable disease, she started looking for spiritual reassurance, knowing her life on earth would soon end and not knowing where she would go from this planet. She was a physician—a specialist caring for many patients—and she knew what was happening in her body, wracked by cancer. With her whole being shaken, she thought seriously about the purpose of life on earth and about her destiny. She knew that there is life after death, and her spiritual needs were so obvious. As a medical professional, she knew that physiologically her cells had started an abnormal proliferation process, dividing uncontrollably and metastasizing in her vital organs, shutting them down and causing multiple organ failures. Science was helpless, and she was hopeless during her dying process. She knew her life was coming to an end but her soul was eternal and she needed to feed her soul with spiritual food.

Broken Heart Syndrome

> The human spirit can endure in sickness, but a crushed spirit who can bear?
> —Proverbs 18:14

Psychological trauma—including the death of a loved one, divorce, children on drugs, abuse, catastrophic loss, and unbearable stress—causes excess catecholamine (adrenaline) to be released in the muscles of the apex of the heart, causing heart attack–like symptoms in many cases. In medicine it is called the "broken heart syndrome" and is similar to emotional brokenness.[44] God may allow you to enter a place of brokenness so you will have compassion for others who have a broken heart, but it is not His will to crush your spirit.

All kinds of physical and emotional diseases are caused by brokenness. A crushed spirit is harder to bear than a physical sickness, as Solomon wrote in Proverbs 18:14 more than twenty-five hundred years ago. Medicine has no cure or answer for a crushed spirit. Educate your soul to let go of everything you cannot control and keep praising God, even in hard times. He will bring healing and hope to your soul supernaturally.

Educate yourself with the promises of God through His powerful Word. Know that the Word has healing power to penetrate your heart, transform you, and bring deliverance from all "the world's noise and bondage." Quiet your soul by shutting down secular music, the internet, Facebook, Instagram, Twitter, the TV, your iPod, your iPhone, and other devices. There is no healing in those atmospheres full of distressing news and distracting information. Comfort your spirit by trusting in the Lord, who can bring healing, salvation, and deliverance. Hope in God's promises, for His Word is the anchor of your soul. You cannot be shaken when you put all your worry, fear, anxiety, and depression in His hands and rest in Him.

God restores your soul. He knows your situation, and He knows you by name. He shows up to give you victory. He is the Creator of heaven and earth, and nothing is too hard for Him. As He asked Jeremiah: "I am the Lord, the God of all mankind. Is anything too hard for me?" (Jer. 32:27). Through the Word, God can perform spiritual surgery in our brains and hearts and bring back to life what was poisoned. (See Hebrews 4:12.) The Word continues to transform lives even today. For spiritual health and fruit of the Spirit we need spiritual surgery by the Word of God and neuroplasticity of the brain from a transformed mind.

Chapter 5

PAIN

The night racks my bones, and the pain that gnaws me takes no rest.
—Job 30:17, ESV

Why is my pain unceasing, my wound incurable, refusing to be healed? Will you be to me like a deceitful brook, like waters that fail?
—Jeremiah 15:18, ESV

Man is also rebuked with pain on his bed and with continual strife in his bones, so that his life loathes bread, and his appetite the choicest food.
—Job 33:19–20, ESV

Pain in any form can increase our stress level. Science has advanced so much and developed myriads of pain medications, methods, and techniques that are used for acute and chronic pain management, especially at the end of life. I know this for a fact, since I have taken care of dying people with multiple chronic conditions since 1990. I joke sometimes with people and tell them that I could have a megachurch by now with how many people passed in my years of caring for them.

But with all the painkillers developed lately, we still do not know how much physical and emotional or spiritual pain a person has when he or she is passing on from this life, even with all our interventions and advanced technologies. According to the Centers for Disease Control, in 2017 there were fifty-eight opioid prescriptions written for every one hundred Americans, and more than 17 percent of Americans filled at least one opioid prescription.[1] Seeking relief, people crave more and more pain medication while ignoring the side effects. As a result, mortality is rising. Even prescription drugs cause addiction, opening the door for illicit drug addictions in huge proportions. Young children and teens are especially vulnerable to addiction to narcotics. Their immature systems metabolize codeine and morphine more quickly, and they easily become over-sedated.[2]

Our Creator designed pain modulators in our nervous systems and receptors for natural chemicals, including endorphins to decrease pain—creating the same effect on pain as synthetic morphine.[3] Fear of pain causes yet more stress. The pain threshold then decreases and even a little pain is felt and perceived as "lots" of pain, leading to overuse of medication.[4]

Scientists do research, trying to discover how much pain a person can endure and what kind of medication will be needed to control that pain to provide maximum comfort. However, they usually conclude that more research is needed. People continue to be afraid of pain and stress themselves, thinking nobody will be able to control their pain. In America an estimated one hundred million people suffer from chronic pain at an annual cost of $635 billion for treatment and lost productivity.[5] Pain results in so much suffering, including fear, anger, guilt, loneliness, helplessness, catastrophizing, limited coping skills, passive thinking, negative emotions, suffering, and more.

In children, perception of pain is a combination of genetic predisposition with environmental influences, such as poor parental support, stress, sexual abuse, and early substance abuse.[6] All of these lead to opioid seeking and craving.[7] This gives euphoria and anhedonia as a reward but also results in dependency, withdrawal symptoms, and depression when drugs are not available—repeating the vicious cycle. Both illicit and chronically used prescription drugs destroy neurons in the brain, disabling them in time.[8]

From Panic to Joy

> He will wipe away every tear from their eyes, and death shall be no more, neither shall there be mourning, nor crying, nor pain anymore, for the former things have passed away.
> —Revelation 21:4, esv

Children suffer complex changes with development, as changing hormones play a huge role in their temperament.[9] If they experience fear or anxiety, they react with fear, which can become chronic, causing chronic post-puberty pain.[10] This can lead to depression and constant doctor shopping. One young girl came to my office after many doctors and multiple visits to the emergency room. Though treated with many medications for different symptoms, she was still afraid and unable to stay in her classroom at school. She was not able to function normally at home or in society due to symptoms of severe panic attacks. After a close examination

I advised her to join a group of young teens at her parents' church. She expressed fear of "not being able to breathe," which others would notice, causing her embarrassment. After many attempts and long discussions she finally attended that group and made some good friends. Now she enjoys a normal adolescent life and is involved in church activities and even an athletic club. I meet her in the community at the gym and other events, and she is a completely different person—happy, joyful, and full of energy and motivation.

Chronic pain in adolescents is often due to stress and anxiety.[11] Anxiety from fear and stress is debilitating for the younger generation. Many adolescents come to our clinic reporting debilitating headaches, abdominal pain, excessive worry about their health, and imagining that they have a horrible illness, such as cancer. Sometimes they worry about not performing well in school, about their parents' financial situation, frequent sleep disturbances, or a lack of ability to succeed. I believe that God is still in the business of managing people's pain, helping them manage their stress effectively, and comforting those who believe in His Word and its supernatural prescriptions.

The Natural Analgesic

Emotional pain from stress causes people to experience more physical pain. Anxiety from fear, anger, and bitterness, and frustration from everyday worries will cause one's brain to release chemicals that tighten the muscles, creating more pain through an inflammatory process.[12] In response the brain will release a chemical from its own natural pharmacy—endorphin, the endogenous morphine, a natural human analgesic, built into our bodies by the super intelligent designer to control the stimuli of pain. God built sensory neurons into our brain structures, in peripheral pathways, to protect us from damage when accidents occur.

Even professionals will often say that the pain "is in your mind." That is a valid comment, in a sense, because the brain interprets the severity of the pain and governs the response to those feelings of pain in our bodies. People can use medications for pain (acetaminophen, ibuprofen, Aleve, Advil, other over-the-counter medications, or prescribed narcotics), but using these for more than two weeks at a time and not carefully following the physician's instructions and the indications on the packages can cause more damage to the body. This may include hepatotoxicity, kidney failure, dependency, and addiction, if patient usage includes narcotics.[13]

Supernatural Pain Modulator

Scientists have discovered that "anandamide is a natural, marijuana-like lipid derivative produced in the human body that provides pain relief. As an endocannabinoid, it binds and activates G protein–coupled cannabinoid receptors (CB) as well as several other targets, both within the plasma membrane and intracellularly."[14] It was also discovered that endorphins are natural pain-killing substances found in the human brain. The name comes from *endogenous* (meaning within) and *morphine* (a painkiller). Endorphins are some of the neurotransmitters in the brain that are released to calm an overacting brain and to help people "feel good," healing emotional pain.[15] Levels of endorphins in the brain may be changed by taking a number of drugs, including alcohol, anabolic steroids, and heroin and other opiates.[16]

As science has proved, our Creator built pain modulators and natural analgesics into our systems, while giving us instructions to pray and meditate on His laws—plus instructions for coping with pain. It is well documented in literature that meditation alters the neural circuits in the brain and reduces chronic pain.[17] Meditating and focusing on God's promises will improve our mood, bringing hope, joy, peace, and happiness. The natural analgesics, such as endorphins, and other natural chemicals released by the brain's natural organic factory also help with healing.

The biggest promise we have is that "with his stripes we are healed" (Isa. 53:5, KJV). The reassurance from God's supernatural promises brings us so much hope. This hope causes more joy, creating the atmosphere in the brain to release more natural analgesics, endorphin and norepinephrine, regulating the pain. It also will change the atmosphere in the amygdala and other structures in the limbic system associated with memories, emotional pain, and mood.

Besides all these natural processes, there is a supernatural resource that can be activated by our faith in Jesus' healing power by the Holy Spirit. As Hebrews 13:8 tells us, He "is the same yesterday and today and forever." He supernaturally healed in the past, is healing in the present, and will do it again in the future. Our hope is in Him, and we do not lose hope in His supernatural power to heal the sick.

PAIN AS GOD'S INSTRUMENT

> No discipline seems pleasant at the time, but painful. Later on, however, it produces a harvest of righteousness and peace for those who have been trained by it.
>
> —HEBREWS 12:11

Popular author and Bible teacher Beth Moore, in her book *Jesus, the One and Only*, wrote:

> Eternal purpose is the central issue involved in whether or not God heals a believing (see Matt. 9:28) and requesting (see James 4:2) Christian's physical illness. Although I don't pretend to understand how and why, some illnesses may serve more eternal purpose than healing, while other healings serve more purpose than illness.
>
> I cannot imagine what purpose some illness and premature deaths serve, but, after years of loving and seeking my God, I trust who He is

even when I have no idea what He is doing. Above all things, I believe God always has purpose in every decision He makes....

Developing the mind-set of one who is continually taking up his cross and following Christ is the heart of having "in mind the things of God" (Matt. 16:23) rather than man.[18]

That is the prescription to live daily a victorious life. People who put their minds on understanding God's heart soon realize that God's love is endless and His last Word is for our benefit.

Do Not Lose Heart in Pain

> After Job had prayed for his friends, the LORD restored his fortunes and gave him twice as much as he had before.
> —Job 42:10

Your pain can be used to glorify God. Do not look back when life hurts the most, but set your eyes on Jesus and eternal life. Christ's heart was touched by people with diseases, disabilities, infirmities, hunger, and loneliness. He went to the cross to endure extraordinary pain in order to free the human race from all pain. Jesus, as a human on earth, had perfect mirror neurons when—with supernatural compassion—He felt the weight of a sinful world. It drove Him to the cross to be crucified and to deliver us from our iniquities.

We read in the Old Testament that after Job lost everything in his troubled time, God restored everything he had lost in double proportion, as noted in Job 42:10. The significance to this is how Job blessed the Lord even in the most painful of situations. Pain is God's instrument to shape us into a shining diamond because He loves us. Do not lose heart when you go through extreme pain or trials. When God is disciplining you, He pours out His great love, and you become stronger.

There is a point when you turn your heart to God, when the pain causes a cry from the bottom of your heart. We read in Mark 10:47 that Bartimaeus was crying out loud, "Jesus, Son of David, have mercy on me!" If Bartimaeus weren't blind, or his blindness did not matter to him or did not bother him enough, he would not have cried out for mercy. God used Bartimaeus' blindness for His glory. Millions (even billions) of people can read his story today and cry out for their own physical needs and for their spiritual blindness to be healed.

Getting Our Attention for Heaven

You might think you can have great thoughts and be transformed in your thinking, finding contentment, peace, joy, and happiness only during good times. People ask, "If God is so good, why does He not spare His children from suffering?" Disaster, trouble, disease, and suffering are common to all people on earth. God allows those conditions to get our attention to prepare us for eternal life. During suffering He makes you feel His love. His peace will come into your heart and open your spiritual eyes. Your positive attitude and reaction to suffering will bring you victory and spiritual health.

Any parent with a disabled child has for that child a unique, extraordinary love and compassion. Any discipline is difficult, but God has a divine plan to shape you. Your final spiritual shape implies physical and emotional suffering. Physical and emotional discipline are painful. Any person on earth knows about pain. Pain is universal. This is a mystery, and God uses suffering and pain to grab our attention for heaven. He wants us for eternity. We are here only temporarily. No one living on earth now will be here 120 years from now. Eternity matters.

Grace to Endure Pain

> A woman in that town who lived a sinful life learned that Jesus was eating at the Pharisee's house, so she came there with an alabaster jar of perfume. As she stood behind him at his feet weeping, she began to wet his feet with her tears. Then she wiped them with her hair, kissed them and poured perfume on them.
>
> —Luke 7:37–38

God's grace blesses everyone who comes into His presence with a broken heart to worship. Worshipping will bring you into the presence of the Almighty and bring healing to your soul. Many fell at His feet and worshipped and were delivered from their inner pain. Brokenness brings you on your knees to a place of worship, as it did Mary Magdalene in the previously mentioned passage from Luke. She needed to break her alabaster jar before the perfume could flow on the Lord's feet.

Mary Magdalene's heart was heavy from the weight of her sins, but her broken heart brought her to a place of weeping (the "good cry" that brings healing[19]), worshipping, and breaking the jar of perfume. Brokenness is needed before the fragrance of anointing for worship flows. In 2 Samuel 6 David's heart grieved after circumstances forced him to take the ark of the covenant to the house of Obed-Edom. After three months, when David was able to return the ark to Jerusalem, he started to worship joyfully with all the assembly. David danced before the Lord with all his might, rejoicing in knowing that the anointing of God was coming back. He knew what it meant to be in God's presence, and he also knew the anguish and pain from being away from God. God's presence brings healing.

Worshipping brings you intimacy with God, and by His grace you can endure the pain. People who worship will prevail because during worship His anointing heals our pain. Paul declared that the anointing is sufficient, because grace was sufficient in his life and gave him the power to endure pain. Jesus took all our pain and suffering because the anointing of the Spirit of God was upon Him. As Isaiah

53:5 teaches, He was wounded for our transgressions. On the cross He conquered our sickness, disease, and pain because He was anointed by God's Spirit. I think of Jesus as experiencing the "broken heart syndrome," with similar signs and symptoms, in order to heal our broken hearts. The latter part of verse 5 says, "By His wounds we are healed." This is the anointing to take the pain away and to heal the sick. The anointing of the Holy Spirit still heals. The spirit of anointing and passion enables us to do our ministry work and ignites a fire inside us to endure the pain. (See Matthew 3:11 and 12:49.)

The Holy Spirit gave the disciples boldness, power, zeal, and passion to speak in the name of Jesus and to heal the sick in His name. The Holy Spirit is working miracles in your life today to heal your brokenness and pain. The Spirit of the Lord makes the difference. You need a holy fire to impassion you to do the services of God. There is a fresh outpouring of the anointing oil in you and in people around you when the holy fire comes upon you. The fragrance in the perfume comes from crushed, bruised leaves. You must bring the fragrance of the anointing to other people's lives after your own soul experiences healing. This is how you help others find peace and grace to endure their pain.

In our facility I have often heard patients' families and health care professionals who have visited our patients say, "This is such a peaceful place. We feel something different that quiets the soul." Now, in our facility we have thirty residents (patients) with Alzheimer's and dementia. Their severely challenging behaviors are difficult to manage. Many facilities in our city and state will not accept them because of their frequent behavioral disturbances. It is the anointing and the grace of God that take the feeling of pain, anxiety, and depression away. People feel the peace of God.

This is beyond science. The miraculous anointing, which quiets the soul of these precious people we care for in their most difficult time, is rejected by many. Specialists have tried many potent treatments with minimal results. Our staff and caregivers notice the changes within a few days after the patients move in. Others from the outside, including health care professionals, often throw their hands in the air, feeling helpless and running out of solutions for these people, who suffer from aggressiveness and neurocognitive disorders. But in our facility they find the peace and grace to endure their pain because of God's anointing.

> We are to God the pleasing aroma of Christ among those who are being saved and those who are perishing.
> —2 Corinthians 2:15

You must have the right response and right attitude to surrender to God for the anointing to work. The anointed ones, the followers of Christ, must respond in the right way and radiate the anointing to be the fragrance of Christ.

The more the apostles were persecuted, the more they spread the fragrance of Christ. As they did, the more the churches multiplied because of the fragrance of the anointing of their brokenness. When I was threatened by communist persecution in Romania, I shared the gospel more with those around me and continually sought God's presence in prayer and fasting. In the midst of your pain you must spread the fragrance. Through pain God creates your destiny.

Sometimes through your pain your destiny is born, as Shaneen Clarke, author of *Dare to Be Great*, says in her speeches around the world. You must show the world the appropriate way to serve God, even in painful situations. The world needs what you have—the hand of God on your life. The world is in terrible pain and turmoil and needs solutions because medication alone cannot cure the world's pain. The Holy Spirit is alive in you. You are anointed to endure the pain and to serve by comforting and helping others in their painful time. You fulfill your destiny when by grace you endure temporary pain and serve others.

Spiritually, pain and fear of death will make you pray more, establishing a deeper relationship with God, the highest power in the universe. You are not the only one to benefit from praying more; so do those around you and society as a whole. You must activate the gift you have inside you to be willing to choose to look for meaning in troubles and pain and use those troubling situations in healthy, positive, and constructive ways.

Dependent on God

> Praise be to the God and Father of our Lord Jesus Christ…who comforts us in all our troubles, so that we can comfort those in any trouble with the comfort we ourselves receive from God.
> —2 Corinthians 1:3–4

Fear of failure comes from a lack of confidence due to our weaknesses. Our weaknesses help us develop a dependence on God and a humility before Him. We read in Isaiah 14 that Lucifer chose to be independent because of a lack of humility, and because of his pride he forever lost his place in heaven. In his book *The Journey: How to Live by Faith in an Uncertain World*, Billy Graham said, "Isaiah's portrait of Lucifer describes Satan's arrogance and rebellion: 'How you have fallen from heaven, O morning star, son of the dawn!…You said in your heart, "I will ascend to heaven; I will raise my throne above the stars of God.…I will make myself like the Most High"' (Isa. 14:12–14)."[20] From this passage we know that Satan in his pride will do anything to destroy God's people on earth. God gives grace to humble people in their weakness. In weakness we choose humility and obedience over pride and we find victory over fear of failure.

All the characters in the Bible teach us dependence on the power of God and increase our faith. We just need to be hungry for knowledge and revelation from the Word of God, from stories of people who lived on earth before us and experienced God's supernatural power. Life is a journey, and we must keep notes of the events in our personal journeys. God is moving through our weaknesses and is working in our hearts, perfecting His power. Fear is not from God, because He did not give us a spirit of fear. The power of God is made perfect in weakness. He is a God of compassion and of all comfort, and He is the One "who comforts us in all our troubles, so that we can comfort those in any trouble with the comfort we ourselves receive from God" (2 Cor. 1:4). The confidence we get when we are comforted in our trouble will increase confidence and faith in God in those around us.

Burnout

When you feel burned-out and extremely weak, accept your imperfections and proactively face your uncertainties, limitations, and mistakes. Stay current, build your skills, and learn something new. Focus on the positive aspects of life, be flexible, and set professional boundaries. Consider what is essential. What are your talents? What are you passionate about? Eliminate old activities before adding new ones, and decide what you would sacrifice for a new opportunity. Strengthen key relationships, prioritize your family and friends who are important, clear your calendar, and make a "do not do" list. In your profession and business you must focus on positive relationships and rewards. And always remember your values.

Redirect your mind with meditation and spirituality, reflecting on good results, setting boundaries, and promoting a work balance. In his book *Free at Last: Removing the Past From Your Future*, Pastor Larry Huch states: "Jesus was anointed with the burden-removing, yoke-destroying power of God to heal the brokenhearted. Why the brokenhearted? Because God desires for His people to live in joy. When we are filled with joy, we have the strength to fight the good fight of faith."[21] Your life has meaning, and you can live a life free of anger, insecurity, abuse, addiction, and depression through Jesus Christ. Fill your heart with joy because "the joy of the Lord is your strength" (Neh. 8:10). Joy is the opposite of depression, with all its signs and symptoms caused by unhealthy neurochemicals. All our physical and emotional damage is repaired through joy, which further prevents stress levels from increasing, causing less of the stress hormone, cortisol, in the body. Thus, fewer neurons die in your brain.

Life Without Dreams

People often live without a dream, focusing more on harmful things than on the power of God. You can read discouragement on the faces of people who have no vision for the future. This is how medical professionals assess the pain level in those with neurocognitive disorders and dementia. We use a chart with sad faces because those patients cannot express themselves verbally. The idea is to read the severity of pain, discomfort, distress, and discouragement on people's faces and to prescribe the right treatment. Discouragement leads to depression.

Discouragement brings bitterness, sadness, and discontent. After times of great success, when your excitement slows down, when you are facing the enemy of your soul and the scene changes, discouragement appears. In 1 Kings 18 we read about Elijah on Mount Carmel. After his great success, when his life was threatened by his enemies, discouragement overwhelmed him.

In his discouragement Elijah did not call upon the name of the Lord. While filled with wrong thoughts and discouragement, Elijah expressed a desire to die. It is hard to believe that this great man of God—one of the boldest prophets, anointed to perform staggering and stupendous miracles through the power of the Holy Spirit—became suicidally discouraged. He was the one whose prayers brought drought and no rain on the earth for three and a half years (1 Kings 17:1; Jas. 5:17). On two other occasions oil and meal were multiplied in the widow's house (1 Kings 17:14), and a widow's child was raised from the dead and restored back to life (1 Kings 17:22)! Even more astounding, through Elijah's prayers sacrifices in a huge trench were consumed by fire on Mount Carmel (1 Kings 18:38), men and captains were slain by fire at his word (2 Kings 1:10), clouds and rain came after three and a half years (1 Kings 18:41), and his mantle divided the waters of the Jordan River (2 Kings 2:8).

Elijah thought and "dreamed" that his enemy, Ahab, would be changed after the confrontation on Mount Carmel, but he needed to change his thinking. A wrong dream will bring discouragement and bitterness. To avoid the emotional pain of disappointment and bitterness, you must change your perspective and get visions and dreams from God's promises. Changes come when you humble yourself, seek the Lord's face, and call upon His name. The Lord is in control. God knows your heart, feelings, thoughts, emotions, and struggles. The One who gives dreams and visions is looking for a heart that is completely loyal to Him. He is the potter, and we are the clay—not the other way around.

FINANCES AND STRESS

> Remember this: whoever sows sparingly will also reap sparingly, and whoever sows generously will also reap generously.
> —2 CORINTHIANS 9:6

> Ship your grain across the sea; after many days you may receive a return.
> —ECCLESIASTES 11:1

People facing serious financial stress suffer worry, fear, and anxiety, with adverse physical and emotional effects. Medication will not always work for those conditions, because psychosocial and emotional distress disrupt neurotransmitters. Your finances will improve when you follow God's prescription (supernatural law) of sowing and reaping. You reap what you sow (Luke 6:38). God is generous and good, according to Matthew 6:25–33. God loves and also rewards you when you give cheerfully, as 2 Corinthians 9:6 assures us.

Be a cheerful, generous giver, and invest in charity. Charity yields high returns in God's economy, as Solomon said in Ecclesiastes 11:1. When you give joyfully, good things happen. Joy and happiness create an atmosphere in the brain that enables it to release neurotransmitters, such as endorphins, dopamine, oxytocin, and serotonin. These help to calm an overactive brain (from high levels of stress, which increases the cortisol level). This also helps, to some extent, to repair and rewire the brain's structures through the process of neuroplasticity, which in turn restores the health of the body, soul, and spirit.

You are able to produce more with a healthy body and mind. True wealth in your internal soul is eternal through God's grace. "For it is by grace you have been saved, through faith—and this is not from yourselves, it is the gift of God" (Eph. 2:8). When you are tired, you are vulnerable and make bad decisions and mistakes in business or family life, affecting your relationships and your finances. A lack of finances will bring more stress, anxiety, worry, bitterness, and anger in your soul, provoking you to think and speak inappropriate words.

You must watch your language during times of financial stress so as not to bring more curses over your financial resources. We know that abundant life and lack of resources (death) are in the power of your tongue: "The tongue has the power of life and death, and those who love it will eat its fruit" (Prov. 18:21). What you say is important, because words have the creative power to activate invisible thoughts in your brain. Words represent things. They put an image in your mind that will become visible when you act on it. Words define your future.

Do not ignore the promises of God about finances and health. When the Word of God abides in you, then you know what to ask according to the will of God, and He will give you everything for His glory (John 15:7). When you receive answers to your prayers, you will be full of joy and glorify God more (John 16:23–24). Just believe when you ask (Matt. 21:22).

God's prescription is to "take delight in the Lord, and he will give you the desires of your heart" (Ps. 37:4). Do what is pleasing in His sight, and then everything you ask according to His will, you will receive (1 John 3:22). The devil is the culprit of all the evil things happening in the world financially. He puts the seed of fear, worry, and discouragement into people's minds. We do not see thoughts, but they control our lives. If we had no thoughts, life would be aimless and purposeless. God's love gives us power to control our thoughts about our finances. Align your thoughts and actions about finances with God's Word, and let the peace of God flood your mind and heart.

STRESS FROM A LACK OF FINANCES

> For the love of money is a root of all kinds of evil. Some people, eager for money, have wandered from the faith and pierced themselves with many griefs.
> —1 Timothy 6:10

> Whoever loves money never has enough; whoever loves wealth is never satisfied with their income.
> —Ecclesiastes 5:10

Wealth does not always make people happy. They think it will, but many wealthy people are emotionally broken, as shown in Ecclesiastes 5:10. Many of those who have lots of money will never have enough and will never be satisfied. First Timothy 6:10 says, "The love of money is a root of all kinds of evil." Money cannot fill an empty heart.

Financial insufficiency does cause a big burden, but there are ways to approach this most unwanted stress. Consider the root cause of financial stress. God's economy is the best economy in the universe. He is the CEO of the universe and established the laws of sowing and reaping. You get what you give; you reap what you sow; whatever you do, you are rewarded according to your deeds on earth—and in eternity. It makes sense that if you give using your skills, talents, and knowledge with effort and passion, you will receive a reward. To receive, you must give. We must be good stewards of our God-given abilities too.

Many times we spend our finances on things that are not strictly necessary, and they will not satisfy our souls. There are financial guidelines in the Word of God. Enjoy the work of your hands. Do not forget that God gives you power to gain wealth—meaning your finances. God has always cared about our finances. More than thirty-four hundred years ago, when Moses wrote the Book of Deuteronomy, he reminded the Israelites: "For it is he who gives you the ability to produce wealth" (Deut. 8:18). The ingredients for maximum potency are contained in His prescriptions for you to prosper financially, physically, and spiritually.

DECISIONS

> Now fear the Lord and serve him with all faithfulness.... But as for me and my household, we will serve the Lord.
> —Joshua 24:14–15

Difficulty making the right decisions can add to your emotional distress. The anterior cingulate cortex in the frontal lobe is associated with making rational decisions.[22] If you decide to spend time in the Word of God, you will have immediate gratification. Rejoicing in the Lord, you can develop a *good addiction* to joy and peace. The healthy amounts of dopamine, serotonin, and endorphins will give you strength and increase your ability to make the right decisions.[23]

When you saturate your brain with the Word of God, all the decisions made in your anterior cingulate cortex will be according to the will of God and you will not be afraid of making the wrong decisions. The "inner voice" in your anterior cingulate cortex will slow down dopamine release and restrain addictive behavior, even to your own epinephrine, from fear and anxiety. The battle is between the dopamine (the perceptions of immediate reward of "feeling good" during addictive behavior) and the anterior cingulate cortex in the frontal lobe (rational reasoning and good decision-making).[24]

Life is the sum of our decisions. The world is where it is today due to the sum of decisions made in the past—at the individual level and at the national level. Blessed is the man who fears the Lord and follows His instructions when making decisions in life (Ps. 128:1). Do not jump to a personal decision without asking God for wisdom. Do not let others make decisions for you on what to eat, where and how long to sleep, how to use your time, how to use your body, how to dress, or how to behave, as that will lead to destruction.

Your decisions determine your quality of life. Choices you make affect your health, finances, family life—your future and your eternity. Make decisions with eternity in mind. Every moment, you make decisions that can affect you and those around you in a healthy way. Physically and spiritually, you have two choices. Choose between good and bad, life and death, as Joshua declared in the passage I just quoted from Joshua 24:14–15. Joshua's decision can be yours too—an unexpired prescription for all of us, even today.

My life now is the result of decisions I made in the past. Like everyone else, I had to make decisions about school, marriage, career, family, business, finances, faith, prayer, and spending my time on useful things. My blessed present is the result of my well-informed decisions in the past, even since childhood, and my future will be determined by decisions I make today. If you choose to serve the Lord, you choose life here on earth, leading to eternity. Follow the Lord with more passion and courage and trust in the Lord.

What is written *will happen*, as the Lord promised in His Word. Decide to serve the Lord continually, in all situations. He will reward your obedience. Life is full of unexpected events and deceptions. They might look good on the surface, but deeper inside they are full of "thorns." That can increase your stress and affect your health. You need help to make good decisions, and only God knows your tomorrow. Ask Him to help you make the right decisions today, and He will. Making wise decisions is a gift, and to have to make a choice is a privilege. (See Genesis 2:16–19.) Many people are not able to make decisions or choices for their lives.

Recently I had the privilege of speaking at a women's conference for mothers of children with disabilities and of visiting a few centers sponsored by Star of Hope in Romania. A few hundred children are brought to those centers by their parents for therapy. It is hard not to weep when you see how those children struggle to live without the ability to make decisions or choices for their lives. You have the ability to choose what kind of stimuli from your five senses will trigger and dictate your thoughts, what kind of thoughts will enter and take residence in your brain, what kind of actions to take, and how to behave. Do not abuse this gift with destructive choices that lead to death. Choices about your relationship with God, your career, whom you should marry, what friends and groups to hang out with, where to live, and how to spend your time can have an enormous impact on your life.

I had to decide whether to follow God's Word instead of the communist, atheistic teaching in Romania. People there taught that there is no God—from first grade until I graduated from the Academy of Economic Studies in Bucharest. Communism led to the destruction of the whole country. Even now, many years after the revolution of 1989, I still see the results of that communist indoctrination when I visit Romania. People are still oppressed and living under the curse from when they denied God's existence. Their anger, anxiety, bitterness, and discontent have been transferred to the younger generation through epigenetics (gene expression) as a generational curse. People are still affected by the teaching that there is no God. The Word of God stated more than three thousand years ago, "The fool says in his heart, 'There is no God.' They are corrupt, their deeds are vile" (Ps. 14:1).

I had to be careful about whom I would marry so that we could live together to the end of our lives in obedience to the will of God, follow the Word of God, be blessed, and avoid stress from unwise decisions. Now, more than thirty years later, we enjoy life together more than ever before, serving the Lord. We are so grateful for all the blessings we have received, beyond what we could ask or think, from our heavenly Father, according to His riches in glory. And together we are able to bless many others in our community and abroad. For me, it was very important to know that I was in the will of God, no matter the circumstances. You may wonder how to know the will of God for your life. Fear God, and desire His will for you with your whole heart. Then He will put an impression in your spirit, and you will know confidently, deep in your heart, what the will of God for you is. God's will and plan for your life is in His Word.

Where do your passions, skills, and abilities converge? Ask God about everything you want to do, or where you want to go. Cling to Him and come close to Him. Transformation starts when you renew your mind and continue making wise decisions. It doesn't happen overnight or automatically. The grace of God works according to our growth. Feed yourself with right information. Read the Bible every day, and memorize and recite the Word. During high school I had to memorize and quote Scriptures, especially from the New Testament, to keep my faith alive in difficult and challenging situations.

We must pray according to the will of God. Jesus prayed in Gethsemane, "Father, if you are willing, take this cup from me; yet not my will, but yours be done" (Luke 22:42). In the Lord's Prayer, Jesus taught us to pray, "Your kingdom come, your will be done, on earth as it is in heaven" (Matt. 6:10). God has the last word in your decisions. How you invest your resources and gifts affects what you receive in the future. Make the right choices for your life, serve selflessly, and ask Jesus to live in you.

People reflect their culture, but if you choose to embrace Christ's culture, having the same thinking as Christ, you will be blessed. Your faith in God should influence your daily decisions for all your problems. Jesus has your solutions. God shows favor to those who walk in obedience. Enjoy the favor of God as a result of wise decisions. I chose to serve the Lord Jesus, even when the communists were against me. For many years they humiliated and mocked me, putting pressure on me to give up my faith and threatening to revoke all my privileges, including opportunities for an education and a job. I did not give up, even though it was painful and hard. Now I reap a great harvest from those decisions. Your attitude toward God must be right at all times. He is watching over you every moment. Pay attention to who guides your decisions and what kinds of decisions you make to prevent unnecessary stress and unwanted consequences.

Depression From Compromise

Don't let society rob you of what is most important in life. Say no to compromise, and say yes to the principles of God. Ignoring God's Word led Solomon to a compromised life, and he became depressed. Against God's advice he married women from nations that worshipped many false gods (1 Kings 11:1–2). He knew he was compromising, and he paid for his mistakes with his life. At the end of Ecclesiastes he says, "Remember your Creator" (Eccles. 12:1). At the end Solomon regretted all he had done. He said God will bring all deeds before the final judgment. Solomon started well but departed from God and ended up with regrets and depression.

David also compromised when he committed adultery, inviting depression as a generational curse. David's sin multiplied and ended up cursing his children's lives. Even though God forgave David of his sins of adultery, with Bathsheba, and the indirect murder of her husband, Uriah, David lost four sons as the consequence of his disobedience to the Lord. Sin brings curses that break hearts and stay in the family "to the fourth generation" if not detected and dealt with. Do your own assessment about sin in your life, and take action to repent and obey the Word. God wants to give you supernatural rest when you are stressed and depressed. Start meditating on the Word of God to be healed from your depression.

When I hear people say, "My life is falling apart," "I am resigning from the human race," or, "I am at my wit's end," I know that depression is setting in. People get discouraged when dark uncertainty overwhelms them. They become disoriented and cannot think clearly. Disappointed, they lose their direction. They feel miserably distressed by all their troubles, lonely, and lost. (See Lamentations 3:19.) Depression overtakes them, bringing more disease in the body and spirit. Jesus promised rest for those who follow His prescriptions and refuse to compromise with sin (Matt. 11:28–30).

If you feel depressed, come to Jesus. He is the light, and you will be able to see where you are going (Ps. 119:105). He will lead you and guide you through your darkness and into light. If you follow Jesus, you will never walk in the dark. Encourage yourself as David did when he was depressed and surrounded by his enemies and his life was falling apart. (See 1 Samuel 30.) Know the Word of God and His promises, and you will be able to unload your burdens. When you lose all your hope, the Lord is near you (Ps. 34:18). I challenge you to encourage yourself to prevent depression.

In my desperation and dark uncertainty I had to unload my burden at the feet of Jesus, calling out for His provisions for my life. When you trust the Lord, He preserves you (Ps. 138:7). God's potent prescription to prevent physical and spiritual disorder: "Do not let your hearts be troubled and do not be afraid" (John 14:27). He is able to deliver you from all your fears, anxiety, and depression when you bring your worry to His feet, at the cross, where He took your burden. "I sought the Lord, and he answered me; he delivered me from all my fears" (Ps. 34:4).

Emotional Pain

People sometimes minimize or disregard emotions when talking about our Creator. But God grieves with us. Allow your heart to be broken, because Jesus' heart was broken. Jesus Christ has emotions about our pain. It is the fellowship of His suffering for our sins, so we suffer in many situations. Jesus in Gethsemane entered the fellowship of His sufferings because of the joy that was before Him, to give us eternal salvation from eternal punishment.

Sometimes we reach a point of desperation, like when I was a teenager in Bucharest without my family, and then again when I left Romania and arrived here in the United States with nothing. Even though I entered the United States legally, I had to wait six years to get my documents ready so I could travel back to Romania to see the rest of my dear family. During this time one of my sisters died at a very young age, and I was not able to attend her funeral. My heart was so broken that I developed "broken heart syndrome" and felt bitterness deep in my soul. To paraphrase Proverbs 17:22, it felt as if my bones were drying from the bitterness and emotional pain. I was depressed and unable to eat or enjoy food.

Later my father and brother died within a six-month period. The events of life can crush your soul. Your hope can disappear when you are devastated by such losses. Emptiness and despair can seem to last forever. But they only last for a season. The Lord is able to lift you out of despair and renew your hope and joy, bringing life back to your "drying bones," as we find in Ezekiel chapter 37.

A passage in Ezekiel 37 tells of scattered dry bones, but the Lord gave instructions to the prophet to speak life over them. The prophet spoke life, as the Lord instructed; the bones started to gather together; flesh began to grow on them; the breath of life entered those bodies; and they received life. That was a prophecy for our lives, to be inspirational speakers. Speak life to yourself and to others, and declare the work of the Lord. You are called to speak life. To receive supernatural power, we must cultivate a sensitive spirit. The Holy Spirit is in rhythm with the hand of God. When the hand of God comes upon you, you can do what other people fail to do. When the hand of the Lord is on you, you function at a higher level and your emotional pain is healed. In the Bible are many stories written as examples for us to follow in our daily lives to help us overcome emotional pain and bitterness.

BITTERNESS

> Get rid of all bitterness, rage and anger, brawling and slander, along with every form of malice. Be kind and compassionate to one another, forgiving each other, just as in Christ God forgave you.
> —EPHESIANS 4:31–32

Our parents described losing everything when the communists came to power in Romania. I remember them talking of their bitterness—and other people's. For example, Elena Răscol-Rady's husband, Vasile, was imprisoned two years for his Christian faith and for supplying Romanians with Bibles. In her book, *Flight to Freedom: God's Faithfulness in Communist Romania*, she stated:

> Everything people had earned up until then, after a lifetime of hard, honest work, was swallowed by that dragon in the name of the Party. People were stripped of their lands, houses, lives, freedom, conscience, joy and peace. Nobody owned anything anymore. The only owner was the State, the fierce dragon embodied by the Communist Party.[25]

Many unjust situations on earth can leave your soul bitter and empty. But that is only for a season when you trust God with your life.

The Bible tells us that after Naomi lost both her sons and her husband after many years in Moab, she returned to Bethlehem and told her friends to call her Mara, which means bitterness. Naomi's situation made her feel empty and bitter (Ruth 1:20–21). When Naomi and Ruth left Moab, bitterness filled their souls, but God ordained their steps and planned a joyful future for them in Bethlehem. God caused Ruth's heart to break Naomi, and Ruth cared for Naomi when she was in great need. Naomi's bitterness started to disappear when she watched how God provided for Ruth and brought Boaz into Ruth's life as a "redeemer." God turned her despair to hope and joy, ending her season of despair and bitterness. Naomi became the great-grandmother of King David when Ruth married and bore a son. That was God's greatest blessing, being placed in the lineage of the Messiah. And

Ruth provided unconditional care for Naomi with gentleness and love, so all the city knew that Ruth cared for Naomi. God compensated Naomi for her years of bitterness.

A godly, committed family and good, godly friends play an important role in turning our despair into joy, but above all, our hope, joy, and strength come from the Lord. Our transformation and renewal will likely take time, as with Naomi, but change will begin as soon as we ask God to renew our hearts. Whatever kind of hurt or hopelessness you might be feeling, turn to God and ask Him to heal your bitterness and restore your joy. God's heart is broken for you.

God does not want you to isolate yourself in your bitterness. He is the One who healed and transformed the poisonous, bitter waters into sweet, drinkable water at Marah when the Israelites were thirsty in the wilderness (Exod. 15:25–26). Jehovah Rapha, our healer, can heal all your emotional pain and transform your bitterness into sweet joy, peace, and hope.

Loneliness

> But one thing I do: Forgetting what is behind and straining toward what is ahead.
>
> —Philippians 3:13

As I mentioned in the previous chapter, loneliness can lead to more bitterness and destruction. Run to God when you are discouraged and lonely. Do not isolate yourself when life is hard and hurtful. Pray as Jesus prayed when He was in the Garden of Gethsemane, when all His disciples left Him by Himself in the hands of the enemy. God's love is the same for everyone in every situation; you have value in God's eyes. Remember, Gideon isolated himself when he felt inadequate, saying (in effect), "I am nobody." But God sent His angel and lifted him from obscurity.

Confess your situation, and talk to the Lord throughout the day. Stay connected with your heavenly Father. He can be your closest friend and comfort you. Elijah was lonely in the cave, but the presence of God came to him there. God's presence will come to you where you are. He is involved in your life, even when you are discouraged.

Inactivity brings loneliness and discouragement. When I arrived in the United States in 1990, I was so discouraged. I started to criticize myself for leaving my family, my profession, my friends, and my home church and coming halfway around the globe (almost six thousand miles) to an unknown situation. But I decided neither to isolate myself nor to let bitterness take residence in my mind. I decided to work two jobs and also to not miss church. I even helped friends paint their houses and took care of the elderly, even though I had no clue about caring for disabled people. As an economist, I had very little knowledge of anatomy and physiology. Working reduces your discouragement because it redirects your brain activity.

God reveals Himself layer by layer when you seek Him in your loneliness. (See Exodus 33:1–6.) Moses asked God not to forsake the nation of Israel. He did not want to move on without God. When God is present, all things become alive. Even dry bones come to life (Ezek. 37:1–14). In your loneliness, always keep on praying. Prayer will bring people who are far away closer to your heart to prevent loneliness.

God will send people to help you in times of need. You cannot be lonely. (See 1 Kings 20.) You must speak out in your anguish of loneliness, as Job did in Job 7:11. There are crises in life, and we all will experience emotional wounds and times of loneliness that need to be addressed and discussed in order to be healed. King David mentioned many times that he had unhealed wounds in his heart. He was desperate for his healer. David lived a busy life surrounded by people but still had emotional pain from loneliness in his spirit (Ps. 109:22). He was running to God constantly for healing in his mind and soul. For emotional and physical healing you must run to God constantly. That is God's prescription for emotional healing. Love those around you, and do not let loneliness ruin your happiness.

Christ accepted you as you are, and you must accept others as they are. Do not run away from people to isolate yourself. (See Romans 15:7.) Believe that God receives and accepts you the way you are as His son or daughter. You do not need to be overcome with fear. Just forgive people who offend you, and ask for forgiveness if you offended them, and your burden will be removed. You will be free in Christ Jesus, saved by grace. Even though we do not understand everything, we must throw away our fears and worries and run to Jesus. We know that blind Bartimaeus lived in bitterness and loneliness due to his disability. He did not understand it, but when he heard Jesus passing by, he threw off his clothes and ran to Him (Mark 10:46–52). You have your "clothing" of fear, blindness, insecurity, bitterness, and loneliness in your darkest moments. Run to Jesus, and ask Him to take them off one by one, even if you do not understand the process. He came to earth just for this. God is giving you new "clothes," a new mind, new thoughts, and a new vision.

Start where you are. Throw away those blankets of fear and insecurity that create bitterness, isolation, and loneliness. Exchange them for the love of Jesus, and you will never be lonely again. The love of Jesus will enable you to love others. Through Jesus' love you can lead other people to Jesus now that you have met Him yourself. Christ's love will help you pray for their needs, their diseases, and their addictions and lead them to Christ. John Hagee, in his book *In Defense of Israel: The Bible's Mandate for Supporting the Jewish State*, explained:

> The Christian doctrine of love was first taught by a Jewish rabbi from Nazareth, who said: "Love your neighbor as yourself" (Matthew 19:19, NIV). "Love one another as I have loved you" (John 15:12). "By this all will know that you are My disciples, if you have love for one another" (John 13:35). "Love your enemies" (Matthew 5:44).[26]

God is constantly restoring our loneliness and those around us through love.

Even in the loneliest time of his life, John the Baptist recognized that Jesus brings Holy Spirit fire. In prison, lonely and isolated from the world, John received a revelation of Jesus. John looked for the Lamb of God even in his lowest moments, and Jesus protected his soul from bitterness in prison. Redirect your focus to what Jesus is doing in other Christians' lives. He is willing to do the same for you.

When you defer hope, you postpone healing of your emotional wounds, and your heart will continue in loneliness, hurt, and isolation. Everyone faces disappointments and losses, but God gives us hope for every day. The challenge we have is to know who God is and *who we are in God*. Know your identity in Christ. Explore the fullness of God to hear His heartbeat. He takes delight in His children and expresses His heart to them in their loneliness.

Many people choose to live in bitterness when things do not go their way. The world all around us is in pain. We can get distracted by the things of life and miss the essential one, Jesus. (See Luke 10.) We must be carriers of Christ, living a life of sacrifice, love, and freedom from bitterness and loneliness.

Leave behind your mistakes and wrong choices. It is never too late. Get a vision for accomplishments and manifestations of the power of God in you. Choose what is important. Do not use your energy on things that will perish or negatively affect your life. Do not miss the best that God has for you. Forget the past, and look forward; as the apostle Paul said, "But one thing I do: Forgetting what is behind and straining toward what is ahead" (Phil. 3:13). You need the power of the Holy Spirit in order to move forward in God's dimension, because "with God all things are possible" (Matt. 19:26). Despise the shame, and anchor your faith in the invisible power of God. With Jesus in your heart, you will never be lonely again.

PART III

GOD'S SUPERNATURAL PRESCRIPTIONS

Chapter 6

CREATING CHEMICAL BALANCE IN YOUR BRAIN

Rejoice in the Lord always. I will say it again: Rejoice!...Do not be anxious about anything, but in every situation, by prayer and petition, with thanksgiving, present your requests to God. And the peace of God, which transcends all understanding, will guard your hearts and your minds in Christ Jesus.
—Philippians 4:4, 6–7

May these words of my mouth and this meditation of my heart be pleasing in your sight, Lord, my Rock and my Redeemer.
—Psalm 19:14

To create the best atmosphere for a healthy chemical balance in your brain, you must prevent anxiety, avoid worry, and change the way you perceive life, following the prescription King David offered in Psalm 19:14. Meditation that pleases the Lord must be increased to preserve our neurons and promote neurogenesis. We want new neurons to be developed to prevent neurocognitive disorders such as dementia and Alzheimer's. Dementia presents with morphological changes in the brain structure, impairing cognition and executive functions.[1]

That is why the Bible teaches us to maintain a joyful attitude. Meditating day and night on the promises of God brings more hope, healthy thoughts, and stronger neurons in our brains. We need to actively rejoice in the Lord of our salvation. The New Testament states God's prescription for neurogenesis—the creation of new neurons—instructing us to rejoice in the Lord at all times, as Philippians 4:4–7 advises. This amazing prescription was written almost two thousand years ago, with no expiration date. Gladness and joy will assist the brain structures to create new neurons, calm an overactive brain, and clear the mind, enabling us to filter out all unhealthy thoughts that would lead to a chemical imbalance in the brain. When you rejoice or feel happy, a healthy atmosphere is created in your brain. Your neurotransmitters (such as oxytocin, endorphin, dopamine, and serotonin) are released in healthy amounts, promoting the healing process.

When you bring all your worry to God in prayer, Philippians 4:7 promises the peace of God will guard your heart and mind. You can see why it is very important to guard your heart and mind in Christ, bringing health to your mind, spirit, and body. Continuous joy, love, peace, trusting God in all things, and avoiding worry are all on God's prescription pad for you. They will reduce anxiety and its symptoms and destructive complications. Do not allow those conditions to prevent you from fulfilling your God-given destiny.

God lovingly wrote another clear prescription more than three thousand years ago, advising us to neither worry nor struggle: "Be still, and know that I am God" (Ps. 46:10). Not only is it good to flood your mind with the Word of God; it is essential. Rest in Him and wait upon Him when you are depressed or anxious. His prescription for renewing our strength appears in Isaiah 40:31: "They that wait upon the Lord shall renew their strength" (kjv). Anxiety and depression from excessive worry can kill you by stealing your strength, but when you wait on God and allow His love to flow over you, your strength will be renewed through new neurons! Meditating on God's promises means growing stronger neurons, having healthier thoughts, and slowing the aging process. Meditation on God's Word is an antiaging therapy and a priceless treatment.

All people on earth should live with this hope. Look in the Word of God. Reaching beyond science, the Bible teaches that we must be filled with faith, peace, compassion, and joy, which will drive out fear and all its consequences. By following God's prescription, you will not lose heart.

Given some of the challenges I had endured, at one time I felt great distress over who would change this world, so full of worry, problems, and stress. Finally I realized that the power that can change the world is a mind renewed through the Word of God, which contains God's supernatural prescriptions, beyond science. Romans 12:1–2 says:

> Therefore, I urge you, brothers and sisters, in view of God's mercy, to offer your bodies as a living sacrifice, holy and pleasing to God—this is your true and proper worship. Do not conform to the pattern of this world, but be transformed by the renewing of your mind. Then you will be able to test and approve what God's will is—his good, pleasing and perfect will.

The perfect will of God is for each person on planet Earth to be healthy and prosper. God wants us to be healthy, so He gave us prescriptions, far above the scope of science, to stay healthy and to prevent diseases at any given time and age. In 3 John 2 we read, "Dear friend, I pray that you may enjoy good health and that all may go well with you, even as your soul is getting along well."

The fear of the Lord, which is the beginning of wisdom, can change you. People who fear the Lord have a treasure—the wisdom to apply God's prescriptions and instructions from His Word in their daily lives. The world will change if each person's mind is renewed by exercising that wisdom. Each person can be transformed through wisdom received from God—His prescriptions in His Word.

RESTORING RIGHT ATTITUDES

> One generation commends your works to another; they tell of your mighty acts. They speak of the glorious splendor of your majesty—and I will meditate on your wonderful works. They tell of the power of your awesome works—and I will proclaim your great deeds. They celebrate your abundant goodness and joyfully sing of your righteousness.
> —PSALM 145:4–7

This generation, the next generation, and the generations after them will be changed if we change our thinking about teenagers' attitudes at home, in school, in the community, and in the world. They are the leaders of tomorrow. Students should be eager to learn with discipline; to gain wisdom, knowledge, and revelation; and to change their attitude in the classroom. This will even improve their exam scores!

What we teach our children at home and in our schools is very important. They need to learn healthy values and beliefs that promote health and prevent disease. What they learn in school, at home, at church, and in their community will remain in their brains (prefrontal cortex, hippocampus, amygdala, nucleus accumbens, and other brain structures[2]), regulating their emotions and memories and dictating their behavior for life. If society allows the education standards to deteriorate, the future will be ruined for our next generation.

I experienced a tremendous earthquake in Bucharest, Romania, on March 4, 1977. Nearly two million people felt the violent tremors, measured at 7.2 on the Richter scale. More than fifteen hundred people died under collapsed buildings, leaving the city devastated and in great turmoil.[3] That fault line traverses Bucharest. Thousands of smaller seismic aftershocks continued all night long and the next day, such that people thought it was the end of the world. Just as a fissure—a fault line deep in the earth—will bring disaster to a city or a nation, so a fault in the education system can ruin the entire future generation.

Misunderstanding true freedom, and lowering moral and educational standards, will degrade a society. Unhealthy behavior, including exposure to movies whose actors live unhealthy lifestyles, should not be promoted in schools. Kids are not supposed to engage in premarital sex. They should not be exposed to teaching that promotes adulterous relationships, drugs, alcohol, pornography, violence, and all the destructive habits popular in modern media.

Vaccination is not the answer to destructive sexual behavior. When taking past histories to decide on the right diagnosis, interventions, and treatment, I see patients who do not even know how many partners they have had. Our schools are preoccupied with providing condoms to boys as early as the sixth grade, and encouraging their use, instead of promoting abstinence and discipline. There is no such thing as "safe sex." Scientifically, only abstinence from unhealthy behavior is 100 percent risk-free from sexually transmitted disease,[4] yet it is seldom taught.

Sex is more than sleeping with another person to satisfy the flesh's momentary desire. Sexuality is not meant for fleeting pleasure. Sex outside of marriage often results in emotional pain, intense psychological distress, and sadness, and can lead to "broken heart syndrome." During episodes of great emotional distress due to broken relationships, toxic levels of neurochemicals are released and affect the left ventricle of the heart, weakening it until it is unable to contract properly. This impairs circulation in the body, with potential long-term, unhealthy consequences.[5] Then we wonder why so many young people are unhealthy. Sex will create a physical and emotional bond, which, when broken, creates deep emotional wounds, high levels of stress, and other complications.

We need serious teaching on this important subject, which affects the body, mind, and spirit of the future generation. Current instruction in our schools on adultery, premarital sex, chemical abuse, pornography, and other unhealthy behaviors is woefully superficial. Students are not taught how to seriously analyze the consequences of their behavior. So many lives are destroyed, costing society a fortune. Our broken human nature was the very reason God gave us His divine instructions and prescriptions. He wants to show us how to prevent those diseases through abstinence and self-control.

Billions of dollars is spent on our military to fight overseas to protect our freedom and preserve our lives. Yet at the same time, we slowly destroy our future generations at home by avoiding teaching abstinence in schools, promoting destructive behaviors, and exposing those generations to a culture of filth. Children are our future, who in turn will influence the next generation coming after them.

Victory in a Changed Attitude

> You were taught, with regard to your former way of life, to put off your old self, which is being corrupted by its deceitful desires; to be made new in the attitude of your minds.
>
> —Ephesians 4:22–23

Attitude is one key for a stress-free life. Changing your attitude will help you reduce your stress level.[6] Nick Vujicic, an Australian man born with no limbs (legs or arms), decided to change his attitude despite his unfortunate condition. Instead of being bitter and angry at God, Nick decided God knew what He was doing. Even though he has neither legs nor arms, today he is involved in more activities than many physically perfect human beings, all because he changed his attitude. He looks not at his disabilities but at all his opportunities and possibilities. He is married to a beautiful wife and has four precious children.[7]

When you go through the fire of trials and discouraging situations, remember that God is in the midst of your problems, working to reveal His glory. His eyes are watching over you day and night, ready to fulfill His plan in your life when you renew your attitude. We often do not see beyond the trial, but as we learn from so many Bible characters' lives, a supernatural intervention is available. The barriers that hinder God's interventions include our old mental attitudes of unforgiveness, bitterness, laziness, narcissism, greediness, fear, doubt, and hopelessness. If left unmanaged, all these degrade our health and leave us unable to function.[8]

You can change things inside you and deal with your circumstances better if you grow in the knowledge of God. Only He will enable you to be the best person, mother, father, sister, brother, friend, colleague, and neighbor possible, despite all your unfavorable circumstances. With that attitude you can move forward. Just open your brain to better visions and dreams. Change your attitude, and find victory in every area.

EPIGENETICS IN THE BIBLE

> For I, the LORD your God, am a jealous God, punishing the children for the sin of the parents to the third and fourth generation of those who hate me, but showing love to a thousand generations of those who love me and keep my commandments.
>
> —EXODUS 20:5–6

Daily environmental stresses, combined with an unhealthy lifestyle, will alter and influence our gene expression through an epigenetic mechanism. Genetic changes (epigenetics) can be passed down through gene expression, affecting the next generation.[9] Everything parents experience in their everyday lives, including memories and associated thoughts related to their emotions, will be transmitted to the next generation through epigenetics, even in utero, through the genes.[10]

Children are the most vulnerable population. As they are exposed to information through the media and the internet, the changes occurring in society now will be carried further to become either a burden or a blessing for the next generation. Bishop T. D. Jakes, pastor of a thirty thousand–member church in Dallas—and whose TV show reaches some sixty-seven million households per month—says in his best-selling book *Reposition Yourself: Living Life Without Limits*: "Repositioning your children and acclimating them to a new financial environment may be the hardest thing you do. As we change, not only financially but morally and socially, don't forget that the children carry the weight of the changes we make."[11] Studies show that the epigenome is influenced by physical and emotional stress, altering the gene expression in the human body. Those changes can be passed down through at least three or four generations.[12]

The study of epigenetics has led to new findings "about the relationship between epigenetic changes and a host of disorders including various cancers, mental retardation associated disorders, immune disorders, neuropsychiatric disorders and pediatric disorders."[13] This discovery confirms what the Bible mentioned more than thirty-four hundred years ago in Exodus 20:5–6, about curses lasting to the third and fourth generation of those who hate God, but great rewards going to those who love Him. God's pure love can reprogram genetic mutations for thousands of generations for those who follow God's supernatural prescriptions. Scientists have also discovered that epigenetic modifications are potentially reversible with healthy lifestyle changes.[14] Using our conscious minds, the prefrontal cortexes, we can modify bad habits.[15] (More about lifestyle changes later.)

As parents, our lifestyles affect our children. Children from divorced families often suffer from poor social development. Poor emotional support and inconsistent role modeling can lead to depression and early-onset personality problems.[16] Seeking relief from worry, anxiety, and depression, children from broken homes may engage in risky behaviors. A 2017 survey showed that in the United States alone within one month about 7.4 million people age twelve to twenty had consumed alcohol and 30.5 million people age twelve or older had used an illicit drug (primarily marijuana).[17]

As low self-esteem and early peer pressures escalate, abstinence is rare, and life becomes complicated by social, medical, and legal expenses for teens and young adults. Some of them inherit that burden from their parents. They go out to have a good time, engage in multiple sexual relationships, and abuse alcohol and drugs for immediate gratification, while this wreaks silent havoc on their dopamine storage at the cellular level. Many times they mirror their parents' behavior, socializing with drinkers, and thus develop a high risk for mortality. Feelings of hopelessness only worsen the situation.

We, as parents, need to tell our children and their generation about God's miracle-working power to transform minds, thoughts, and lives. We need to pay attention to the exhortation from Psalm 145:4–7 (which I quoted earlier in this chapter) to tell of God's great works, meditate on them, and proclaim them to others. These positive habits are learned by reinforcement, and internally, dopamine is released throughout our systems. What healing power is hidden in God's prescriptions for joy and His abundant goodness!

May the Word of God be known to the next generation, and may His promises permeate their brain structures. Addictions have a neurobiological origin in the limbic system (hippocampus and amygdala). This plays a huge role in the storage of emotions and memories.[18]

Bad habits need to be replaced with healthy habits. Anxiety, and all the emotions and memories from a dysfunctional family life, can be replaced with the powerful promises in God's Word. His restoration power brings glorious hope, casting out fear and worry and reducing anxiety and depression from feelings of neglect, rejection, isolation, exploitation, humiliation, and terror. Children in an abusive, chaotic environment often overreact. They adopt unhealthy, risky behaviors and develop diseases and disabilities and possibly suffer an early death.[19] Kids under stress will have nightmares.[20] They will eat more for comfort to soothe their emotions. This causes weight gain, then diabetes, hypertension, high cholesterol, metabolic syndrome, and sleep apnea.[21]

Following a healthy lifestyle will activate healthy epigenetics. Your lifestyle can either optimize your health or contribute to disease development, which will carry on into future generations. It is your choice.

Intrinsic Motivation

> "For I know the plans I have for you," declares the Lord, "plans to prosper you and not to harm you, *plans to give you hope and a future*."
> —Jeremiah 29:11, emphasis added

Building intrinsic motivation and regulation in our brains is crucial to the restoration of relationships in families with children, in schools, and in society. Children need healthy challenges, realistic expectations, and encouragement. Memories of appropriate rewards and punishments will empower children to develop useful skills. We have already seen that the neurotransmitter dopamine in the brain is associated with the reward, gratification, and expectation of reinforcement. In the brain the limbic system (including the amygdala, associated with emotional and behavioral responses to memories stored in the hippocampus, interconnected with other brain structures) will store those memories of reward or punishment.[22]

Raising our children in a healthy emotional environment will bring the future generation to higher standards of behavior. This is one way to prepare them for a promising future, as promised in Jeremiah 29:11. God has set high standards for us. These are meant to protect us and ensure a higher quality of life. His standards also demand immediate obedience. God's supernatural prescriptions (laws and promises) protect us from the adverse effects of disobedience. Those who follow neither biblical guidelines nor the Lord's superior standards will suffer harmful consequences. Thankfully the Holy Spirit works in the believer's conscience, motivating us to fulfill God's superior standards. God's Spirit in us becomes our intrinsic motivation. Then we make better choices that will set us on the right path for a meaningful life—if we are willing to listen and obey.

Considering where the future generation will arrive, and laying the foundations for our own children, what principles do we promote? Our whole culture today is globalized; countless cultures intermingle. Furthermore, cultures and technologies change continually. The question is, Whose culture do we follow, and what are the immediate and eternal consequences? Pursuing a biblical culture will build a strong foundation for the future. That is the antidote to disaster for the future generation.

Our bodies are gifts from God and temples of the Holy Spirit. The Holy Spirit within us helps us develop an intrinsic motivation to honor God with our lifestyle. We honor Him through praying, fasting, reading the Word of God regularly, exercising, eating healthy, helping others, and making good decisions to protect our future from dangerous diseases. Positive attitudes increase healthy dopamine activity.[23] Do not use substances or foods that poison your body and brain. Elevate the way you manage your body, your heart, and your mind by following the world's most powerful wisdom—the Word of God—through the power of the Holy Spirit. That gives us hope for the future.

Honor God From Generation to Generation

> Know therefore that the Lord your God is God; he is the faithful God, keeping his covenant of love to a thousand generations of those who love him and keep his commandments.
> —Deuteronomy 7:9

He lifts the poor from the dust and raises the needy from their misery. I grew up under communism but still felt God's invisible grace. I remained in awe of God because of the passion of my parents to keep us true to the knowledge of God and His miracles. When you teach your children God's Word and to set their hope in God, He will put you in a place of honor. I recently learned that my paternal grandfather was a very rich Jew. He owned farms and forests, but the communists took everything away and left the family in poverty, even though we worked hard. Many days we had only polenta or simple crackers to eat for breakfast, lunch, and dinner. We girls had only one dress and one pair of worn-out shoes, but our hearts were filled with joy because we had God on our side.

With God's help I finished my secondary education in Bucharest, Romania. Then He brought me to the United States, where many doors opened for me to learn English and find jobs. I had jobs even before I could speak English! I worked extra hard so people would let me keep the job. Then I started taking care of elderly people. I went back to school and got my associate's, bachelor's, master's, and then my doctorate degree. God gave me favor everywhere I went, a fulfillment of 1 Samuel 2:8, which says God "raises up the poor from the dust...to make them sit with princes and inherit a seat of honor" (ESV). God did that for me. He literally moved me from the dust and poverty of a small village in northern Romania, oppressed under a brutal communist regime, to freedom, a high position, and riches in the city of Portland, Oregon. That is a place of honor, where only God could position me. Since my childhood I have followed God's prescriptions for living—long before I was a health care provider—because I believed obedience would bring great rewards here on earth and for eternity. Everything I have gained came only through prayer, obedience to the Word of God and His prescriptions, and the Lord's grace. He is able to do it for you too, and for your children, and your children's children. Why would anyone choose disobedience, with its dreadful consequences of chronic stress and physical and spiritual damage?

THE MOST POWERFUL FORCE ON EARTH

> These are the things God has revealed to us by his Spirit. The Spirit searches all things, even the deep things of God.
> —1 CORINTHIANS 2:10

The Spirit searches all things visible and invisible. He is searching your heart, mind, and thoughts, and His thoughts about you are overwhelming. God has been thinking about you forever. He has dreams for your life that you can see only with your spiritual eyes. To see what He sees, you must recognize God's presence in your life. He is speaking directly to you. You can recognize the voice of God, speaking directly to you through the power of the Holy Spirit, through your conscious mind.

The Spirit who resurrected Jesus Christ from death lives in you, if you believe in Jesus and have received His forgiveness of sins. Jesus is the Lord of all creation. Pray through the Holy Spirit for transformation to reach a new level. Revelation will come through obedience and prayer. God expects us to act responsibly and obey His Word. Wisdom from the Holy Spirit, and a revelation of Jesus, will bring transformation and breakthrough in your thinking process.

Don't let unhealthy thoughts invade your brain. Tune in to His spiritual realm to discern the truth and reach wise decisions. The human mind in tune with the Holy Spirit is a powerful engine, through which God accomplishes His work on earth and fulfills His plan in our lives. The Holy Spirit–renewed mind has indescribable power.

Guard God's prescriptions for decision-making, and His instruction, deep in your heart. Understanding the mystery of the work of the Holy Spirit in people's lives can empower educational reforms to change the next generation. The concept of an eternal soul must be understood in our society so people can make wiser decisions. Lack of wisdom brings destruction.

Our education system is failing to teach children the truth about the human spirit, soul, and body. We must filter our thoughts, discard negative thoughts, and focus on what is necessary to accomplish our daily tasks. If we are honest, we recognize that we are eternal, spiritual beings living in temporary physical bodies. Our physical bodies are only the temporary homes of our eternal spirits, temples of the Holy Spirit. God's spirit of wisdom and revelation is waiting to be released in our minds, but lack of knowledge brings destruction. Hosea tells us, "My people are destroyed from lack of knowledge" (Hos. 4:6). Let your soul and spirit be hungry for more knowledge, revelation, and understanding to live a healthy life, physically and spiritually, on earth.

Parameters of Our Prescriptions

> Fear not, for I am with you; be not dismayed, for I am your God; I will strengthen you, I will help you, I will uphold you with my righteous right hand.
>
> —Isaiah 41:10, ESV

God gave people clear parameters in His written prescriptions in the Word in order to function and live a healthy life. In medicine if you do not follow the parameters for your treatment you do not obtain the desired therapeutic, expected outcomes. People can die if they ignore medical advice and do not take what their doctors prescribe.

Here is a very simple example of parameters for an over-the-counter pain medication: acetaminophen (Tylenol). The prescription is: "Acetaminophen 325 mg tab, 1–2 tablets every 4 to 6 hours for pain, as needed, for two weeks. Do not use more than 3,000 mg of acetaminophen in 24 hours." Taking more than 3,000 mg in twenty-four hours for several days can cause liver toxicity, even without a history of liver disease.[24] For some patients, acetaminophen is not enough to control pain, and they need to talk to their health care professional for further interventions. They must seek advice from their medical provider to prevent liver damage. Some who already have liver disease or allergies cannot use this medication at all.

Another parameter, for a common nonsteroidal anti-inflammatory medication, is: "Ibuprofen 200 mg tablets; use 1–2 tablets by mouth every 4 to 6 hours as needed for pain for two weeks. Do not use more than 1,800 mg in 24 hours." Using more than 3,200 mg prescription-strength or 1,200 mg over-the-counter medication in twenty-four hours for longer than two weeks can cause water retention, kidney damage, and heart disease.[25] Some people cannot use this medication at all. Always check for adverse reactions, side effects, and allergies—for any kind of medication you take. Always communicate with your primary care provider for clear instructions for any medical advice and intervention.

Clear Parameters for a Renewed Life

Spiritually you need to seek knowledge from the Word of God. In the Bible we find prescriptions with clear instructions and parameters for spiritual therapy that benefit our bodies, souls, and spirits for eternity. The Bible is full of written prescriptions that need to be followed correctly to bring spiritual health and prevent spiritual diseases, because our bodies benefit from spiritual decisions here on earth.

God's revelations are a vast resource. They are available to everyone but must be respected and obeyed to fulfill their potential, which is divinely imprinted in each individual's DNA.

Through the supernatural power of the Holy Spirit, we access God's knowledge by faith—beyond science, beyond natural circumstances, and beyond the world's understanding. There is a realm of revelation through divine inspiration for medical professionals, businesspeople, politicians, educators, ministers—everyone. Revelation is given by divine grace for us to accomplish the will of God on earth, for His purpose and His glory. The Word and its clear parameters will transform and modify your thinking process, transforming your unhealthy thinking into healthy, productive thinking according to the promises of God. Healthy, normal levels of neurotransmitters and chemical messengers will prevent toxicity in your soul and body. Allow godly thinking to trigger the right emotions in your brain. This is the blessing of a transformed mind.

Fasting and prayer have incredible power to help us transform our minds. When we pray and fast, we humble ourselves before God, meditating on what is good and bad. Redirecting our thoughts, we can then make well-informed decisions.

Good Seed, Good Harvest

With the seed of the Word deep in your heart and mind, new neurons develop and your life is transformed.[26] There is a supernatural law about sowing and reaping. The unhealed areas of your life do not allow the Word of God to penetrate the callous, hidden places of your soul. First a cleaning process, a healing of your emotions and your memories, must take place. The soil must be fertile and well prepared—a healthy mind and body and a new life—for the seed to bring forth a good harvest. The brain's amygdala can protect your emotions from stress, but you must allow the Word of God (the seed) to penetrate the deepest place of your mind to clean out old, hidden thoughts of rejection, bitterness, unforgiveness, anger, anxiety, depression, and low self-esteem.

The Word of God is powerful beyond imagination. The universe was created through God's Word, and this same Word of God has the power to align your thoughts with the Father's divine purpose. Many people think evil is stronger than the power of God, but we have power over evil through the Word of God when it fills our minds through the Spirit of God.

Shift Your Priorities

Create in me a pure heart, O God, and renew a steadfast spirit within me.
—Psalm 51:10

Renewing our minds means a shift of all our values and our belief system, starting inside. Do not set your mind on earthly things that influence you in an unhealthy way. Change your values. Shift your priorities. The Word of God, changing hearts one by one, will reshape history. Lives are transformed because of God's grace, freely given, and He will raise you up. Live your divine destiny by deciding every day to transform your thinking and obey the Word of God.

Obedience brings miracles. God will bless not only you but your children and your children's children—even those not yet born. The epigenetic process through gene expression in the next generations will continue to work both physically and spiritually until His coming. In Psalm 51:10 King David asked God for a transformed heart and a spirit of wisdom. David shifted his priorities because he learned how much destruction and disaster a selfish, sinful heart could bring, even to an innocent soul. He also realized that the heart without the spirit cannot change.

Desperate for God's Presence

> Now show me your glory.
> —Exodus 33:18

Where there is sin and unbelief, there is no presence of God. There is emptiness, loneliness, depression, fear, worry of uncertainty, anxiety—and the stress level rises. This is a serious situation. We must be desperate for God's presence, like Moses in Exodus 33:18–19, crying out for God to show him His glory, which prompted God to bring His presence and goodness. You will be a different person when the Holy Spirit comes to live in you. It dispels fear, worry, and anxiety from your body and restores your soul and spirit. In God's presence you experience His supernatural power—joy in sadness, peace in crisis, and strength in weaknesses. God is full of compassion. He is angry for a moment when we are disobedient, but He is always merciful. God's heart is moved because of your situation. God feels the effect of our sins, and He wants us to feel His goodness. God is a covenant keeper, without boundaries, infinite. Let His presence invade your mind and change your destiny.

Chapter 7

EVERYTHING STARTS IN THE BRAIN

My people are destroyed from lack of knowledge.
—Hosea 4:6

YOUR PHYSICAL AND emotional health begin in your brain, which receives information from the outside world and interprets those messages. Drawing on prior knowledge, experiences, emotions, and memories, your thoughts form instantly. The more knowledge you have, the better you can interpret the threats you receive and formulate better responses. As mentioned before, the Bible (in Hosea 4:6) explained the consequences of a lack of knowledge thousands of years before Christ came to earth.

Clearly, in order to thrive you need to understand what happens in your brain. Information processed there can prevent the destruction of your body, mind, and spirit. The brain needs the right food (good thoughts and healthy emotions) to stay healthy and avoid mental decline, neurocognitive disorders, and other physical and spiritual illnesses. Positive affirmations found in the promises of God throughout the Bible create healthy thoughts and positive attitudes that strengthen your neurons and brain structures.

As your knowledge grows, your faith will increase. Faith creates confidence in God's promises and affects your mental and physical being in a healthy way. Fearfulness and worry are destructive thoughts, causing anxiety because of a wrong thinking process. This affects your whole being. It decreases your quality of life, leading to physical and spiritual damage to your body, mind, and spirit. To be healthy, your body, mind, and spirit must be in harmony. (See Exodus 23–25.)

Detoxify your emotions and thoughts by renewing your mind through a healthy thinking process. A clear mind and clean thoughts will bring health to your entire being. Submission to the Word of God will bring life, healing, and deliverance from the strongholds of fear, worry, anxiety, and depression. Be desperate for a visitation from God and the manifestation of His power in your life. When you have a visitation from God, your life is changed and your spirit comes alive. He will breathe from His spirit into your spirit so you can worship Him in spirit and truth. Worship is a great weapon in your daily battle with the worries of the world. Adoring God and worshipping Jesus restore your heart, your emotions, and your spirit and calm your overacting brain. What God is doing in your heart and mind is supernatural. (See Isaiah 40:29–31.)

God's Healing Presence

In our postmodern era pressure is increasing in all areas of life. Get smart and protect your body, mind, and spirit through healthy thoughts. God holds the answer to your fear and worry. He wants your heart to be entirely His. Get closer to Him because in His presence is fullness of joy. He wants to draw you into His presence to be fully transformed. Many times I have felt the joy of His presence in my life, even in the midst of struggles. He wants to fill your heart with joy too. Love and joy will sustain you in a broken world by reprogramming your brain with healthy neurotransmitters.[1] Reprogram your brain by praising God and drawing near to His presence, and joy will overtake you and elevate your thinking process. Believe in His mighty power. God moves supernaturally on behalf of His people.

You can find refuge in the Word of God with *prescriptions beyond science* to manage your fear, worry, and stress. Keep reading, and you will realize that Jesus Christ, the Son of God, is the answer to all the problems people around the world have, especially those in countless terrible, uncontrollable, unpredictable, and disastrous situations. Knowing that here on this planet we live as visitors with "a temporary visa" will reduce your stress. You cannot control everything, but you can control your decisions and your attitude. What you believe, and whose prescriptions and instructions you follow, will determine your quality of life on earth and in your eternal home in heaven.

Managing Pressure

Worry, fear, and anxiety overwhelm so many people. God created us to be able to manage life's pressures one day at time. You cannot correct the past, but by faith you can look to the future with joy, hope, and love. David prayed to be cleansed from problems inside him. There are things inside your subconscious, stored deep inside your memory, that create inner pressures when triggered by unhealthy thoughts. God, however, has access to your subconscious areas and can heal them right now. Release every unhealthy, threatening thought, and concentrate on God's instructions. Embracing godly thoughts and obeying God are renewing and create a healthy lifestyle.

Low self-esteem can make peer pressure feel even worse. When your peers in school try to humiliate you, declare the Word of God. You are truly a unique creature on earth, "fearfully and wonderfully made" (Ps. 139:14). God knew exactly who He wanted you to be—your hair, skin, eyes, nose, ears, and height, whether short or tall. You were created for His purpose, to glorify His name. Everything was deliberately placed in your DNA and your genes.

Peer pressure can isolate us in loneliness. Some young people, trying to escape peer pressure, loneliness, anxiety, depression, boredom, stress, or relationship problems, become addicted to the internet. To cope with loneliness, they seek refuge in games, social media, or chat rooms, to the point of addiction. Statistics show that before age eighteen, 93 percent of boys and 62 percent of girls have seen internet pornography,[2] another destructive habit.

RENEW YOUR JOY

We have the ability in our conscious minds, through the prefrontal cortex and other brain structures, to reason with our thoughts and decide how to act.[3] For example, maybe you used to be active in church and enjoyed group activities but have lost interest in going out and sharing your thoughts with others. Maybe you feel depressed, not even wanting to leave your house. Use your frontal lobe, and think about what made you so devoted and passionate in the past for the Word of God—and what changed. Reflect on your positive experience with God in the past, and revive your passion. Find joy with God and His Word in your life again. Even specialists and psychologists will tell you to count your blessings to prevent pressure caused by depressive thinking.

The Word of God that we hear, meditate on, and memorize is converted in our brains into electrical impulses. These trigger neurons to release neurochemicals, according to the intensity and quality of those impulses. When we meditate on the Word of God, we receive wisdom and clarity to interpret information received from our environment through the five senses. When we encounter problems and temptations, we can then reject unhealthy thoughts, reflect on God's prescriptions for the situation, and focus on the promises of God to bring us hope, joy, and happiness.[4] The Bible has an answer for every situation, but we must train our brains to reason according to what God says about those situations.

Bring any problem to the Lord, let your request be known to God, and you will find peace. God's strongest prescription for worry, with a maximum potency, is far beyond the scope of science. As Philippians 4:6 says, "Do not be anxious about anything, but in every situation, by prayer and petition, with thanksgiving, present your requests to God." Follow that instruction in the Bible, and you will find the result is that "the peace of God, which transcends all understanding, will guard your hearts and your minds in Christ Jesus" (v. 7).

It is well documented that peace decreases anxiety, calms an overactive brain, helps us relax, and allows our brains to release healthy neurotransmitters into our bodies, starting the healing process and preventing illness.

DIVINE PRESCRIPTIONS IN THE BIBLE

> Do not fear, for I redeemed you; I have summoned you by name; you are mine. When you pass through the waters, I will be with you; and when you pass through the rivers, they will not sweep over you. When you walk through the fire, you will not be burned; the flames will not set you ablaze.
>
> —Isaiah 43:1–2

Fear, worry, anxiety and stress can kill. It is impossible to overcome all the stressors in the world without following the principles of God and His prescriptions for supernatural solutions. Only the Bible has the right prescriptions to treat this paralyzing pandemic. As I've already mentioned, the Bible contains God's prescriptions, but it also offers numerous directions, instructions, and recommendations. Its effectiveness reaches far beyond science. Instead of pills to cover worry and pain, God's divine prescriptions prevent spiritual and physical diseases and promote spiritual and physical health. God exhorts and instructs us repeatedly in His Word to not fear, as illustrated by the previous passage from Isaiah.

PREVENT WORRY AND ANXIETY

Worrying about the future triggers thoughts of fear and anxiety, which affect the thinking process. This impairs your cognition and interferes with your ability to make decisions. Even scientists agree that lack of knowledge, feelings of rejection, unforgiveness, financial problems, sickness, and loneliness will trigger more worry and increase your level of stress, affecting your entire well-being.

Recognize what kind of worry is triggering the stress in your life. Is it fear of losing your job, losing your loved one, being rejected, facing a lack of money, or suffering from poor health? The Word of God gives you God's remedies and His prescriptions and antidotes for worry of all kinds.

When you are worried about being rejected, you need to know that you are accepted! God predestined you for adoption. You can be adopted into God's family at any time. You only need to say yes to Jesus Christ as your Lord and Savior. As Ephesians 1:5–6 says, "He predestined us for adoption to sonship through Jesus Christ, in accordance with his pleasure and will—to the praise of his glorious grace, which he has freely given us in the One he loves." It is God's will for you to be His son or daughter through Jesus Christ. My heart is always touched and my spirit moved by adopted children, even when they are very old. I have known many patients in my practice who were adopted; they automatically receive a special place in my heart. I go the extra mile for them because I realize how their adoption changed their destiny. Our own worldly and eternal destiny is changed by our Lord Jesus Christ, through whom we are adopted by God. We receive special attention from heaven as adopted sons and daughters for eternity.

Pastor Larry Huch, in his book *Free at Last: Removing the Past From Your Future*, stated:

> Our finances, marriages, homes, emotions, and minds have been kidnapped by the devil. But Jesus came and paid the ransom for every area of our lives in full and has brought us back to the way we are supposed to be....
>
> There is a transformation that takes place by the renewing of our minds. It is a spiritual metamorphosis. When we think right, our words are right; when our words are right, our actions are right. Our potential is multiplied hundreds of times beyond anything we can think, but it happens through a metamorphosis of God's Spirit changing us by the renewing of our minds.[5]

Due to the changes in your brain structures and the healthy amounts of neurochemicals released, you regain power to live with real hope, joy, peace, healed relationships, restored health, and a prosperous spirit, mind, and body.

Discover Your Destiny

The power of the Holy Spirit can help change your image of yourself, your attitude and your destiny. The Book of Acts (chapter 2) describes how the Holy Spirit came as a mighty rushing wind and touched everybody who was there, both before and after Peter's preaching. Their thinking changed instantly, and their lives were transformed forever. Their worries and fears were gone because they discovered their destiny. Likewise when the Holy Spirit comes upon you, your spiritual eyes will be opened, and you will be convinced that you need to repent and be baptized. You will become a new creature, with new thoughts and a new view of yourself. Your low self-esteem will be gone forever. But you need to collaborate with the Spirit of God.

Even if you feel no motivation or do not see any reason to change your thinking and attitude, do it anyway. You will benefit the most. When God put the thoughts in my mind and desire in my heart to leave Romania, it did not make sense to me. Better circumstances existed after the revolution in December 1989. I knew how to live a simple life. I had my family, many friends, a house, my education, a job, and a good church, and I spoke my native language and practiced the profession I had studied for so many years. But I followed my God-given instincts and His instructions step by step until I finally became what I am today, even though it was an extremely difficult process.

Now I know why I needed to be in the United States. I am glad that I listened to the small voice inside of me and obeyed the Holy Spirit, who has guided and instructed me all these years. The small voice inside me reassured me all the time that all was right with my soul, even though I often felt like I was walking in the valley of the shadow of death. It was tough, but everything that I perceived as impossible in the beginning, with God, became possible in every way.

Change your attitude and start to work even though you feel like you are in the "desert with no water" or in the "valley of the shadow of death," like I felt when I arrived in the United States—knowing no English, having no plans, and not knowing what to do next. For months I did not know where I would sleep or where I would eat my next meal. Honestly speaking, I was homeless. God prepared "angels"—good friends who took care of me. I will mention their names so you will know they were real people: Arina, Nely, Maria, Marcela, and many others. Through them, God was working out my destiny.

I knew the Word of God and His promises, and I believed He had a destiny for me and my family, but that was a difficult time. People were giving me instructions to go to the left, and I was going to the right, because I did not understand a word in English. I can make fun of this now, but at that time it wasn't fun at all. Going to work and not being able to communicate with those around me was like going to a "funeral service," with sadness in my heart. I was afraid of failure and couldn't see myself succeeding in my own power and abilities. But I trusted God always.

See yourself through God's eyes to increase your self-esteem, and your dreams will become true when you start to work, continue to serve others, and pray and fast even though you do not feel like it. Your work may be hard, but be faithful in small things, even though they seem unimportant—even if bitterness floods your soul. Remember that God's eyes are always watching over you to fulfill your destiny.

GOD'S GLOBAL HEALTH PRESCRIPTION

> If my people who are called by my name, will humble themselves and pray and seek my face and turn from their wicked ways, then I will hear from heaven, and I will forgive their sin and will heal their land.
> —2 CHRONICLES 7:14

God is in the business of healing and He wants the human race to be healthy. From creation God has shared divine, unexpired prescriptions in His Word for all His creation. His provision is made clear in 2 Chronicles 7:14.

What I want to convey in this book is that God gave us instructions from the beginning on how to behave, how to stay healthy, and how to regain our health if we become ill. In the Ten Commandments, God gave clear directions about right attitudes toward God, our neighbors, and ourselves. He set forth rules on what to eat, how to dress, and how to behave in any situation. The Word of God taught us from the beginning how to react in stressful and uncontrollable circumstances. We cannot control death, but we can control the way we react when facing death.

The Word of God ultimately is written to prevent spiritual diseases and the eternal death of our spirit.

There are still opportunities to return to God's instructions and restore healthy thoughts by renewing our minds and hearts to follow a healthy lifestyle, physically and spiritually. Many times we complicate things by trying to solve problems in our own strength. We don't want to follow God's instructions. God who created us knows our capacity to cope with situations. But many deceptions in the world blind people's eyes, so they cannot see God's plan or His desire for them to follow His divine prescriptions to stay healthy and prosperous.

The devil used evolutionists and atheistic communists to distract millions of people with lies about the non-existence of God, insulting the Creator of the universe. This dogma confused the people, who gave up believing in the Word of God for physical and spiritual healing. I experienced this when living in a country victimized for several decades by the lies of a communist regime. It tortured me to constantly hear communist lies.

People turning their back on a sovereign God think they can control everything. I remember as a student in high school, and at the university in Bucharest, how atheists taught us there is no God. The entire country was hopelessly deceived under the brutal, ruthless, false teaching for more than forty years.

Their false teaching disturbed me. I had experienced God's supernatural power and treasured His Word, which transformed my life at a young age. Many times in class, hearing the atheistic affirmation about an orphan planet with no Creator, I had to quote Scriptures and write Bible verses in my notebook to maintain my hope, stay strong, and preserve my faith. The false doctrine and lies in the educational system continued in Romania until 1989, but the confusion remains. Communist indoctrination put the whole nation under a curse, leaving people in terrible, hopeless distress. Each time I visit Romania I see the consequences of those curses from the communist generations that reverberate even today in the lives of many people, both in Romania and other nations.

God's ways are the best plan for managing stress on a global scale. Stress is a root cause of all disease and turmoil. Stress levels will decrease when you refuse to let your heart be troubled by bad thoughts and bad circumstances. Our thoughts and actions will shape our future and our eternity. Do you know God's prescriptions for your life? How carefully do you follow His instructions for a future that is safe and secure in His hand?

Chapter 8

UNEXPIRED, DIVINE PRESCRIPTIONS

A cheerful heart is good medicine, but a crushed spirit dries up the bones.
—Proverbs 17:22

I rejoice in following your statutes as one rejoices in great riches. I meditate on your precepts and consider your ways. I delight in your decrees.
—Psalm 119:14–16

Proverbs 17:22 verifies there is a medicine that makes a merry heart—the joy that fills our spirit. Healthy thoughts and the fruit of the Spirit are able to reprogram our brains to release healthy amounts of neurochemicals and neurotransmitters throughout our systems to heal our bodies, minds, and spirits. Scientists are now studying this ancient prescription from the Word of God. The best medicine of all—a merry heart—has the highest potency.[1]

DIVINE GUARD

Our hearts and minds are protected only when we follow God's prescriptions. Earlier I quoted Philippians 4:6, about making your requests to God. Verse 7 adds: "And the peace of God, which transcends all understanding, will guard your hearts and your minds in Christ Jesus." The Creator knew that only the peace of God could guard our minds, calm an overactive brain from stressful thoughts, and relieve our hearts of emotional distress. About three thousand years ago, after years of war, turmoil, and depression, King David realized that only God's principles and prescriptions for a cheerful heart could heal his body and restore his crushed spirit. He valued God's prescriptions more than great riches. Prophetically David knew the blessing of being physically healthy. The health of our bodies, minds, and souls depends on meditating on God's instructions.

Meditation is a helpful treatment for high levels of stress from fear, worry, anxiety, and depression. David, the strongest man of war against God's enemies, often meditated on God's precepts to receive peace and divine protection for the wars in his mind. (See Psalms 39:3; 143:3; and 145:5.) It was the tool God recommended in the Old Testament for people to use to win physical and spiritual wars.

Around the beginning of the twenty-first century, scientists discovered that meditation can reduce stress and promote neurogenesis.[2] New neurons created during meditation strengthen our thinking, providing a "divine guard" for the mind and releasing healing neurotransmitters. The Word of God that effectively healed people in ancient times works the same today. It also helps us discover who and what we are, who we can become, and how we can fulfill our destiny.

God created us with unimaginable power and built-in creativity. Our skills to cope with high levels of stress are amazing. God included in our DNA everything we need to reach our full potential. When we follow God's divine prescriptions, through the power of the Holy Spirit we experience the peace that guards our heart and spirit in Christ Jesus.

Our DNA is the creative fingerprint of God in us. It is the language of the divine Designer in each person, with all the characteristics God encoded in our genes. We just need to let the Holy Spirit transform our thinking and renew our spiritual DNA through His supernatural power.

DNA gives instructions to the cells in order to maintain life. In the same nucleus where the DNA resides, a smaller organelle called the nucleolus contains RNA (ribonucleic acid), with a genetic message to create proteins specified by messenger RNA for gene expression. Its thousands of amino acids are arranged in complex, precise sequences.[3] This genetic life blueprint packed into the DNA carries genetic information, which I believe is God's language in our human chromosomes. It gives instructions for life to each cell in the body. How can a human being's character be transformed and modified when our physical DNA intertwines with new spiritual DNA? Let's see how that can be possible.

NEW SPIRITUAL DNA

> You should not be surprised at my saying, "You must be born again." The wind blows wherever it pleases. You hear its sound, but you cannot tell where it comes from or where it is going. So it is with everyone born of the Spirit.
>
> —JOHN 3:7–8

> I will put My laws in their minds and write them on their hearts. I will be their God, and they will be my people.
>
> —HEBREWS 8:10

The first passage above comes from the story of Nicodemus, a member of the Jewish ruling council. It appears in the third chapter of John, telling how Nicodemus came to Jesus to ask how to get into the kingdom of God. The Lord Jesus replied, giving him (beyond science) the same a spiritual prescription we need today: "You must be born again" (v. 7).

In my opinion, the "breeze" of the Spirit of God "blows" through our brains' cortexes with "the forest" of our neurons—the "tree" configuration—to renew our thoughts and change our attitude, personality, and identity. As a born-again believer you become a godly, spiritual person with new thoughts, attitudes, character, and life.

When you are born again by the blood of Jesus, it completely changes your personality. When Jesus Christ lives in you, your spirit is reborn, affecting your personality by activating Jesus' DNA in you. You are prone to righteousness, because the nature of Christ, who knew no sin, is righteous. Your personality is changed through His new covenant in His blood, shed on the cross. Even when Jesus was living on earth as in human form, He possessed God's "spiritual DNA."

I like to imagine that He enters from His spiritual realm, crossing (as the Spirit of the Lord did when Jesus was conceived in Mary's body) into your physical body through the "buffering zone" of the subatomic quantum world (as described by Australian pastor and theologian Phil Mason in his book, *Quantum Glory*).[4] You do not want to live in sin anymore; as God said, "I will put my laws in their minds and write them on their heart. I will be their God, and they will be my people" (Heb. 8:10). The Word of God in our minds and His prescription in our lives will change our thinking and behavior. The new spiritual life will become part of our personality. The ability to obey the Lord and follow His law is built into our spiritual-biological DNA.

We just need to activate what He wrote on our heart and mind by the power of the Holy Spirit and the new covenant through the blood of Jesus. No one else can know your thoughts and heart, only God. Through advanced imaging technology scientists can observe the electrical impulses and the gene expression through the proteins that are created in our brains,[5] but they cannot know our thoughts. When Christ died on the cross, through God's grace humanity gained new "spiritual DNA" for a new destiny. The Lord will extend His grace to anyone.

Desperate Inner Cry for Spiritual Health

O Lord my God, I cried to you for help, and you have healed me.
—Psalm 30:2, esv

Sir, give me this water so that I won't get thirsty and have to keep coming here to draw water.
—John 4:15

Besides physical health, it is important to be aware of your need for spiritual health. God built the need for spiritual health into our unconscious mind, but in our consciousness we do not always want to listen to the Master. If we quiet our souls and listen to the small inner voice that seeks our attention, we realize that we need a healthy spirit to have a healthy body. There are no exceptions. There has always been a cry deep inside me for integrity, purity, honesty, emotional health, and problem-solving abilities. I always wanted to know who I was created to be, what God wanted me to be, and what I needed to learn from my experiences. Many times I have literally cried out to God for a healthy spiritual life. That "good cry" always brought healing to my life.

The Holy Spirit knows our inner cry for a restoration of our relationship with the divine, and this will come when we turn our hearts and minds toward God. God will restore your relationship with the Father, the Creator of heaven and earth, and with your Savior, the Son of God, who died on the cross for the sins of the world. Through daily repentance, you receive the power to restore your relationships with God and everyone around you, through the power of forgiveness and divine love.

Even on the cross Jesus prayed for His enemies. They mocked Him, spit on Him, perforated His hands and feet with sharp nails, and His forehead with sharp thorns, and beat Him with heavy whips. Then they pierced His ribs and heart with a sharp spear and made Him suffer and hang on the cross in indescribable pain. Dying in agony, He prayed for them, "Father forgive them, for they do not know what they are doing" (Luke 23:34). He restored our relationship with the Father through the power of His crucifixion. Jesus took the weight of your sins on Himself, dying on the cross to bring deliverance of sin, and to give spiritual DNA to the entire world. You receive forgiveness for all your sins when you invite Jesus in to take control of your life, and return to the Father who deeply loves you.

Getting in line with the Word of God and His prescriptions for your life will deliver you from the stress of sin. Jesus died to restore you to what God planned for your life. You are the unique creation of God. God was thinking about you, even before the foundation of the world. The Father is looking for people to love Him back, who are sold out for Him, and thirsty for the "living water."

PRESCRIPTION FOR LIVING WATER

> Repent and be baptized, every one of you, in the name of Jesus Christ for the forgiveness of your sins. And you will receive the gift of the Holy Spirit. The promise is for you and your children and for all who are far off—for all whom the Lord our God will call.
>
> —ACTS 2:38–39

Are you thirsty for the "living water" deep in your soul? John 4 shows how a Samaritan woman was thirsty for more in her life. She wanted the "living water" to quench her spiritual thirst. In her conversation with Jesus at the well, she reacted to His statement about living water by saying, "Sir, give me this water so that I won't get thirsty and have to keep coming here to draw water" (v. 15). Her deep inner needs made her thirsty for the living water. Nothing she had done in her life, including having five husbands, had satisfied her. However, when she met the Lord Jesus, who gave her the "living water," her life changed. Instantly, it began bubbling inside her. She had to tell others that she had found Jesus, and people followed her because they saw the change in her. You need to meet Jesus, who can change your thoughts, attitudes, and character. When your life is completely changed, people around you will see Jesus' work in you, and they will want to meet Jesus too.

People want to see an honest businessperson, a loving husband, a submissive wife, obedient children, or a young couple living in purity, living a life of redemption, with beauty and humility and no contamination from the secular world. You must develop an identity that will draw people to Jesus. Sinners are attracted to people who are living an uncompromised life. The Word of God is the uncontaminated "living water" that will restore individuals, families, communities, societies, and nations. This is God's vision for global health.

The Book of Acts describes how on the day of Pentecost 120 people were drinking the uncontaminated "living water" from the Holy Spirit and about three thousand sinners cried out for restoration of their spiritual health. After being touched by the power of the Holy Spirit, they cried, "What should we do?" and were immediately saved through the "living water." The same answer is available today for anyone who cries out for spiritual transformation—the call in Acts 2:38–39, which opened this section.

You are called to be forgiven of your sins and to receive eternal life. Follow God's prescription that transforms lives. He intercedes for you even in this moment because of His covenant of relationship through the blood of Jesus. He will redeem your spiritual health for the sake of His love for you and He will not abandon the work of His hands (Ps. 138:8).

LEARN TO HEAR GOD'S VOICE

> Although the Lord gives you the bread of adversity and the water of affliction, your teachers will be hidden no more; with your own eyes you will see them. Whether you turn to the right or to the left, your ears will hear a voice behind you, saying, "This is the way; walk in it."
> —ISAIAH 30:20–21

The promises of God will transform you, even when you are in despair, and without hope. Search the Scriptures to find Jesus. Jesus has transformed billions of lives and hearts, and He can transform yours too. You must train your eyes to see the things of God and train your ears to hear His voice. Early in my career I was listening carefully with my stethoscope to an eighty-three-year-old woman's heart.

It sounded normal but there was a mild regurgitation from a mild stenosis in her aorta (a grade I/VI murmur on a scale of 1 to 4), so quiet I couldn't hear it, even with my stethoscope in my ears. I asked the cardiologist why, and she explained that my ears were not trained to hear such a quiet murmur in a healthy heart. I later learned that, because of their specialty and experience, only a cardiologist can hear that heart murmur.[6] Their ears are trained.

When you study the Word of God every day, you will begin to recognize His voice every day in your life. It is important to get the Word of God into your mind and heart and to train your "spiritual ears" to hear His voice. Nobody can take away things hidden in your heart. During the communist regime we couldn't carry a Bible in our purse or take one to work. For the inner voice to be easily activated, we had to learn the Word, memorize verses, and recite them in hidden places so as not to forget them. Many Christians, if discovered reading the Bible or talking about God's goodness with others, lost their jobs. They relied on Christian friends to secretly feed them and their family. Communists did not provide social services or food stamp coupons, nor did they encourage charity work. It was a difficult time, but I was able to train my ears to hear Jesus' call through His Word. Everything changes when you hear His voice in your heart. In the toughest circumstances, it will bring you joy, love, peace, faith, and hope that will last forever.

The Word of God transforms lives. If you meditate on the Word of God your thinking process will be changed, and your brain will be reprogrammed to think differently. Hope originates in the Word of God, which must become part of our daily life. You must invest time in the Word of God and pray for revelation and knowledge to be able to hear His voice. The Word gives you clear directions for eternal life. When the world around you falls apart, it provides hope. Humans live by every word that comes from the mouth of God. Continue to train your ears to hear the voice of the Lord through the Word.

THE SMALL VOICE

> And after the earthquake a fire; but the LORD was not in the fire: and after the fire a still small voice.
> —1 KINGS 19:12, KJV

There is a still, small voice inside your spirit. How amazing that the Creator placed in our brains the capacity to physiologically release GABA neurotransmitters into our physical bodies, as a biological response, to protect us from harm.[7] In the same way spiritually, the small voice is built into our spirit to protect us from physical and spiritual harm.

A few years ago, close to midnight, one of my friends called me to consult about a new client who had just been admitted to her personal care home. She asked me to assess this new patient the next day and make the necessary recommendations.

I was in bed, in my pajamas, ready to fall asleep! But after I hung up, the small voice inside me spoke to my heart that something was not right. In that moment, my mirror neurons were activated to respond to someone's needs. I got up from my comfortable bed (after a long day of caring for many patients), changed my clothes, jumped into my car, and drove to my friend's house. We resumed our conversation, but just when I got ready to leave her house the small voice returned. I knew I had to go back to the patient's room, even though the business owner assured me that the patient was sleeping quietly in her room and that I could see her the next day during my normal visit.

Once in the doorway, I scanned the room and the bed where the patient was lying. The old woman's skin was pale; when I got near and touched it, it was cool and clammy. The linens were soaking wet. Immediately I began interventions to wake her up, and got the stat order to check her blood sugar level, a very low 37 mg/dl level, indicating hypoglycemia. Though semi-comatose, after arousing her, I gave her the right treatment. I observed her until she had fully recovered from her symptoms, and then went home. My friend was shocked. She had never seen someone in this condition before. But she was even more shocked when she saw me show up at her door at midnight!

The small voice led me to save the life of the old woman, who could have died that night from a hypoglycemic reaction. Health care professionals are often in the position to rely on the inner, small voice, when interventions are needed to save lives. Everyone on earth has an inner voice and the mirror neurons, but they need to be activated by the Spirit of God.

GOD'S SPIRIT ENVELOPS OUR SPIRIT

> For the Lord is the Spirit, and wherever the Spirit of the Lord is, there is freedom.
> —2 CORINTHIANS 3:17, NLT

> Nothing in all creation is hidden from God's sight. Everything is uncovered and laid bare before the eyes of him to whom we must give account.
> —HEBREWS 4:13

In our genes, God designed everything we need to help us reach our full potential and fulfill our divine assignment. We must let the Spirit of God envelop our spirit to activate our God-given ability. We have God's Spirit in us and we must live in obedience to the will of God to fulfill our destiny. Imagine if the more than seven billion people on earth at this moment carried with them the Spirit of God. "What, then, shall we say in response to these things? If God is for us, who can be against us?" (Rom. 8:31). Recite this verse when uncertainty and fear flood your heart, mind, and soul. Your future will explode with blessings when He pours out His promises in your life.

God is Jehovah El Roi, who sees everything in the universe. We must give account to Him because "nothing in all creation is hidden from God's sight. Everything is uncovered and laid bare before the eyes of him to whom we must give account" (Heb. 4:13). He gave us His own breath and life, and we must be responsible before Him. He gave us His Spirit to envelop our spirit, to carry out God's plan for our lives in spiritual health.

Manage Stress Through Repentance

> Surely the arm of the LORD is not too short to save, nor his ear too dull to hear. But your iniquities have separated you from your God; your sins have hidden his face from you.
>
> —Isaiah 59:1–2

Sin consumes people. Sin and accompanying feelings of guilt have consumed people since creation; sin ultimately leads to death. God felt the pain of our sin, and longed for reconciliation with people. Jesus came to earth to bring us back into relationship with our Creator and to bring us the joy of salvation. We need Christ's continuous presence. He promised that He would be with us every day. (See Matthew 28:5–20.) Trials will come, but through them He is in us, and with us always.

Life is empty without Jesus, for even the wealthiest person. Sin and guilt make us feel separated from our Creator, as Isaiah 59:2 tells us: "But your iniquities have separated you from your God; your sins have hidden his face from you" (Isa. 59:1–2). Yet that which separates us from God is invisible, "for our struggle is not against flesh and blood, but against the rulers, against the authorities, against the powers of this dark world and against the spiritual forces of evil in the heavenly realms" (Eph. 6:12). The invisible spiritual forces of evil tempt people to sin, including unhealthy thoughts and actions, bad habits, and unhealthy levels of stress.

With his hideous strategies, Satan wants to separate us from God completely. Sin can creep into our lives slowly and bring so much harm. Yet God, who is holy, does not tolerate sin. It is easy to become hardened by sin and stray far away from our Creator. Only through repentance and obedience to God's Word can we find our way back to His plan for our lives. God is fighting for us to fulfill our destiny, by providing a way to bring us back to Him when we repent of our sins. Obey, walk in the spirit, trust God and believe His Word, and you will overcome stress from sin. Obedience leads to intimacy with God.

Biblical Evidence

> Now these things happened to them as an example, and they were written for our instruction, upon whom the ends of the ages have come.
> —1 Corinthians 10:11, ESV

> For whatever was written in earlier times was written for our instruction.
> —Romans 15:4, NASB

Apply the Word of God, with total repentance, fervent prayer, and disciplined fasting to prevent the contamination of sin, paying careful attention to any destructive behaviors. Use the Word like a shield against sin, which can radiate through your entire body with "harmful chemicals" leading to incurable spiritual "cancer."

All things become new when you return to the Word of God, obey the Lord, hunger to know Him more, and follow God's prescriptions. King Solomon had great wisdom, but chose to live outside godly boundaries, consumed by lust and materialism. A good man separates himself from the world, does not associate with sinners, nor listens to ungodly advice, nor does he sit in the seat of mockers. He is like a tree planted by the water; his works prosper when he "drinks" from the Word of God. (See Psalm 1.)

The Word of God is valid. Though an exact number of copies worldwide is difficult to determine, the *Guinness Book of World Records* says five billion copies of the Bible were printed between 1815 and 1975. Its sixty-six books were written by forty different authors with different backgrounds over the span of about 1,500 years. What a miracle book.

The Old Testament looks forward to the cross, and the New Testament looks back at the cross, representing God's truth. You shall know the truth, and the truth will set you free of all unhealthy, contaminated behavior. When people engage in destructive behavior, it is usually due to the lack of knowledge of God's Word and His supernatural prescriptions. The choice you make about the Word of God is the prognosis of your destiny, on earth and for eternity.

I used to study Bible characters' testimonies, hoping to learn how to cope with my own issues. As the two verses cited above say, the biblical records were written for our instruction. God speaks to us every day through His Word.

When I was lonely, with no family or friends around me, I was extremely worried. What if something happened to my husband and my daughter back in Romania? Many times I read, memorized, and recited Jacob's story in Genesis and how Jacob, in his loneliness, cried to the Lord, and the Lord revealed Himself to him. What a spectacular scene—he was lonely in a desert place, and God sent angels to ascend and descend on a ladder in Jacob's dream as he slept with his head resting on a stone: "He had a dream in which he saw a stairway resting on the earth, with its top reaching to heaven, and the angels of God were ascending and descending on it. There above it stood the Lord, and he said: 'I am the Lord'" (Gen. 28:12–13). That gave me so much hope, knowing that God also sends His angels to surround me. Each time I felt lonely and depressed I knelt before the Lord. I often read the Psalms that King David—inspired by the Holy Spirit—wrote when he was depressed, discouraged, and lonely. Just as God fulfilled His promises to David, He answered my prayers.

Holy "Macrophage"...for Spiritual Diseases

In the Bible God's heart was moved when a nation repented, as personified by the people of Nineveh responding to Jonah's message. (See Jonah 3.) The people changed the way they were thinking, from the king on down to the least citizen, and when they repented before God the whole city was saved from destruction. Likewise, today you should not take a neutral position about a moral crisis in your personal life, your community, or your nation. John F. Kennedy, the thirty-fifth US president, warned: "Dante once said that the hottest places in hell are reserved for those who in a period of moral crises maintain their neutrality."[8]

People need deliverance from all kinds of bondage. Put your deliverance in God's hands. In a moral crisis the battle rages in your thoughts, with the "forest" of neurons. Romans 12:1–2 tells us we must renew our thoughts to be transformed. When you change your mind and become a new creation, your attitudes and thoughts change.

You have what I call "holy macrophages" in your spirit, given by the Holy Spirit when you renew your mind and become a new creation in Christ. In microbiology, macrophages engulf and destroy cells that are enemies of the body. These large white blood cells, which are part of the immune system, locate the foreign bodies, engulf their microscopic particles through the process of phagocytosis, and destroy them.[9] In the invisible spiritual world, a similar action occurs by "spiritual macrophages" that engulf and dissolve thoughts of anger, depression, bitterness, ungratefulness, and other negative thoughts, which create so much stress and damage your spirit and your body. Continual repentance will amplify your "spiritual phagocytosis" and allow you to experience victory. Do not remain bound by the past. If you are bound and spiritually debilitated, that will destroy your relationship with your Father. Do not wait until you go to heaven. Repentance will guarantee your salvation, and you will be free of the stress of unforgiven sins.

Jesus is our Redeemer from any kind of sin. He became sin for us so we could become righteous. Jesus was cursed for us so we could be blessed.

Repentance Brings Forgiveness

> If we confess our sins, he is faithful and just and will forgive us our sins and purify us from all unrighteousness.
>
> —1 John 1:9

Sincerely forgive everyone who has sinned against you. "Necrosis" happens in your soul when you cannot forgive. Physically, necrosis means dead tissues, devoid of life or circulation, which create more damage and disease.[10] Your brain, affected by unforgiveness, gets damaged. Unforgiveness causes feelings of anger, increasing your cortisol level, shrinking the dendrites of your nerve cells in your hippocampus, and killing neurons. Unhealthy levels of neurochemicals and neurotransmitters are released in the body, causing physical disease. You are not even able to make right decisions because your thinking process is further affected, creating imbalances in the chemical messengers and damaging your body, mind, and spirit.[11]

The Holy Spirit in you works to regenerate your soul. Get rid of the sin of unforgiveness. When you pray for forgiveness of sin, you must forgive others too.

David changed his attitude through repentance. Sin had brought disaster to his and Bathsheba's life when they lost their son. He needed deliverance from the bondage of sin to be able to move on in life and accomplish his assignment as king. He needed God to help him change. These examples are in the Bible to get our attention. Just as Bible characters had to follow God's prescriptions for healing, so do we.

Recent scientific discoveries show that the human heart has nerve cells (neurons) that control the electrical impulses in the heart.[12] In order for you to turn your heart toward God, so your thoughts become actions, you must obey Christ's commandments. Let the power of the Holy Spirit change your mind and your heart.

Repentance Brings Peace

> I am the Lord your God, who teaches you what is the best for you, who directs you in the way you should go. If only you had paid attention to my commands, your peace would have been like a river, your well-being like the waves of the sea.
> —Isaiah 48:17–18

> If it is possible, as far as it depends on you, live at peace with everyone.
> —Romans 12:18

As Peter said in Acts 2:38, you are called to turn to God, repent, and be baptized. When you get baptized, all the sins that tormented you day and night—even in your unconscious mind—are forgiven. Then you receive the gift of the Holy Spirit to empower you to follow God's Word.

You are not alone in fighting your battle with sin. You will receive a peace that passes all understanding. It will bring healing and restore your spirit, soul, and body. That is the promise we have if we bring all our worries and problems to God: "Do not be anxious about anything, but in every situation, by prayer and petition, with thanksgiving, present your requests to God. And the peace of God which transcends all understanding will guard your hearts and your minds in Christ Jesus" (Phil. 4:6–7). The Lord remembers your prayers, and you will be the only one to see the supernatural power of God working in your life. Others will not see the same things you do. Behind the veil, supernatural things happen. You are chosen the see the glory of God. Pursue God with a renewed heart for a successful life, and know that only God exercises kindness, justice, and righteousness on the earth. (See Jeremiah 9:23–24.)

Trust in Jesus

> In Him we have redemption through His blood, the forgiveness of sins, in accordance with the riches of God's grace that He lavished on us.
> —Ephesians 1:7–8

You must find fulfillment in God and His Son Jesus Christ. Jesus' thoughts were 100 percent about you and me. Before the foundation of the world, He chose to love us so much that He took our sins to the cross. He eliminated sin by asking from the cross, "Father, forgive them, for they do not know what they are doing" (Luke 23:34). He finished paying for our sins when, on the cross, He cried out to heaven, "It is finished" (John 19:30). There is no more separation between us and the Father, but many still live in doubt and unbelief and separate themselves from God, the source of life.

People are looking for reassurance and approval, but fail to find them outside of the Word of God. Yet true confirmation and approval come from the Lord. You are not perfect, so surrender and trust completely in the Lord Jesus. If you do not trust the One who died for you, whom do you trust? He is the only refuge for lost sinners. Only God can bring revival in your spirit and soul. Only Jesus can reveal Himself to you, relieve your stress, and reveal God's calling for you. Your expectations are in Jesus.

Chapter 9

FORGIVENESS BRINGS JOY

The joy of the Lord is your strength.
—Nehemiah 8:10

God's design is perfect. His prescription is: Trust in the Lord and in His power to receive His joy. If you accept His Word, it goes into your mind (brain). Our Maker built joy, and the power to love and trust, into our spiritual DNA. Sin hardens our heart and robs us of joy, but peace and joy are ours when we confess our sins and ask to be forgiven.

Every day we must embrace God's forgiveness. Only joy can help soften the calluses in our heart. Do not give power to things that steal your joy. A joyful heart should be our goal, for that is exactly what God desires for us. Only through joy can we achieve strength physically and spiritually, for "the joy of the Lord is your strength" (Neh. 8:10). Jesus' death and resurrection brought us the new covenant, and the joy of salvation is for every heart whose sins are forgiven. Through Christ the whole world has access to the joy of the Lord and God's kingdom. Take a megadose of joy daily, because your sins are forgiven!

ALL YOUR SIN DEBTS ARE PAID

You forgave the iniquity of your people and covered all their sins.
—Psalm 85:2

Did you ever receive bills that were more than you could pay that month? Do you remember the butterfly feelings in your stomach when anxiety surged as you read the bad news that your balance was due before you got your paycheck? In response to your worry, fear, and anxiety, your neurotransmitters were released in unhealthy amounts. You created that atmosphere in your brain with worried, fearful thoughts and anger. Spiritually, our Father paid the bills for our sins in full with His Son's blood and sacrifice. We must listen to His voice, obey Him, trust His promises to take care of our needs, and receive His joy.

Declaring God's promises out loud with your voice will embed positive thoughts in your brain, affecting your physical body, because "death and life are in the power of the tongue" (Prov. 18:21, ESV). The promises of God are the seeds for your thoughts. His Word produces and develops thoughts that give life. Healthy levels of neurochemicals in your brain promote restoration and healing in your spirit, soul, and body.

RECEIVE FORGIVENESS

> As far as the east is from the west, so far has he removed our transgressions from us.
> —PSALM 103:12

Change your thinking and receive forgiveness for your sins through the power of the blood of Jesus who died on the cross. You need a relationship with the Father through Him. Your life no longer belongs to you. Reading the Word of God daily can wash you clean and refresh your soul, just like taking a shower every day makes you feel and smell fresh. You can develop a sweet aroma with your Christlike attitude and become more like Jesus, when you are washed in the Word of God daily.

The stress from the weight of sin will dissipate when you are cleansed in the blood of the Lamb of God, who took the sins of the world and is willing to give you forgiveness. Receive the gift of forgiveness by the unmerited grace of God: "In Him we have redemption through His blood, the forgiveness of sins, in accordance with the riches of God's grace that He lavished on us" (Eph. 1:7–8). The psalmist said, "You forgave the iniquity of your people and covered all their sins" (Ps. 85:2) and "As far as the east is from the west, so far has he removed our transgressions from us" (Ps. 103:12).

To reduce stress and eliminate its consequences, you must not live in sin. First John 2:1 describes how we can be free from sins and their punishment: "I write this to you so that you will not sin. But if anybody does sin, we have an advocate with the Father—Jesus Christ, the Righteous One," the One who died on the cross for the sins of the whole world. Confess your sin and you will receive forgiveness, a truth expressed in 1 John 1:9 (which I quoted in the previous chapter). By being purified from all your sins and unrighteousness, your spiritual health is completely restored through His unfailing love.

Train Your Mind for Change

> Dear friend, I pray that you may enjoy good health and that all may go well with you, even as your soul is getting along well.
> —3 John 2

We must train our minds and change our thinking habits by meditating day and night on the Word of God and His promises. With new neurons, we can think clearly and make the right decisions during various crises. When you meditate on the Word of God, intrusive thoughts dissipate. Our Lord Jesus Christ wants us to be healthy and stress-free, which we know from 3 John 2. Now, He does allow problems in our lives so we can learn patience, perseverance, and complete dependence on Him. He delays for a season, but His promises will be fulfilled. Just be patient.

Do not miss the opportunities in your trials. One of my friends, a divorced single mother, prayed for more time after being diagnosed with cancer. Her children were young, and there was no one else to provide for them. God answered her prayer by prolonging her life for more than three years—instead of the projected four to six months—so her children could get a little older, make decisions for themselves, get an education, and find jobs. They were surrounded by godly advisers who helped them until they were able to work and make their own living. (You ask why God did not heal her completely. That I do not know. That is beyond my comprehension. Many things in life are a mystery.)

Trust God in Any Situation

> Be still, and know that I am God.
> —Psalm 46:10

Trust God even though it seems that He delays answering your prayers. Many times we are in the shadow of thick, gray clouds and it is hard to believe the sun is shining somewhere else. Even in your seasons of doubt and unbelief, you must know that God's love shines on you continuously and He has a plan and a purpose for your life. His light is shining, even in the darkest hour of your life. I cannot emphasize enough the importance of following the words of Psalm 46:10. As you meditate on that verse, let hope arise inside you. The Son is shining for you, even though the clouds appear to be thick and dark and you cannot see light on the horizon. In God there is no limit, so do not limit His options. God has a purpose, so wait for His timing, and He will fulfill His plan and His purpose in your life.

He has given me victory many times, in the darkest moments of my life. He brought me out of many wilderness trials in greater measure than anything I could have asked or imagined. He did it for me and my family and He will do it for you. Trust Him and be still.

REPENTANCE BRINGS RESTORATION

> Blessed is the one whose transgressions are forgiven, whose sins are covered.
>
> —Psalm 32:1

Physiological and psychological crises are born from fear and worry. Fear of punishment and of the unknown can be major factors in creating high levels of stress, resulting in emotional and physical conditions. That is the time to seek God. Remember my earlier reference to Jonah, and how everyone in the city of Nineveh who heard the prophet's warning feared punishment for their sins, sought God and turned away from their evils—through fasting and repentance? Fasting brings solutions in your spiritual and physical being, promoting spiritual and physical restoration and health and preventing spiritual and physical disaster.[1]

Through crisis, God creates a necessity so you will seek Him. He promised that when you seek Him, you will find Him. When you ask of Him, He will answer your requests. When you knock, He will open the doors for you. The breath in our lungs and the heartbeats of our heart are from God, to sustain this body that carries the eternal soul and spirit. When we are touched by the power of God and by His Holy Spirit, and when the Holy Spirit collides with our spirit threshold, we instantly get His spiritual DNA.

Repentance restores and regenerates your entire well-being. Physically we carry our parents' DNA in our bodies, and our children carry our DNA. Spiritually when we become God's children, we receive His Spirit, and we carry our heavenly Father's DNA intertwined with our DNA. God is love. Our hearts are filled with supernatural love. Being born of God through His supernatural power brings unspeakable joy that reprograms activities in our brains for healthy amounts of neurotransmitters to be released. We enjoy physical and spiritual healing, and restoration.

When people repent, God acts. He revokes the punishment of their sins and shows mercy and saves their lives. God's compassion for people is tremendous. He is a holy God, waiting for people to follow His instructions for consecration and repentance.

Scientists and psychologists talk about the importance of forgiveness in our physical health.[2] It is human nature that, when somebody is doing something wrong to us, we wish they would get what they deserve. However, we can then accumulate destructive thoughts of anger and bitterness in our minds and souls. As a result, the stress hormone cortisol increases to unhealthy levels, shrinking the hippocampus area and impairing other structures of the brain.[3] The hypothalamus (the pleasure center) deprives our whole being of joy and happiness, leading to depression.[4]

To prevent this process, we must follow Jesus' example of forgiveness. At the worst times, when life hurts the most, you must pray for the power to forgive. When you forgive, deliverance comes. You will feel relief and peace, and love will replace your bitterness and anger. The people you forgave will change. God advises us that "if it is possible, as far as it depends on you, live at peace with everyone" (Rom. 12:18). Peace is an extremely important part of restoring your emotional and physical health.

Confession Brings Health

> When I kept silent, my bones wasted away through my groaning all day long.
>
> —Psalm 32:3

Although the psalmist started chapter 32 talking about the blessings of forgiveness, just two verses later he was lamenting his sinful condition. As long as he did not confess his sins, even his bones were affected. When you confess your sins before God and are forgiven, your soul is restored and your health improves! Healthy means a healthy heart, with no high blood pressure, no palpitations, no cardiovascular diseases, no diabetes, no high cholesterol, no anxiety, no depression, and no other diseases related to high levels of stress. All those can be avoided when we are free from internal sins, unrighteous thoughts, unnecessary worry, fear, and high stress.

Spiritually Redeemed DNA

> Very truly I tell you, no one can see the kingdom of God unless they are born again.
>
> —John 3:3

> Though your sins are like scarlet, they shall be as white as snow; though they are red as crimson, they shall be like wool.
>
> —Isaiah 1:18

Only by being born again can you renew your mind, as John 3:3 says. To be born again means you become a new creation spiritually, which transforms your thinking and changes your lifestyle completely. This happens only when you accept Jesus Christ as your Lord and Savior, and His spirit takes residency in you. You let the Holy Spirit take control over your mind and spirit, which further controls your entire being.

Supernaturally, He will give you a new beginning, and unspeakable joy will fill your heart and soul. The burden and stress from past sins will fall away. Your life will be led by the Spirit, and you will be careful not to grieve the Holy Spirit with worldly thinking, actions, and unhealthy choices. Now you will focus on things above, where Christ is seated at the right hand of the Father. You will think more about your purpose in life. Now your desire will be to do good deeds, and you will have great rewards, on earth and in heaven.

Jesus was born in a humble place—a manger—to show the world that He did not need a fancy birthplace, even though He came from the glories of heaven. He wanted to show mankind that He could be born in anyone's heart—even the most miserable heart, full of sin and oppression—through His Holy Spirit. This is the promise of Isaiah 1:18 (above). Even though Jesus was the Son of God, He died on the cross among thieves and murderers, demonstrating that any person, with any kind of sin, can receive salvation through His precious holy blood. No sin is too big for Him to forgive, or too dirty to wash it clean.

A Supernatural Event

You will receive power when the Holy Spirit comes on you.
—Acts 1:8

When you become a child of God, your entire mind and soul are instantly and supernaturally transformed. I experienced this incredible process through the power of the Holy Spirit. Prior to that, I sensed the emptiness in my heart, even at an early age. When I was thirteen, God touched my heart during a prayer time with a small group of friends. They were on their knees praying in the small house where we met regularly for worship. I did not know how to pray, having only heard my parents and older sisters and brothers pray. At that meeting my uncle, a devoted Christian, asked me to pray out loud. Shy because of my low self-esteem, when he called on me to pray, I shook with fear, not knowing what to say. All the other children were on their knees, quietly waiting. To their surprise (and mine), I opened my mouth and the words started to flow—in a loud and passionate voice. It was a sincere, fervent prayer from the bottom of my heart, because I wanted to know God for myself. From then on, my heart changed and I wanted to pray more as I became hungry for more of Jesus in my life.

Through that prayer, God touched my heart. Each time I heard about a prayer meeting I wanted to be there, even though it was dangerous to attend such sessions because of the communist regime. We usually met secretly in different houses, because it was against the law to meet for prayer or even discuss prayer or talk about God. We often had to walk two or three kilometers to meetings since we didn't have cars or access to public transportation.

A New Year's Eve to Remember

I vividly remember New Year's Eve of 1974, a few years after my first encounter with God. We met in a widow's house in another village to pray. That night, I walked in the snow about three kilometers to the meeting. This widow had stuffed pillows in the windows, and blocked the doors with wood for secrecy and protection from the authorities. A poor widow with five children, to pray at her home we knelt on a dirt floor. Despite the modest surroundings, you could feel the warmth of their hearts. When they started to pray, it was like the house was "on fire." During prayer that night, I was filled with the power of the Holy Spirit.

I will never forget feeling overwhelmed and enveloped in the power of the Holy Spirit. It was a supernatural experience. I felt His presence when the power of the Lord fell on me and the Holy Spirit joined my spirit. God made me consciously aware of His presence. Immersed in the power of the Holy Spirit, a shift took place in my whole being. The power of God was so intense it overwhelmed my soul and spirit; exceeding joy flooded my soul. At that moment the Holy Spirit crossed the threshold into my physical being from the spiritual realm. The Spirit of God collided with my spirit. Being born again changed me into a different person. Something supernatural happened in my soul.

Invasion of the Supernatural

> You must be born again. The wind blows wherever it pleases. You hear its sound, but you cannot tell where it comes from or where it is going. So it is with everyone born of the Spirit.
> —John 3:7–8

Phil Mason, an author, theologian, and pastor from Australia, describes in *Quantum Glory* how the relationship between electricity and natural light parallel the glory and power of God. He stated:

> Individual quanta of natural light travel as a wave of electromagnetic radiation. A photon leaves the sun as a particle, it travels through space as a wave, but it arrives at its destination as a particle. The wave-particle duality of photons is a property of all quanta, including electrons....
>
> Photons actually carry electrical charges so that when a photon collides with a metallic surface such as in a solar panel the energy of the photon is absorbed by the electrons and an electrical current is created as electrons break away from atoms. That is why solar panels can convert photons into electrical power. In a similar manner the supernatural light of God energizes those who are radiated by the glory of God. God's glory is extremely powerful. It is not an inert substance; it actually imparts spiritual power or energy.[5]

I love the science of quantum physics because it explains what happens in the subatomic, invisible world—the building blocks for the physical, visible world. Using our imagination and intuition we can imagine and understand how it is possible for the invisible supernatural world to invade our physical world.

Divine Touch

When the Spirit of the Lord came to dwell in my spirit, it crossed from the invisible spiritual world to my physical being. How can that be? One example is the threshold crossed when ice becomes water. Zero degrees Celsius is the freezing threshold of ice. Above that, the ice molecules become water (liquid), and water molecules become steam at one hundred degrees Celsius. Using our gift of intuition, we can imagine a threshold in the spiritual realm. The power of the Holy Spirit breaks out from the invisible world and crosses into the threshold of our physical world faster than the speed of light. Invading our souls, the Holy Spirit transforms our old person into a new, spiritually redeemed creation.[6]

Our universe has many forms of invisible waves that comprise electromagnetic radiation, including microwaves, X-rays, radio waves, gamma waves, infrared light, and ultraviolet light. All the seen and unseen elements of the universe interact in complete harmony. Why not invisible spiritual waves too, that are often felt as an "electrical" force when Christians experience the power of the Holy Spirit? Our physical world interacts constantly with the spiritual world. The Spirit of God sustains all things in perfect harmony. He is communicating to us when He pours out His Spirit and allows us to feel His divine touch through a deep joy, peace, and happiness.

Transformation Through Spiritual "Electrocution"

It is hard to describe the feelings and emotions that rushed through my body like an electrical current, sending warmth from the top of my head to the tip of my toes. I sensed a divine transformation through God's supernatural power. It was like the ceiling disappeared and heaven opened wide over me, immersing my soul in a heavenly realm. Never before had I felt such a sensation of God's power touching me. I felt connected to supernatural power, prompting me to cry, "I was touched by God!" I started to glorify God like never before. Nobody could stop me. Everyone around me felt the same touch, and all cried for joy. My thoughts and emotions were different under the Holy Spirit's control, instantly changing the chemistry of my thinking. Every cell inside received a "transplant" of my new spiritual DNA. Everything became new—I had new thoughts, new character, and a new personality. I was born of the Spirit. It was a *supernatural* event, similar to the description Jesus gave Nicodemus in John 3:5–8, where He said those born of the Spirit were like the wind: we can hear it and see it, but not be able to tell where it came or where it's headed. That was exactly what I experienced. God's spirit gave birth to my spirit through the "wind" of the Holy Spirit.

In his book, *Good Morning Holy Spirit*, Benny Hinn—founder of the World Healing Center Church in Grapevine, Texas, and host of the *This Is Your Day* TV program—describes his feeling when he met the Holy Spirit:

> Like a jolt of electricity, my body began to vibrate all over—exactly as it had through the two hours I waited to get into the church. It was the same shaking I had felt for another hour once inside...vibrating from my head to my toes...I was shaking, but at the same time I again felt that warm blanket of God's power wrapped all around me. I felt as if I had been translated to heaven.[7]

It amazed me to later learn while reading this book that the same feelings and symptoms Benny Hinn felt in December of 1973 in Toronto, Canada, were the same I experienced just weeks later on New Year's Eve, despite the distance of about 4,720 miles between Toronto and our poor village in northern Romania. This discovery profoundly moved me. I realized this was no coincidence, but the manifestation of God's presence. Perhaps it is a kind of spiritual electrical discharge, from the invisible spiritual realm into billions of neurons in our brains. Firing through trillions of synapses, they release an optimal amount of healthy neurotransmitters, making us feel incredible joy, peace, and happiness. We who are touched by Him experience a divine, indescribable phenomenon. It is both a mystery and a reality.

At that time I did not know anything about Christians elsewhere in the world. In Romania we were not allowed to read Christian literature. Our TV programs only featured communist personalities. We couldn't watch any internationally broadcast TV shows, and I had never heard any talk about other Christians receiving the power of the Holy Spirit. Now, when I hear about other Christians' encounters with the Holy Spirit, I connect the dots. I can see the links between the Jesus movement of the 1970s and Christians all over the world sensing the Holy Spirit's power and the revival, even in the spiritually dark, far corners of communist countries.

HOLY SPIRIT THINKING

What Jesus explained to Nicodemus so long ago happened to me nearly two thousand years later. While I was fervently praying on my knees I felt the sudden power, the electricity, the unusual warmth, and a great joy flooded my soul with feelings that words cannot describe. I felt like a fire was burning in my body. The Spirit gave birth to me spiritually. Before that happened my heart was so cold. My brain brimmed with unclean thoughts of doubt and unbelief. But when Jesus was born in my heart, the miracle took place suddenly through the power of the Holy Spirit. My life has been changed completely. From that moment on I did not want to grieve the Holy Spirit through my thinking or behavior. My mind has been reprogrammed with the desire to learn the Word of God, to saturate my soul with His presence, His instructions, His prescriptions—beyond science—and His promises for life. I now desire to be filled with the fruit of the Spirit: joy, love, happiness, kindness, patience, gentleness, and self-control. I want to do good deeds all the time for those around me.

Now I understand how all the clean thoughts started to flow through the billions of dendrites of my brain cells with a "tree" configuration and brought forth the fruits of spiritual thinking, as joy, love, and peace flooded my soul. I became more patient with everybody. My friends, colleagues and everyone noticed a radical change in my character and personality. They liked seeing more kindness, gentleness, faithfulness, goodness, and self-control in my behavior. I was a different person, born in the spirit, just like Jesus told Nicodemus. All things became new. I had to say no to all intrusive thoughts and distractions. Immediately I started to focus on what the Word of God says about living a new life in Christ.

I know that with God, all things are possible. I lived that experience. I know that millions of Christians have experienced the power of God in their lives, but only a few are actively sharing it. The supernatural power of the Holy Spirit is working in people's lives today. "Jesus Christ is the same yesterday and today and forever" (Heb. 13:8). The Holy Spirit is real.

Access to Jesus

You can consciously experience—literally, beyond science—the power of God through the Holy Spirit's power. If you draw near to Him, He will draw near to you. The Holy Spirit interferes with our conscious mind in the prefrontal cortex and makes us conscious of His presence.[8] Our spiritual eyes are opened so we can see ourselves and the world around us through the eyes of Jesus, changing our thoughts through His divine power when we access Him.

Holy Spirit—Beyond Science

> If you then, though you are evil, know how to give good gifts to your children, how much more will your Father in heaven give the Holy Spirit to those who ask him!
> —Luke 11:13

Though we live in a visible world, we can communicate with the invisible spiritual world when there is a true burning desire in our heart. I have heard neuroscientists lecture on how the mind's conscious and unconscious states are completely hidden, and we are strangers to ourselves.[9] Scientists have no direct access to a conscious human mind or to unconscious experiences. But the Holy Spirit has *always* been giving humans life-changing, amazing, divine experiences.

The Holy Spirit, God's supernatural power working on earth today, can come and change your thinking completely if you ask God the Father. The Holy Spirit will not come if you do not ask in prayer. As Luke 11:13 says, all you have to do is ask.

It is God's pleasure to give the Holy Spirit to those who ask Him, just like earthly fathers like to give good gifts to their children. We have one daughter, Andreea. I don't remember one time when she asked us for something she wanted that was useful to her, that we as her parents said no. Many times we did express our rules, such as be a good student, do what is right, be home no later than 10:00 p.m., and be obedient. But everything we asked her to do was for her benefit, especially as a teenager. She willingly followed the rules, and we gave her the things she asked for with so much pleasure. This is exactly the same thing Jesus taught us in Luke. Jesus knew how we were created. God put that desire in our DNA and gave us mirror neurons to bless our children and meet their needs and their heart's desires.

The relationship between parents and children illustrates the relationship of our Father in heaven with us, His children, who are desperately in need of the power of the Holy Spirit to change our thoughts and to restore and heal our emotional and physical needs.

Supernatural Prescription Inside Us

Even when we eat there is a physical prescription inside us in our satiety center that enables us to ingest what is necessary.[10] There is also a *spiritual prescription* inside us to make us hungry for spiritual food, so our souls can be satisfied and we can function spiritually. With all our advanced technology and scientific information about the human body and DNA, it takes more faith to believe the world happened by accident than to believe we were created by the Creator, whose love for us put inside us a hunger to seek Him. He does not force His ways on us. We must choose to follow Him. Everything that exists in nature has a mirror in the spiritual realm. That is why we have unsatisfied spiritual needs, just as we have physical needs waiting for His power to satisfy them.

Obey the Holy Spirit

> If you love me, keep My commands. And I will ask the Father, and He will give you another advocate to help you and be with you forever—the Spirit of truth. The world cannot accept him, because it neither

> sees him nor knows him. But you know him, for he lives with you and will be in you.
> —John 14:15–17

The Holy Spirit is talking to you all the time. He is talking about your future; you just need to listen. The promise of God to give us the Holy Spirit has been fulfilled. In John 14:15–17, Jesus promised that the Father would give another Comforter. He gives the Holy Spirit to those who ask for Him to be their Counselor, Helper, Intercessor, Advocate, and strength.

The Holy Spirit activated thoughts of eternity in me. Without the Holy Spirit I could never have coped with all the stressful situations in Bucharest under communism, much less when I immigrated to a strange country, not speaking the language. All our success came about through the power of the Holy Spirit who guided us, helped us, advocated for us, and strengthened us. I challenge you to invite the Holy Spirit into your heart. You will have a supernatural adventure, experiencing the presence of God as never before. He will help you more than you can imagine.

Connect With God's Supernatural Power

> Not by might nor by power, but by my Spirit, says the Lord Almighty.
> —Zechariah 4:6

In a moment, with one touch, you can connect with the supernatural power of God and be transformed. His supernatural power is like a magnet. His heart is filled with compassion for a broken world. He can open your spiritual and physical eyes. God will never withhold things from us. He gave His One and only Son to save the world. He did not send an angel or some special mortal. He gave us His Son, who stepped onto Earth from eternity, and He promised to give us the Holy Spirit. God's power breaks all the chains—addictions of any kind: like drugs, alcohol, or adultery—as well as ailments such as cancer, depression, poverty, deception, doubt, unbelief, fear, or anxiety.

People are transformed through the power of God's Word, the power of the name of Jesus, and the power of the Holy Spirit. Just wait for God to show up in your life, giving you power to face temptations. Many human traditions lead to destruction. You can overcome those human traditions only through the power of God from above. It is a spiritual battle that you can win only through the power of the Holy Spirit, which Jesus promised we would receive in Acts 1:8.

The power you receive will help you do great things. But you cannot do it alone. Ask God to fill you with His Spirit. His promise connects you with His supernatural spiritual realm. God is with you! The psalmist said, "By this I will know that God is for me" (Ps. 56:9), and Paul added, "If God is for us, who can be against us?" (Rom. 8:31). Your stress level will decrease and your brain will calm down from worry, fear, and anxiety through the power of God's Spirit, when you believe the truth of Zechariah 4:6, which I quoted above.

THE WORD CHANGES BEHAVIOR

> For this reason I kneel before the Father, from whom every family in heaven and on earth derives its name. I pray that out of his glorious riches he may strengthen you with power through his Spirit in your inner being, so that Christ may dwell in your hearts through faith. And I pray that you, being rooted and established in love, may have power, together with all the Lord's holy people, to grasp how wide and long and deep is the love of Christ, and to know this love that surpasses knowledge—that you may be filled to the measure of all the fullness of God. Now to Him who is able to do immeasurably more than all we ask or imagine, according to his power that is at work within us.
> —EPHESIANS 3:14–20

Even behavioral scientists use biblical principles[11] to change people's behavior when they are desperate and uncertain of their future. The principles from the Bible work to change our behavior while they give us assurance. Many scientists feel powerless to change people's behavior, but the Bible is the foundation for hope. Even though there is no hope here on earth, there is hope for eternity for suffering people, and for everyone when it is our time to leave this planet.

I have worked with patients with serious behavior problems, mental conditions, and neurocognitive disorders for nearly three decades, and I use non-pharmacological and pharmacological interventions to manage their behavior. Specialists recognize that medications alone have limited results.[12] Many mental conditions are developed as a result of bad behaviors earlier in life, such as drugs, alcohol, or pornography.[13] Science is often powerless to help people with mental diseases. Even with medications, in many cases we see little improvement or none at all. I advise you to visit a few memory care units, psychiatric units in geriatric and state hospitals, or nursing homes to get some insights and reevaluate your belief systems and values.

The most often used non-pharmacological methods are love, prayer, and the promises in the Word of God. I was impressed with one scientist's method to treat the symptoms from fear, anxiety, and depression that one of his patients had experienced for years. After extensive treatments, therapy sessions, multiple ER visits, and hospitalizations, with the same signs and symptoms but no physiological diseases, the specialist decided to have the patient reflect on his past relationship with his parents. That was what seemed to trigger the patient's symptoms.

This highly specialized physician asked the patient to forgive his parents for abusing him as a child, and to ask his parents for forgiveness. He was reluctant—afraid of worsening the relationship, and his symptoms as well. For many years he had suppressed his harmful feelings, being afraid to expose them. The physician asked his patient to write his issues on paper and read it to him over the phone, but the patient declined that too. The physician insisted that he write all his feelings on the paper, and then next, read out loud the conversation he wished to have with his mother. Finally, the patient agreed to follow his doctor's recommendation. After he wrote the letter, pouring out his heart and mind to his parents, his symptoms disappeared.

When David was in great distress he wrote Psalms, pouring out his heart to God, His Creator. This gave him peace and joy, healing his broken heart and restoring his soul. If you are in psychological distress, which causes physical symptoms, write down your feelings and pour out your heart. Ask God for forgiveness, and then forgive whomever you need to forgive. (Read all 150 Psalms, many of them written by David. It will do so much good for your body, mind, and soul.) This supernatural prescription also applies to future unborn generations. "Let this be written for a future generation, that a people not yet created may praise the Lord" (Ps. 102:18).

Remember, joy is also transferable. Empty your brain of those hidden, harmful emotional triggers and memories, and renew your thoughts with the Word of God. Exchange anger and fear with joy. Recognize that you have been offended in the past, write a letter to that offending person, and read it out loud as you imagine having that person in front of you. A better way is to address that letter to God and read it to Him in prayer. He will hear from heaven and will heal your emotions.

It is well documented that when people write a letter to the person who offended them, and read out it loud, there is a huge therapeutic effect, which prevents further physical and psychological damage. Harmful emotions and thoughts are replaced with peaceful thoughts that bring joy and hope.

Confidence Comes From God

> Let us then approach God's throne of grace with confidence, so that we may receive mercy and find grace to help us in our time of need.
> —Hebrews 4:16

Because of worry, pessimism, depression, and anxiety, our confidence and vision are stolen and our minds are often "clouded," further increasing our stress level. As we continue to struggle with our emotions, our inner being is further harmed. God has the answers to all the puzzles in His almighty hand. If you look at your circumstances, your spirit will suffocate. Jesus is ready to rebuke the "wind" of worry and calm the "storms" in your life if you trust Him, obey Him, wait for Him to intervene, and rest confidently in Him.

Confidence is a very important element in reducing stress and accomplishing our daily tasks. We need confidence to have a clear vision for our future. Joyce Meyer, a *New York Times* best-selling author, says in her book *Power Thoughts: 12*

Strategies to Win the Battle of the Mind, that one way to defeat fear is to be confident, even if you do not feel that way. She states:

> I have decided that I *am* confident, whether I happen to feel confident or not. Sometimes I feel more confident than I do at other times, but I go out every day confident that God is with me and because of that I can do whatever I need to do and enjoy the process. I choose to be confident instead of fearful, even when potentially fearful situations arise.[14]

That confidence comes from God alone, as we read in Hebrews: "Let us then approach God's throne of grace with confidence, so that we may receive mercy and find grace to help us in our time of need" (Heb. 4:16). You must know God, open your heart, and talk to Him. Rest in Him and have confidence that He is ready to help you in small and big things. Each time you have a victory, write it down. When you feel worried and anxious about your future, look at those notes and regain your confidence.

On December 18, 2008 we opened our thirty-bed health care facility for the first time in the United States. That was such a great accomplishment for my husband and me. Looking back, we had come into this country with empty hands, speaking no English. We had no money and were basically homeless, sleeping in different friends' houses, and not knowing where we would eat our next meal. So when we opened our facility we literally put a stone of remembrance right on our desks with a verse from 1 Samuel 7:12: "Thus far the LORD has helped us." That gave us confidence, knowing He had helped us so far, and would do so for the rest of our lives. What an encouragement!

Each time a thought of discouragement crosses our minds and worry tries to "cloud" our vision for future projects, we are reminded that God helped us so far, and He will do it again. Our confidence in God's power increases, and His promises strengthen us every day. We cannot do anything without God. We must trust Him in every situation. He can bring restoration of your visions and dreams miraculously when you have confidence in His unfailing love and mighty power to do everything above what you can ask or think. When you trust in the Lord He will fight for you and bring you peace. God is faithful to fulfill, for you, all the promises written in His Word, like He did for me and my family. Supernatural power can touch your life when your hope is in Him. You must forget what is behind you and move on with confidence, motivation, and perseverance. You must persist and ask God to touch you again with His power. He will do it if you hunger to know Him and His mighty power with all your heart.

Not Your Own Understanding

> Trust in the Lord with all your heart and lean not on your own understanding; in all your ways submit to him, and he will make your paths straight. Do not be wise in your own eyes; fear the Lord and shun evil. This will bring health to your body and nourishment to your bones.
> —Proverbs 3:5–8

People who lean on their own understanding are more stressed. The world will blind our spiritual eyes, limiting our ability to cope with stress. Facing unknown situations is stressful. For many, just hearing about a crisis situation makes their heart pound. Neurochemicals are released in uncontrollable amounts at the first thought of it, knowing that there is no logical solution for the problem. People crave reassurance to cope with high levels of stress from the unknown.

We need to trust in the Creator of the universe, the omniscient Jehovah El Roi, who knows the solutions for all our problems. As Proverbs 3:5–8 advises, we cannot trust in our own understanding, intelligence, or accomplishments.

I learned to trust God through faith and follow His prescriptions for supernatural solutions, and I received health in my body and overflowing blessings. This is how it works. In any given situation you trust that He is in control. The fear is gone, the neurotransmitter level is normalized, and the parasympathetic system will help your body to maintain a homeostatic balance. You relax and return to a normal blood pressure, normal heart rate, normal breathing, and normal digestive function. We have God's prescriptions inside us to maintain our health, because He knows how we are created, and what state of mind and what kind of thoughts we need for homeostasis (balance). He knows what happens in our bodies, even our bones, when there is an imbalance. All our hairs are numbered by Him. "Indeed, the very hairs of your head are all numbered. Don't be afraid; you are worth more than many sparrows" (Luke 12:7). You are precious in His eyes. If you believe this, it will bring you hope and unspeakable joy.

Chapter 10

IDENTITY

Behold, what manner of love the Father hath bestowed upon us, that we should be called the sons of God: therefore the world knoweth us not, because it knew him not.
—1 John 3:1, kjv

WEAKNESSES AND FAILURES in our lives develop our dependence on God and change our identity, allowing us, as 1 John 3:1 says, "to be called the sons (and daughters) of God." People who choose to live independently of God will continuously fail. Those who humble themselves and obey God's instruction will have victory, even in their weaknesses. God's strength changes brain structures, hearts, and identities. He will use our weaknesses for His purpose. The stories of Bible characters are in the Word of God to increase our faith and teach us to depend on God, just as they did. We must be hungry for His Word and learn to follow His prescriptions and directions in everyday life. God is working in our heart when we read His book. God is changing your identity and giving you the right to be called the son or daughter of God for your benefit, just as He changed those believers who lived before us.

When we hear the Word of God, it is transformed into electrical impulses in our neurons, passes the threshold of the cochlear nerve into our brain cortex, and becomes powerful thoughts that will change our behavior, habits, and identity for eternity. Without the Word, people are heading for destruction. With it, they will find encouragement, strength, and boldness. Get into the Word and let it change your identity and lead you in the way you should go. Sin leads to destruction and death, but the Word of God gives life. It is the very power of God to change our destiny.

WITH GOD IT IS IMPOSSIBLE TO FAIL

> And the LORD God formed man of the dust of the ground, and breathed into his nostrils the breath of life; and man became a living soul.
> —GENESIS 2:7, KJV

Fear of failure can wrap you in a cocoon when you feel weak, preventing you from moving ahead. When your heart is gripped by fear, do not forget that in God's eyes you are strong. You carry the breath of life from Him. Your weakness can be an opportunity to experience God's hand and His power in your life. I have experienced God's hand many times in my weakness. When I thought my life was ruined, God showed His power and lifted me up far more than I could ask or imagine.

Your weakness can be the key to open up heaven for you. God can show Himself strong on your behalf when your heart is entirely His. Fear of failure is not from God; with God it is impossible to fail. He did not give us a spirit of fear. Jesus Christ walked in courage to the cross, to finish His call on earth for the world's salvation from sin, including yours and mine. Walk in confidence to fulfill your calling and purpose, because His victory on the cross outlines your destiny and your victory.

GOD GIVES YOU STRENGTH

Recognize who is giving you strength and power. It is all from the hand of God. Genesis 31:1–32 tells us that Jacob returned home from his uncle's house strong and rich, even though he had left his homeland weak and empty-handed. God gave him strength all the years he was away from his parents' home. He learned on the job, and matured in his walk with God. I often think about how I came to the United States with empty hands. When I was at work, I knew 100 percent that it was God who gave me strength every single day, in every area of my life.

When I first arrived in the United States, I felt like a failure in every way. I didn't know the language; I worried about leaving my young husband by himself (I was the first one in my family to get a visa to come to the United States); I was a young woman in a foreign land; I worried about leaving behind my two year-old, fragile child in a very poor village; I regretted leaving the profession I had worked so hard for in Bucharest; I had no house; no friends; I missed my church. I had nothing but God. I just trusted Him totally, and recognized His supernatural power every day. Recognize who God is in your life. Do not lose heart.

Discouragement will make you afraid of losing everything, increasing your stress even more. But remember the Lord your God, who is willing to bless you. Only God can give you power in everything you do. Do not listen to deceitful thoughts that everything is a failure. It is written in the Book of Jeremiah: "The heart is deceitful above all things and beyond cure. Who can understand it? I the LORD search the heart and examine the mind" (Jer. 17:9–10). God knows the inclination of the human heart, so He gave us spiritual prescriptions with supernatural solutions to strengthen us.

Insecurity is quite common, but God's strength is perfect in our weaknesses. God can change our hearts and our minds, even in our weakness. He uses our weaknesses for this purpose. God changed Gideon's identity when he identified with "the least," and He can change yours in your humble state. Weakness is the key to unlocking God's strength! Weakness can be a gift from God, unleashing an unprecedented experiment in your life.

Chapter 11

FAITH

Truly I tell you, if you have faith as small as a mustard seed, you can say to this mountain, "Move from here to there," and it will move. Nothing will be impossible for you.
—Matthew 17:20

When Christ gives you a renewed mind, it transforms your thinking. Having faith to follow God's prescriptions and instructions will transform your life. Faith in Jesus transformed my life, and now I look at life through heaven's eyes, not from the world's point of view. Looking at life from the world's point of view, we tend to forget God's purpose for our lives. Looking from a human point of view, we set ourselves up for failure and destruction, missing opportunities to accomplish our God-given assignment.

From heaven's point of view, we have the promise in Jesus Christ that we will inherit eternal life after this short life on earth is over. We do not need to worry about houses or properties, because we do have real estate in heaven through Jesus Christ. We are heirs with Christ, on earth and in heaven.

Faith that "moves mountains" and makes the impossible possible is required if we want to enjoy God's promises. This requires a radical change in our point of view, and we must adopt God's viewpoint and adapt to heaven's culture. Our assurance comes from verses like Matthew 17:20 (above). Throughout my life I have had to face many figurative "mountains" that required great faith to move them out of my way. I had to exercise unconditional faith. Even though things did not always go the way I wanted, I believed that God would work in my favor behind the scenes, even though I didn't know how.

God had an algorithm for all the difficult situations I had to go through to bring me to this point in life, and to take me where He wants me to be. In every situation I believed that God would guide my steps according to His promises, and that the Holy Spirit would guide me in all truth. You will need the supernatural power of the Holy Spirit (beyond science) to be able to follow God's prescriptions and to be in God's will. Have the faith that can move all the "mountains" and don't let worldly obstacles keep you from accomplishing your heart's desires. Persevere through your trials and pursue your God-given vision.

When you exercise your faith, there is a reward here on earth, and later in heaven. I believe that in heaven there is a crown waiting for you and me, and for all who believe and live according to the Word of God. Do not let circumstances and "mountains" of this earth steal your crown. The crown is promised to those who persevere in their faith, as we read in James: "Blessed is the one who perseveres under trial because, having stood the test, that person will receive the crown of life that the Lord has promised to those who love Him" (Jas. 1:12).

You have inherited faith, because God put the seed of faith in your DNA. Faith was built into your genetic make-up to enable you to "stand the test." That is why faith is required in difficult situations. In the natural, you cannot take a single step without faith. God gave everyone free will, and it is your choice whether or not to believe in God. Let your faith arise and continue to grow. "Your faith is growing more and more, and the love all of you have for one another is increasing" (2 Thess. 1:3). Impossible situations will become possible, because everything is possible for those who believe when they allow their faith to increase. As 1 Corinthians 13:13 tells us, faith will always remain with love and hope.

Believe in the power of the Holy Spirit, your helper, who is hovering over us continuously. Expect miracles when the Spirit of God touches your life. The Spirit convinces you about your sinful nature, and convinces you about salvation and righteousness through Jesus Christ and His resurrection power, when you let Him merge with your spirit through faith.

Genesis tells us that in the beginning the Spirit of God was moving over the water. He is moving over us continually—we just don't see Him. The "wind" blows where it wants, but nobody knows where it is coming from. It is the energy of God. People are hungry for that energy, but many are blinded by their unbelief. And without faith we cannot perceive the Holy Spirit. Before our character and personality can be transformed, before we can cope effectively with problems and crises, real faith must fill our minds, consciously and unconsciously.

With the Holy Spirit in us, we have a closer relationship with our heavenly Father, through His power, the breath of God: "But when he, the Spirit of truth, comes, he will guide you into all the truth" (John 16:13). Many people treat the Holy Spirit superficially, but you should avoid this: "Do not grieve the Holy Spirit of God, with whom you were sealed for the day of redemption. Get rid of all bitterness, rage and anger, brawling and slander, along with every form of malice. Be kind and compassionate to one another, forgiving each other, just as in Christ God forgave you" (Eph. 4:30–32). This amazing supernatural prescription can transform our thinking and bring physical and spiritual health through faith.

Through faith you must trust that He will protect you always. He will never forsake you or leave you, no matter what your circumstances. He is your King, reigning in your life. He is the King of kings, everlasting. Nobody can save you from your sin but Christ. Go to the cross for forgiveness, where Christ regenerates your soul with new spiritual DNA, a new personality, new faith, and new life. Your past is erased by the blood of Jesus. "In him we have redemption through his blood, the forgiveness of sins, in accordance with the riches of God's grace that he lavished on us" (Eph. 1:7–8).

Believe that God knows your past, present, and future, and He has a wonderful plan for your life. We are God's handiwork. He is the superintelligent designer, the beginning and the end. He knows all things, even from before creation. He knows the end of any situation, right from the beginning. God is never surprised by events in your life, but He is always there to guide you. He *creates* events for you. He is Yahweh. He *is*. He is self-existing. He gives you confidence, even when you are not sure about your circumstances.

When you try to run from God to ignore Him, He sees you. You cannot run from Him. He is not surprised by your ignorance, but He does have a plan for your life. He sees everything and knows everything—beyond any science. Just believe God and His Word. Remember the story of the apostle Peter. He ran when Jesus was on trial, and he denied Jesus right before the crucifixion, but Jesus was not surprised by Peter's denial. (See John 18:15–27.) The Spirit of God uses our conscience to remind us about our wrongdoing, whether we face our mountains or try to avoid them.

Have faith that God is the source of all blessings in life. All heavenly and earthly gifts come from the God of light. He prepares gifts before we ask for them to build our faith. Our very life is a gift from God. We were chosen before the foundation of the world, and all our days are written in the Book of Life. David exclaimed, "Your eyes saw my unformed body; all the days ordained for me were written in your book before one of them came to be" (Ps. 139:16).

Modern embryology classes now teach what was written in the Bible more than three thousand years ago—beyond science—about how our lives begin in our mothers' wombs. It is a mystery how a baby girl can have over six million eggs in her ovaries, when she is not even born yet.[1] God works in miraculous ways, creating new life. Each baby begins when a microscopic cell from a female and another cell from a male combine, joining their invisible thoughts and desires together to conceive a new human being. Just embrace God's mysterious hand at work and believe that everybody's days are numbered since before their life began. In the same amazing way, mountains of impossibilities in your life will be moved according to God's plan, when you obey His Word and believe. Nothing is impossible with God, and nothing is too hard for Him.

Believe that His plan is better than your plan. His agenda is better than your agenda. He said, "I am the Lord your God, who teaches you what is the best for you, who directs you in the way you should go. If only you had paid attention to my commands, your peace would have been like a river, your well-being like the waves of the sea" (Isa. 48:17–18). When you have God's peace, your health will flourish. Your brain relaxes, your stress decreases, and homeostasis in your brain and body systems will prevent sickness and disease. God is teaching you the way you should go for your well-being. He is showing you your path, and if you follow His instructions you need not worry. Your peace will be "like a river."

Nothing to Fear

> So if the Son sets you free, you will be free indeed.
> —John 8:36

To overcome fear, remember that you are His son or daughter and belong to God. You are His creation, and you are forgiven from your sins. There is nothing to be afraid of. The old life is gone. "Therefore, if anyone is in Christ, the new creation has come: The old is gone, the new is here!" (2 Cor. 5:17). You have new spiritual DNA, reprogrammed by the Lord. Your healthy level of neurochemicals in your nervous system is maximized, and the balance is shifting in your favor because the Son sets you free.

You are now heavenly minded, because this life is short. Thinking about your future with the Lord in heaven takes away all your fears. Looking at life from heaven's perspective, your direction changes and you walk on a new path. Be careful not to fall into temptation. You are still responsible for your conduct, and carry your own responsibilities. As Galatians 6:4–5 says, "Each one should test their own actions. Then they can take pride in themselves alone, without comparing themselves to someone else, for each one should carry their own load."

Do not deceive yourselves with unhealthy thoughts. Galatians 6 continues: "Do not be deceived: God cannot be mocked. A man reaps what he sows. Whoever sows to please their flesh, from the flesh will reap destruction; whoever sows to please the Spirit, from the Spirit will reap eternal life" (vv. 7–8). You are now freed from your old fleshly desires. "So if the Son sets you free, you will be free indeed" (John 8:36). When your mind is renewed, you have new spiritual DNA. You are free of the old bondage and fear of the past.

Faith for Supernatural Restoration

> The fear of the Lord adds length to life.
> —Proverbs 10:27

All things are possible when you believe. Restoration is coming, and even in tough times your health can be restored. Amazingly, Solomon wrote more than 2,500 years ago in the Word of God—beyond science—the words of Proverbs

10:27. God gives you instructions for your life through His Word. His words of hope bring restoration, healing, and a prolonged life when you overcome fear, worry, and anxiety by fearing the Lord and following His commandments. The Word of God has the power to "detoxify" your soul from spiritual contamination and diseases—the power to clean, transform, change, and add years to it.

Faith gives you hope for supernatural restoration. When you said yes to Jesus Christ as your personal Savior, you got a "spiritual DNA transplant," as I like to call it. This helps you to function according to His will. He will add length to your life. Otherwise, under extreme physical stress the structure of your DNA can be altered. The cell can divide uncontrollably, leading to cancerous tumors and shortening your life.[2]

When you pray, asking God to come into your life and change your thinking, read His Word and memorize Scriptures and quote and declare the promises of God, your thinking is reprogrammed. There is a spiritual change in your mind and your DNA. You become what the Word says. You start to think like Christ. Every thought becomes captive to Him and your mind is renewed. (See Romans 12:1–2.) You can change the world around you, because you are a new creature. You act, talk, and walk differently. You now represent another kingdom here on the earth, your heavenly Father's kingdom.

Faith Like a Little Child

> He called a little child to him, and placed the child among them. And he said: "Truly I tell you, unless you change and become like little children, you will never enter the kingdom of heaven. Therefore, whoever takes the lowly position of this child is the greatest in the kingdom of heaven."
>
> —Matthew 18:2–4

Children believe everything you tell them. Their brains are not contaminated until they are exposed to ugly things on TV or the internet or in books and magazines, or bad influences from peers or dysfunctional family behavior. We must protect our innocent children from frightening news and evil influences. God wants us to be like children in our faith, to believe God's Word and receive the kingdom of God like a little child. God expects honor and reverence from His children, who live by faith.

When you worship Him with a sincere heart like a child and give Him honor, the veil is pushed away. You start to express your heartfelt praises and recognize His role in your life. He is pleased when you praise Him, and when you have faith like a child. When I spend more time in prayer on my knees worshipping God, I feel closer to Him. It is like the roof of the house disappears, heaven opens up above me, and I am soaked in His presence. I had that kind of experience in my childhood, which refreshed, renewed, and restored me. I received revelation, inspiration, and discernment for my daily assignments.

If you want to see God more clearly, you must read and study His Book, the Bible. The more you read the Word of God, the clearer picture you will get of the spiritual world. More wisdom, knowledge, and understanding will benefit your body, mind, and soul. Worry, fear, and discouragement will disappear. You will feel the love of your heavenly Father in your heart. "He will be the sure foundation for your times, a rich store of salvation and wisdom and knowledge; the fear of the Lord is the key to this treasure" (Isa. 33:6).

People who do not fear the Lord carry fears around in their heart and mind, allowing sin to bring disaster. God has a plan to destroy those who refuse His directions, commandments, instructions, and prescriptions, as stated in the Book of Jeremiah. "This is what the Lord says: 'Look! I am preparing a disaster for you and devising a plan against you. So turn from your evil ways, each one of you, and reform your ways and your actions'" (Jer. 18:11). The divine prescription is to turn from your evil way to prevent disaster. As Matthew 18:2–4 teaches, God wants you to have faith like child and be a part of His kingdom.

Chapter 12

DREAMS

We also glory in our sufferings, because we know that suffering produces perseverance; perseverance, character; and character, hope.
—Romans 5:3–4

You were born with God-given dreams in your DNA—yes, in your very thoughts. Nothing can get in the way of your dreams and visions. You were born with healthy dreams. God gives good ideas, to be implemented at the right times, with the right people in the right places. Jentezen Franklin, senior pastor of Free Chapel, a multicampus church based in Gainesville, Georgia; said in his book, *Right People, Right Place, Right Plan: Discerning the Voice of God*:

> There is a right plan. One idea from God can change your life. Thomas Edison had one idea, and today we have the electric lightbulb. The Wright brothers had one idea, and now we have aviation. Bill Gates had one idea, and today we have the personal computer. There are "good ideas," and there are "God ideas." The Holy Spirit wants you to discern the difference between the two.[1]

God allows you to discern His voice and gives you favor in your life to fulfill your dreams. Do not be afraid, do not be discouraged, and do not lose heart. Step into the things God wants you to do, according to His plan and purpose for you. Do not waste time where God does not want you to waste time. Quit things that do not please God. Be involved in things that bring pleasure to the Lord, because things you are going through will work together for your good when you love God and do what pleases Him.

God allows difficult things in your life so you can learn from them. He delays for a season, but He will fulfill His promises if you follow His instructions. Do not miss the opportunity to pray when trials come. Trust God even if He delays working on your dreams. Even through seasons of doubt, even though your heart is broken and you are discouraged, God sees your trouble. Stay still and know that God loves you and He will accomplish the dream inside you. Let hope arise, for in God there is no limit. At the right time He will intervene on your behalf to finish what He started in you.

In Romans 5:3–4, Paul talked about the process of suffering leading to hope. God is always working in your life, building your character to become what He wants you to be, in order to fulfill your dream and visions. Hope working in your brain structures builds healthy thoughts.[2] Gifts and skills are important, but character with healthy thinking is vital. The Holy Spirit helps you change your attitude. As Paul added in Romans 5:5: "Hope does not put us to shame, because God's love has been poured out into our hearts through the Holy Spirit, who has been given to us."

With help from the Holy Spirit, the potential in your DNA is activated and you make progress toward your destiny. The supernatural power of God will activate your DNA, the fingerprint of God, and your genetic code will enable your true character. You become the person God predestined you to be from the foundation of the world, to participate in building His kingdom. This is amazing. God, through the power of the Holy Spirit, decodes your genes to display who you were created to be through your changed attitude for His glory.

Invisible Imagination

> For as he thinketh in his heart, so is he.
> —Proverbs 23:7, kjv

God speaks to us through dreams, visions, and signs, but most of the time through His Word. When God speaks to you, your thoughts are aligned with His vision for your life. Your thoughts are the recipe for your personality. Proverbs 23:7 clearly explains that your thoughts dictate who you are. Your thinking is assisted by your imagination. You first see things in the "imaging center" (occipital lobe) in your brain,[3] then your thoughts develop the person that you will be. God created you in His image. He used imagination when He created the universe, and man, after His own image.

Use your imagination about the promises of God, and who God wants you to be through the power of His Word. Everything man has created, and all our advanced technology, comes from a God-given ability to think, imagine, and create. As I said earlier, when you meditate on the promises of God—in His Word—you create new neurons, which enable healthier thinking and create an atmosphere in your brain for God's promises. You empty your unconscious mind of all unhealthy thoughts, bad memories, and negative emotions, and replace them with joy, peace, happiness, and hope for your future. Anointing for breakthrough and solutions for your dreams happen through prayer, fasting, giving, and believing God's Word for your life.

DREAMS FROM THE FOUNDATION OF THE WORLD

Dreams always amazed me. Like my parents, I could have remained in my small village, farming and owning a few cows, and sheep, and some chickens. (There is nothing wrong with farming, but at that time in Romania you had to work the ground manually with your hands to feed your animals, as we had no machinery at all.) I could have kept working the ground with my hands and living a primitive life, if God had not worked on my mind and given me the desire for more education and a different future. To fulfill the dream God had for me from the foundation of the world, I simply had to follow a desire for higher achievements that God put in my imagination. So I went to the capital city for vocational school when I was not yet fifteen years old, then finished high school and university in Bucharest. In God's timing, I decided I must do something more to be able to help others.

One day God brought a Christian lady to find me in that big city of nearly two million people. She obeyed the voice of God to come back to Bucharest from the United States after ten years of living in exile. She called me to talk about an invitation to come to the United States. I'd forgotten that she even existed. When I heard her voice on the phone, the Holy Spirit reminded me who she was. In just a few minutes we reconnected, refreshing our memories and making new plans for the future. God orchestrates things in ways we cannot even imagine. He does more than we can ask or think, while making plans totally different from ours. We must keep our minds open and be receptive to His call.

The most powerful engines in the world are our brains—our unconscious and conscious minds, influenced by our senses.[4] We must guard the quality of the thoughts we allow to take residence in our brains' image centers. You have the power to be the gatekeeper of your five senses. Use them well when you need to make decisions and do not contaminate the image centers. Job knew that we have the power to control what gets in our brains through our senses and the ability to exercise self-control. He stated, "I made a covenant with my eyes not to look lustfully at a young woman" (Job 31:1), because Job knew that through his eyes his brain could get a message to lust, contaminating his image center and bringing spiritual disaster.

Be discerning about the thoughts you allow into your mind from movies, books, magazines, TV shows, ads, or events in your community. Make a covenant with your eyes and ears to avoid those things that promote unhealthy thoughts. God honors our attitude to promote healthy thinking. There are no limitations in creating healthy and useful things. God gives desires, dreams, and visions, and only God can breathe life on your dreams to bring them alive for His glory.

Keep your dreams alive. There is pain in death. I see people dying all the time, and their dreams die with them. But heaven's supernatural hope is superior to earthly hope. Through faith, God can do anything through your dreams. God will do greater things, because Jesus changes everything, bringing you life. The gift of the Holy Spirit can breathe life into your dreams. Live up to the biblical standards and your God-given dreams will be fulfilled.

Your Dream Can Be Restored

> When I heard these things, I sat down and wept. For some days I mourned and fasted and prayed before the God of heaven.
> —Nehemiah 1:4

In the Old Testament we read about Nehemiah's dream: to rebuild the walls of his city, the old Jerusalem. So he fasted and prayed day and night to fulfill this desire. (See Nehemiah 1:5–11.) Circumstances were against his dream, but God gave him supernatural favor with the king where he was living in exile, and the governor provided materials and resources to build the walls. Even an army to protect him. God even changed the law for Nehemiah to fulfill his heart's desire, according to God's purpose for his life.

God works the same today to fulfill your dreams. He worked in my dreams in Romania, and beyond. I wanted to get an education and a job during the communist regime, marry the right man, have a child, come to the United States, continue my education, finish my degrees, operate and own a business, help needy people, serve the Lord, write a book, and speak at professional and spiritual conferences—and more. All of these were my dreams at one point in time, and yes, they became reality by God's grace.

He can change laws and people's hearts for you to fulfill your dreams, visions, and destiny on this earth, according to His will. God's will is to bless you, and when God's hand is with you, He will protect you and give you victory. There will be challenges, but have patience for the right timing and persevere in your prayer and fasting. Do not give up in the hard moments. God will send the right person for the right plan, as He did for so many people in the Bible, and as He has done for me and for countless other Christians.

God gave victory to Gideon even though he was so afraid of the enemy and hid himself; to Esther, an orphan who became a queen and was the instrument to save the entire Jewish nation; to Nehemiah who rebuilt Jerusalem's ruins; to Joseph in Egypt—rejected and sold by his brothers and falsely accused by his boss—who was used to save the life of his own nation, and to enable the Egyptian nation to survive a severe famine; to Jacob, threatened by his brother and deceived by his father-in-law, but used by God as a key patriarch of a great nation. The Bible is full of stories of dreams becoming reality, and God is still working for us, in our time, for His glory. In times of distress I like to recite Habakkuk's prayer: "Lord, I have heard of your fame; I stand in awe of your deeds, Lord. Repeat them in our days, in our time make them known; in wrath remember mercy" (Hab. 3:2).

All these persons I just mentioned had to face fear, worry, and distress in their particular unfavorable circumstances, but they stayed strong in their faith, and fear vanished through God's supernatural power and miraculous work. Do not give up the dream God put in your heart because of fear. All fearful circumstances are temporary. Jacob's dream was to be blessed. He started to manipulate things around him to fulfill his dream, and it took twenty years of serving his father-in-law to get all the blessings God prepared for him. God gave him favor, and when he was really blessed, his brother wanted to kill him. Jacob's only choice was to fight in prayer, and his dream was restored in one night while he was wrestling with an angel (Gen. 32:22–32). In one night prayer changed everything, and Jacob was blessed indeed and became the nation Israel.

Jabez, another biblical example, was afraid of suffering because he was born in pain. But his dream was to be blessed and free of pain. He prayed a bold prayer to be blessed, for God to enlarge his territory, and for God's hands to be upon him to protect him from evil and to prevent disaster in his life (1 Chron. 4:10). So many examples in the Bible record situations when natural fear, worry, and anxiety were overcome with supernatural interventions and brought purposeful victory when people believed, prayed, and obeyed. Many people in the Bible went through terrible circumstances that caused excessive fear in their lives, but through prayer they became strong and overcame fear under the powerful hand of Almighty God.

When you face big challenges in your life, you must pray as Hezekiah did to surrender his future to the Lord when the enemy sent him a threatening message to destroy the people of Israel (2 Kings 19:14). Take your "letter from the enemy" with bad news that tries to bring you fear, worry, and anxiety, and spread it out before the Lord. Tell Him why you are afraid. When fear paralyzes you, you must seek God as Hezekiah did when the enemy threatened his life and the life of his nation. Bring your situation before the Lord in prayer. He hears your prayer and intervenes on your behalf, as He did in all the above examples.

THE PROMISES OF GOD ARE YOUR DREAMS FULFILLED

To fulfill your dream, start your day with the promises of God. Tiz Huch, in her book, *No Limits, No Boundaries: Praying Dynamic Change Into Your Life, Family, and Finances*, wrote:

> Always try to make your first and last appointments of the day with the Lord. As soon as you wake up in the morning, allow His Spirit to instill in you a sense of expectancy and a faith for the plans He has in store for you that day. Let Him pour into your mind and spirit His joy, confidence, strength, wisdom, and insight to equip you to serve Him

and others. Then, at the end of the day, just before you go to sleep, let His Spirit fill you with peace, calm, hope, and rest.[5]

Cast out fear and increase your faith. Let the promises of God frame your life and your world. Let your brain's structures (with the "forest of neurons" and the limbic system, involved in your thinking, emotions, mood, and memories) be filled with the Word of God and His promises for any situation. I wake up every morning and start my day by declaring God's promises over my life and over those around me and far away, even for the entire world.

I start with the Lord's Prayer and acknowledge who God is for me. I tell Him in my prayer, "Father God, You are Jehovah Elohim, the Creator of heaven and earth. You made us in Your image, and I carry Your breath in my lungs every single moment. You are Jehovah Tsidkenu, the Lord my righteousness, through the power of Jesus Christ, Your only Son, who shed His blood on the cross when He died for my sins. I acknowledge that all my sins are forgiven and I am not stressed anymore by the weight of my past sins. You are Jehovah Mekoddishkem, the Lord who sanctifies me and gives me power over temptations and sins every single moment. By the authority of Christ's sacrifice on the cross I have the authority over all evil thoughts today, and over any bad habits and attitudes.

"You are Jehovah Shalom, the Lord who gives me peace that passes all understanding in a world of uncertainty, worry, and fear. My thoughts are submitted to Jesus. I declare that I am covered with the blood of Jesus by faith, and I have authority over all the wicked spirits. You are Jehovah Shammah, the Lord who is present, self-existent. You are always there when I need You. You are from eternity to eternity the everlasting Father, the great I Am. In Your presence is peace, joy, and happiness. In Your presence all demonic spirits faint. What You speak will be created. Nothing is impossible for You. You have solutions for all my problems today. You are Jehovah Rapha, the Lord my Healer, who heals all my diseases. I declare that by the stripes of Your Son, Jesus, I am healed completely. Jesus' body was broken so there will be no diseases, no pain, no brokenness, no bruises, no infirmity, no disability, no abnormality in my body.

"Each cell in my body will function perfectly according to Your divine programming. Father God, I declare that in my body there are no abnormal genetic mutations or uncontrolled cell divisions. I declare divine health and complete healing in Jesus' mighty name.

"I proclaim that You are Jehovah Jireh, the Lord my Provider, who provides all my needs. You have blessed and You continue to bless me and my family so much more than I could ask or think. You enlarged my territories in every area, Your divine hands are upon me to protect me from evil, and nothing will harm me. You bless me at home and in society, when I go out and when I come in. Everything I put my hands to, You will cause to prosper. You give me favor with all whom I speak with and come in contact with today.

"You are Jehovah Nissi, the Lord who is my victory and my protection from my enemy. You send Your angel ahead of me, and Your angels surround me and fight for me. All the demonic strategies are in vain. I declare that You, Lord, fight for me. Your plans and Your will are done in my life to fulfill my dreams, visions, and destiny, and to help me reach my full potential. I declare that no weapon formed against me shall prosper, and any language against me is condemned, according to Isaiah 54:17.

"My heavenly Father, You are Jehovah Rohi, the Lord my Shepherd, my guide. I shall not want. You cover my head with oil and my cup is overflowing. You give me inspiration, revelation, clear thoughts, and discernment, and I do not make any decision without You. You give me wisdom from heaven, and the Holy Spirit takes control over my life, my emotions, my feelings, my thoughts, my entire being. You fill me with the Holy Spirit, take possession of all my being, and I surrender to You.

"You are Jehovah El Roi, the Lord who sees me when I stand up and when I sit down. You know all my deep thoughts. Nothing is hidden from You.

"My heavenly Father, You are El Elyon, the Most High God, and in the shadow of Your wing I find divine protection. I rest because You put my enemies under my feet."

Those are my declarations in my morning prayers, which flood my soul and spirit with unspeakable joy. Then I worship Him, bringing my petitions one by one. Then the Holy Spirit starts to intercede through me for my family, friends, business, city, nation, and the world with prayers and intercessions. God will work with you to stay in His way, when you declare His promises. He desires that none of His creation should perish, but have eternal life.

PURPOSE OF VISIONS AND DREAMS

> I keep asking that the God of our Lord Jesus Christ, the glorious Father, may give you the Spirit of wisdom and revelation, so that you may know him better. I pray that the eyes of your heart may be enlightened in order that you may know the hope to which He has called you, the riches of his glorious inheritance in his holy people.
> —EPHESIANS 1:17–18

Your fear starts to dissolve when you believe in the promises of God and trust in Him. Keep declaring His promises over your life and fear will evaporate. When you laugh at fear, you achieve a breakthrough. God honors your faith and raises you up to a new level to fulfill your dreams. You are on the path that will take you to your godly destiny. The enemy will fight your visions and dreams with fear of failure. But stay connected to Jesus and stay focused, and your visions and dreams will be accomplished. God orders your steps. Be determined to trust God to get where God wants you to be. God is giving you wisdom, revelation, and understanding to know the hope of His glory, as assured in Ephesians 1:17–18.

God's dream is to use you to bring hope to a broken and dying world. Everything in your life can change in one day at God's command. Just be faithful. Genesis 28:10–22 records Jacob's dream, and in Genesis 37–50 we read about Joseph's dream from God, confirming His will for Jacob and Joseph each to fulfill their personal destiny. Both men had an eternal impact on the nation of Israel and the entire world. When your dream is from God, you will know it. It lifts you up and preserves lives either physically, emotionally, or spiritually. My dream was to be successful and to help needy families and poor people left behind in Romania. Here in the United States, I dreamed of helping God's kingdom expand. He has fulfilled my dream and continues to do so.

No Harmful Thinking, No Discouragements

Renew your mind with new thoughts, and believe that God will bring solutions to your problems. "Do not conform to the pattern of this world, but be transformed by the renewing of your mind. Then you will be able to test and approve what God's will is—his good, pleasing and perfect will" (Rom. 12:2). Jesus wants you to be like Him. God sees us as His children. Open your spiritual eyes to see the invisible spiritual realm and start thinking differently. Pursue God. When you make that determination in your heart, things start to change in your life. Learn how to see God with your mind's eye. When you have that desire, you will picture things differently, with no harmful thinking or discouragements.

When we hear something, it often triggers our vivid imagination. We start to see things in our minds based on our imagination and our past experiences. If bad news arrives, you start to picture those bad things and fear invades your brain. Bad memories and emotions stored in your brain structures conjure up more fear associated with the bad news in your conscious mind. God can open your spiritual eyes to see Him working in your life; this can replace those bad memories and emotions with good memories and good thoughts of love, joy, peace, goodness, kindness, and happiness, and dissipate harmful thoughts.

When bad news comes, confront it with the promises of God, and healthy thoughts will form based on His promises. God is always with us, but our natural eyes are limited. God can open your spiritual eyes to see what you were not able to see before. The spiritual eyes will give you hope, courage, confidence, contentment, and healing. God wants to work miracles in your life.

Many times the eyes of our minds—especially when our cortisol level is very high—are clouded by anger, unforgiveness, envy, jealousy, immorality, or pride. All our flesh that triggers unhealthy levels of neurochemicals makes those clouds even thicker, causing more discouragement. Cleanse your heart, and honor God in your daily life. In order to see with your spiritual eyes you need a close relationship with God the Father and Jesus Christ, His Son. We are broken people due to the sin in which we were born. You start the repair process when you confess your sins and begin to live in purity and be honest with yourself. That will give you a clearer vision to see God working in your life. As Jesus promised: "Blessed are the pure in heart, for they will see God" (Matt. 5:8). Your discouragement will be replaced with hope.

FROM NOBODY TO THE KING'S TABLE

> Since you are precious and honored in my sight, and because I love you, I will give people in exchange for you, nations in exchange for your life.
> —ISAIAH 43:4

God made us in His own image, which means *you carry God's image.* You are descended from a royal family. You are His child. Your heavenly Father cares about you more than you care about yourself. When our daughter was living with us, even from her birth, we as parents were more worried for her and loved her more than she knew. Your heavenly Father's heart is touched by your problems. Jesus wept for the city of Jerusalem (Luke 19:41), and He weeps for you too. Your soul is precious to God, more than all the wealth of the world.

God wants to raise you up, as He did for Jonathan's son: "Jonathan, son of Saul, had a son who was lame in both feet. He was five years old when the news about Saul and Jonathan came from Jezreel. His nurse picked him up and fled, but as she hurried to leave, he fell and became disabled. His name was Mephibosheth" (2 Sam. 4:4). King David rescued Mephibosheth from disaster and set him at the king's table for the rest of his life. You and I are victims of another kind of fall—a spiritual fall. The prescription for your spiritual fall is, "Go, and sin no more" (John 8:11, KJV). Once you are forgiven, you can follow God's prescription for a new life. You have the Holy Spirit to lead you, guide you, and give you directions. God wants to wash your sins away with the blood of Jesus and to put "holy oil" on your emotional wounds to heal them. God wants to lift you up from your failure and bring you into fellowship with the King at His divine table.

> My son, pay attention to what I say; turn your ear to my words. Do not let them out of your sight, keep them within your heart; for they are life to those who find them and health to one's whole body. Above all else, guard your heart, for everything you do flows from it.
> —PROVERBS 4:20–23

Physically our bodies cannot function without the heart. Amazingly the heart is situated upside down, with the base of the heart up and the apex down, and twisted to the left in order to function well.[6] This position regulates and oxygenates the blood flow to the lungs before it is pumped throughout the body.[7] To cope with stress God's way and be healthy so blessings will overflow in your life, you must follow God's prescriptions for a clean heart in a right position, spiritually. Be humble, joyful, thankful, kind, trusting, open, forgiving, confident, pure, wise, sincere, sensitive, and happy. You can have that kind of heart through consistent time in the Word, prayer, and fasting. As Proverbs 4:20–23 says, the heart is deceitful. Pay attention to God's Rx for a healthy spiritual heart and guard it from evil so you can feast at the King's table forever.

Chapter 13

SUPERNATURAL HEALING

Praise the Lord, my soul, and forget not all his benefits—who forgives all your sins and heals all your diseases.
—Psalm 103:2–3

It is better to stay healthy than to seek healing. God designed us to walk and function in health. Sickness, then, can be devastating. Chronic medical conditions create not only emotional pain, anxiety, and depression, but impaired physical abilities. One of the most prevalent diseases today is metabolic syndrome (a cluster of related diseases: hypertension, diabetes, dyslipidemia—high lipid levels, and obesity), which leads to cardiovascular disease, heart attack, and stroke.[1] The best way to prevent complications from these diseases is a change in thinking and a healthier lifestyle. The power for physical and spiritual healing comes from God through His powerful Word.

Sickness can make life miserable. If you feel miserable in your sickness and bondage, Jesus is there to lift you up. It is His will to heal you. Take it to Him in prayer with childlike faith. Jesus was God in a human body but fully anointed by the Holy Spirit. He completely understands your situation. You can go to Him in prayer and ask for His mercy and healing.

The Lord also gave us instructions to go into the entire world to spread the good news and heal the sick. All the mirror neurons and compassion cells in our brains were created by God to help us feel others' pain.[2] We were created to serve with the same passion and compassion as Jesus, whose passion and compassion for lost souls drove Him to the cross. He suffered and paid with His holy blood for each person on earth, because He cares for each one of us more than we do for ourselves. He forgives our sins and heals our diseases. Forgiveness and worship come first, then healing. Jesus always addressed the sinful nature of the soul, and then the healing of the body. He is interested first in our eternal soul, and then in our temporary body. The biggest miracle is the transformation of the human mind through renewed thinking. Scientifically, as I described before, many diseases are caused by emotional pain in our souls: fear, worry, anxiety, depression, and high levels of stress due to unhealthy and corrupted thinking. It is extremely important in medicine to address the spiritual sickness first, then the physical condition.

JESUS HEALS PHYSICALLY AND SPIRITUALLY

> He sent out his Word and healed them; he rescued them from the grave.
> —PSALM 107:20

The body's healing process is astonishing. Surgeons are amazed by the healing process that takes place in the body after surgery. The programming and built-in features in our DNA repair damaged cells and heal them, as described by Dr. Michael Mercandetti, who stated:

> Within these broad phases are a complex and coordinated series of events that includes chemotaxis, phagocytosis, neocollagenesis, collagen degradation, and collagen remodeling. In addition, angiogenesis, epithelization, and the production of new glycosaminoglycans (GAGs) and proteoglycans are vital to the wound healing milieu. The culmination of these biological processes results in the replacement of normal skin structures with fibroblastic mediated scar tissue.[3]

This is just a short description of what scientists have discovered about the healing process at the cell level, without mankind's intervention. That natural healing process after surgery is God's programming in our DNA.

Jesus' desire to heal was so strong that even after His death and resurrection, He gave instructions to His disciples to go into all the world to heal the sick in His name. This has never changed. Jesus wants to heal the sick today too through believers. He spent about two-thirds of His ministry on earth healing people and delivering them from oppression. People's faith made them whole. The blind were able to see, the mute were able to speak, the deaf were able to hear, the lame were able to walk, leprosy was cleansed, and the demon-possessed were delivered. You need to believe that Jesus is willing and able when you need a miracle. He heals through believers by laying on hands. He said in the Book of Mark that believers "will place their hands on sick people, and they will get well" (Mark 16:18).

Laying on of hands is in the Scriptures. When we practice laying on of hands there is nothing magic about it. It is a way of activating the faith that is in one's mind and heart, as we focus on God's Word that brings healing miracles. We are reassured of Christ's will to heal, because through His Word people were healed and rescued from the grave. As it says in Psalm 107:20: "He sent out his Word and healed them; he rescued them from the grave." You need a point of contact that will release faith. Jesus had authority and He had the power of the Holy Spirit. People who were healed had faith. (See Matthew 8; Mark 2; Mark 10; and Luke 6.) Anointing with oil is God's stamp (Jas. 5) and the symbol of the Holy Spirit (Mark 6). The New Testament speaks of people using handkerchiefs touched by the disciples, as a sign of their faith in God's healing power. All are biblical and useful when people have faith in God for signs, miracles, and wonders through the power of the Holy Spirit. (See Acts 19.)

This command is for all those born-again Christians who believe in the gifts of the Holy Spirit to heal the sick. You can do greater works as Jesus said, "Very truly I tell you, whoever believes in me will do the works I have been doing, and they will do even greater things than these" (John 14:12). You are the instrument to bring healing through your hands and faith. You just need to lay your hands on the person and pray in Jesus' name. As Matthew 19:26 teaches, nothing is impossible with God.

Scientists know there is power in touching someone, especially when praying for the sick. Physical touch increases endorphins, and oxytocin is released.[4] This neurochemical in the brain is a natural chemical from the brain's natural pharmacy, with power to restore and heal the body.[5] God knows the chemistry of our bodies, how our bodies function, and what touching does to the physical body. His invisible supernatural touch from the spiritual realm will collide with our physical natural touch, causing faith to increase and healing to occur.

Passion and compassion are important ingredients in God's healing power. Humans have spindle neurons—special cells residing in the anterior cingulate in the brain—which are activated through prayer and meditation to increase compassion for sick and needy people. When we are afraid, have no faith, and are anxious and stressed out, these cells in the anterior cingulate responsible for compassion will be deactivated.[6] Passion changes the brain's function and the heart's condition. Watch out for demonic spirits that come to steal, kill, and destroy by distorting your perceptions about external and internal stimuli. They are driven out by the supernatural power of God when you use God's "lenses" through faith. Stay in the Word, and the supernatural power of the Holy Spirit will be at work for you.

PRESCRIPTION WITH NO EXPIRATION

> The grass withers and the flowers fall, but the word of our God endures forever.
>
> —Isaiah 40:8

You need to know God, have a relationship with Him, and go deeper than ever before in order to receive emotional and physical healing. Be courageous and optimistic in all circumstances. Take courage, not only in your daily routine but also in challenging situations. Do not be discouraged in times of terrible sickness or severe emotional distress, for the Lord is with you. Even in ancient times God's prescription was to be brave in tough situations. "Have I not commanded you? Be strong and courageous. Do not be afraid; do not be discouraged, for the LORD your God will be with you wherever you go" (Josh. 1:9). This prescription has never expired, and is available for your soul today.

Because God's Word and His love endures forever, we can be strong, live in victory, and be filled with joy and gladness. Feed your mind with God's prescriptions for supernatural power from supernatural ingredients every day, to live a victorious life and enjoy divine interventions when you need them the most. God wants His Word and promises to be fulfilled in His creation, including you. Be sensitive to the Holy Spirit and agree with His treatment and supernatural therapy for your emotional, spiritual, and physical diseases, preventing complications and promoting spiritual and physical health.

In my clinical practice many patients remain sick despite the best treatment, primarily because of their noncompliance with instructions. Noncompliance is detrimental in any intervention. Nothing is too hard for God when you comply. You can rely on God in any situation when you follow His instructions. Do not give up in prayer, meditating on God's instructions and promises as long as it takes until you see God moving. Prayer will cause a shift in your heart and mind, and your perceptions of things around you, so God will receive all the glory. You will recognize that truly this is the hand of God. God will fulfill His promises so we can give Him glory through Jesus Christ, His Son.

God fights for you, and Jesus—your Advocate in heaven—intercedes for you. The Holy Spirit intercedes for us also, so keep praying, fasting, giving, working, helping, loving, and believing. God is a miracle worker and you will see His miracles in your life. God is doing a new thing in your heart right now. He makes a way in "the desert" of your life, and your "dry places" will flourish when you trust in Him completely. His promises will last forever.

The United States became a great country by following God's prescriptions for success. In the midst of the Civil War, then president Abraham Lincoln realized the country's great spiritual and emotional needs when he proclaimed a day of prayer and fasting on March 30, 1863:

> And whereas it is the duty of nations as well as of men, to own their dependence upon the overruling power of God, to confess their sins and transgressions, in humble sorrow, yet with assured hope that genuine repentance will lead to mercy and pardon; and to recognize the sublime truth, announced in the Holy Scriptures and proven by all history, that those nations only are blessed whose God is the Lord.
>
> And, insomuch as we know that, by His divine law, nations like individuals are subjected to punishments and chastisements in this world, may we not justly fear that the awful calamity of civil war, which

now desolates the land, may be but a punishment, inflicted upon us, for our presumptuous sins, to the needful end of our national reformation as a whole People? We have been the recipients of the choicest bounties of Heaven. We have been preserved, these many years, in peace and prosperity. We have grown in numbers, wealth and power, as no other nation has ever grown. But we have forgotten God. We have forgotten the gracious hand which preserved us in peace, and multiplied and enriched and strengthened us; and we have vainly imagined, in the deceitfulness of our hearts, that all these blessings were produced by some superior wisdom and virtue of our own. Intoxicated with unbroken success, we have become too self-sufficient to feel the necessity of redeeming and preserving grace, too proud to pray to the God that made us!

It behooves us then, to humble ourselves before the offended Power, to confess our national sins, and to pray for clemency and forgiveness.

Now, therefore, in compliance with the request, and fully concurring in the views of the Senate, I do, by this my proclamation, designate and set apart Thursday, the 30th day of April, 1863, as a day of national humiliation, fasting and prayer. And I do hereby request all the People to abstain, on that day, from their ordinary secular pursuits, and to unite, at their several places of public worship and their respective homes, in keeping the day holy to the Lord, and devoted to the humble discharge of the religious duties proper to that solemn occasion.

All this being done, in sincerity and truth, let us then rest humbly in the hope authorized by the Divine teachings, that the united cry of the Nation will be heard on high, and answered with blessings, no less than the pardon of our national sins, and the restoration of our now divided and suffering Country, to its former happy condition of unity and peace.[7]

THE HOLY SPIRIT SETS US FREE

In order to truly repent, and seek forgiveness through prayer and fasting, we need the Holy Spirit's supernatural anointing. God tells us to pay very close attention to specific ingredients of His prescription for anointing. (See Exodus 30.) God's Word and the anointing never change. The Word of God and the Holy Spirit always remain the same. In the New Testament, the acts of the apostles were accomplished through the Holy Spirit. God anointed Jesus and the apostles, and the same anointing is still available. Jesus told His disciples to not depart from Jerusalem until they received the anointing of the Holy Spirit (Acts 1:4–5). God wants perfection for the Holy Spirit to work in our lives. He gives us the clear instruction (to paraphrase Joshua 1:8): "Do not depart from the Word." The Holy

Spirit wants to flow freely as a divine invasion in people's hearts. Be open to the Holy Spirit to have His way. (See Isaiah 61:1–2 and Luke 4:11.) The anointing breaks bondage and chains. One touch from God destroys the work of the enemy in your life, and changes the chemistry in your brain.

When I was a child, I had the opportunity to spend time at my grandfather's house. He was a strong believer and very strict in teaching us the Word. He had zero tolerance for sin. He had so much passion for God that people in the village would pass his house from a distance and sense that the presence of God was there. He would point out things in the Bible that still remain with me after more than fifty years. We did not like his discipline for our bad behavior as children, but I still treasure his life-giving teaching about the anointing that set me free.

Chapter 14

STRATEGIC CHOICES FOR A HEALTHY LIFESTYLE

For as he thinketh in his heart, so is he.
—Proverbs 23:7, KJV

PHYSICALLY YOU MUST choose to follow a healthy diet, exercise regularly, and follow appropriate stress management to prevent disease. Through self-control and discipline, you must train your body and reprogram your brain to follow a healthy lifestyle. The Holy Spirit will give you power to make the right decisions and overcome temptation. For example, in fasting and praying, if I decide to drink only liquids for three days, I program my brain to accept that for three days I will not touch food. You must have discernment; you must plan ahead and prepare your body, soul, and mind to be preserved. Take action and just do it. If you do nothing, nothing happens. It is the same in health as in business, family life, education, and society. You need wisdom to make the right decisions, take the right actions, grow in the knowledge of God, and engage in actions for a healthy lifestyle.

Your actions reflect what decisions you have made, as well as your personality. As Proverbs 23:7 says, they reveal what kinds of thoughts are circulating in your brain structures! What thoughts you put in your brain, and what you feel in your heart, will come out. Thoughts that are critical, judgmental, envious, resentful, jealous, or negative are harmful for your body. Harmful thoughts will negatively affect your brain's pleasure center, causing compulsive eating and other compulsive behaviors to find just a little pleasure.[1] Avoid making decisions when harmful thoughts fill your mind. Make decisions only when you are at peace and your thoughts are in line with the Word of God.

To have the gift of self-control and discipline, you need Jesus in your heart. The right basis for a healthy lifestyle comes from a heart and mind filled with knowledge and wisdom from God's Word. Be filled with knowledge, understanding, wisdom, and revelation of the Word of God in order to have discernment when deciding how to pursue a healthy lifestyle.

> Do not waste time arguing over godless ideas and old wives' tales. Instead, train yourself to be godly. "Physical training is good, but training for godliness is much better, promising benefits in this life and in the life to come." This is a trustworthy saying, and everyone should accept it.
>
> —1 Timothy 4:7–9, nlt

Lifestyle modifications for weight loss and stress management are required across the board for preventing diseases. Unhealthy habits result in atherosclerosis, hypertension, heart disease, fatty liver, fibrosis, cirrhosis, depression, dementia, and other diseases. Lifestyle changes are preferable to medication. Atherosclerotic diseases are brought on by food high in cholesterol, proteins mainly from animal products, and lack of activity.[2] Drugs, such as statins and other medications, are used in conjunction with healthy diet and regular exercise to prevent heart attack and strokes. But all medications must be combined with lifestyle changes for efficient results.

High Cholesterol — Talk to your doctor about treatment for your high cholesterol if you previously had an unhealthy diet and a sedentary lifestyle. You may need to take medication if the benefits outweigh the risks from side effects and adverse reactions. Many patients with cardiovascular diseases also have metabolic syndrome, which is preventable, and reversible to some degree when correct actions are taken. People with metabolic syndrome have a 50–60 percent higher cardiovascular risk that those without.[3]

Hypertension — Uncontrolled hypertension increases the risk for cerebrovascular events known as stroke, as well as damage to the heart leading to cardiac dysfunction, congestive heart failure, and death.[4] Prevention is the key. Your heart will benefit from any exercise, including walking, or when the good parking spots are all taken and you need to park farther out and walk more. Instead of getting angry in those situations, think about the benefit. Weight loss is key in reducing risks for metabolic syndrome and its complications and comorbidities. Even a 10 percent weight reduction can benefit.[5]

Overweight — Losing weight is a big problem. A heavy flow of hormones and neurotransmitters circulate in the body when you lose weight too fast, such as a low calorie intake of 800–900 calories per day.[6] Through prolonged starvation you can develop a fatty liver, which can lead to fibrosis and cirrhosis of the liver.[7] The healthiest way to lose weight is to lose one to two pounds a week.[8] You can calculate the calories you need daily, then eat 300–500 calories less per day to prevent weight gain and lose some weight if you need to. Exercise daily and be active, and you will start to lose weight.

My friend Emy, a cardiologist, stated in her speech at a "Healthy Heart" seminar that overweight people eat three times more than one should normally eat. She also advised her audience to skip some meals during the week, save money, and buy food for the hungry. Another cardiologist stated that nowadays the new way to stay healthy is by "going hungry." It is a new paradigm in the health system to carefully watch what we eat and count the calories. One professor of medicine was teaching his patients that "every crumb counts," so if you are overweight you really need to watch what you put in your mouth. Several years ago at a medical conference I heard another specialist declare, "Everything that tastes good, you should spit it out," because food that tastes good often makes you gain weight.

Sedentary — A sedentary lifestyle is another culprit leading to weight gain, metabolic syndrome, and heart disease. With ever newer technologies and the "disuse" syndrome, people become less and less active.[9] The same professor of medicine advised all his patients to keep moving, and not to underestimate any activities. Among them:

- getting mail from your mailbox
- going back upstairs when you forget something
- intentionally parking farther away from the store
- meditating or singing joyfully to create a healthy atmosphere in your brain that will release more healthy neurochemicals

Scientists recognize that many weight-loss drugs are not safe, and the side effects cause more harm than good.[10] Even herbal compounds can cause liver and kidney damage.[11] Our built-in free will plays a huge role in our lifestyle choices for healthy diet and weight loss. Take back your free will and gain control of your body, mind, and soul. People are looking for psychological treatments: cognitive behavioral therapy and relapse prevention, behavioral strategies, cognitive strategies, coping with craving, and helping us to reflect on the why, what, when, where, and who questions. All of them are beneficial, but when put your trust in God, your Creator, you will have better results. He wants to lift you up from where you are and bring you where you need to be with your health, if you simply *follow His divine, eternal prescriptions.*

A Healthy Lifestyle Starts in Childhood

Start children off on the way they should go, and even when they are old they will not turn from it.

—Proverbs 22:6

In the early 2000s, American public schools talked about "No Child Left Behind," but more recently pediatricians talk about "No child left on his or her behind." Every child must be active to prevent a sedentary life—not sitting in front of a TV set or constantly staring at an iPhone, iPad, iPod, gaming screen, or computer. Children can easily become obese and develop diabetes with complications from a very early age. Fat deposits on the aorta can begin at age two if children are fed a high fat diet, such as french fries and fast foods.[12] Children under stress develop compulsive eating disorders to deal with their emotions—gaining weight and developing metabolic syndrome.[13] Obesity causes obstructive sleep apnea when the tissues around the neck restrict the air flow, compromising the airway and the oxygenation of the brain and other body tissues.[14]

In order to prevent diseases and promote physical and spiritual health, follow the wisdom of God's spiritual prescriptions. In any disease we must first address behavior management before prescribing medication, starting with children, as Proverbs 22:6 tells us.

High levels of stress and unmanaged behavior often lead to depression. Depressed people eat more and gain weight early in life, increasing the risk of developing dementia later on.[15] In 2011 more than sixteen million Americans had cognitive impairment and neurocognitive disorders. Much work and more study needs to be done in the health field regarding stress management and lifestyle changes.

A simple dietary plan is to divide the food you consume on your plate so that half of your plate is vegetables, one quarter of your plate is healthy, high-fiber carbohydrates (fruits, multi-grain bread, whole grains, oatmeal, brown rice, or sweet potatoes), and the other quarter is healthy protein (fish, eggs, white meat), plus some healthy fats, such as nuts, avocado, and olive oil, with the latter used sparingly.

There is no better time than now to start adjusting your diet and your activities, and managing your stressors. People everywhere need an awakening to protect against preventable diseases.

Chapter 15

GOD'S WORD REPROGRAMS YOUR BRAIN

All Scripture is God-breathed and is useful for teaching, rebuking, correcting and training in righteousness.
—2 Timothy 3:16

For the word of God is alive and active. Sharper than any double-edged sword, it penetrates even to dividing soul and spirit, joints and marrow; it judges the thoughts and attitudes of the heart.
—Hebrews 4:12

God's prescriptions work for all ages and for all physical, mental, and spiritual health conditions. Through the power of the Holy Spirit the Bible penetrates the deepest part of the soul to preserve it. The Word of God preserved my life under a communist regime, even when the destruction of my soul seemed eminent. The power of the Word of God has often restored my soul, changing my life forever. I was hungry and thirsty for the Word of God, and it fed my mind, bringing confidence in God's power to restore and preserve my life from my enemies. "When your words came, I ate them; they were my joy and my heart's delight, for I bear your name, Lord God Almighty" (Jer. 15:16).

God's Prescriptions for Neurogenesis

> But they that wait upon the LORD shall renew their strength; they shall mount up with wings as eagles; they shall run and not be weary; and they shall walk, and not faint.
>
> —Isaiah 40:31, KJV

Scientific research has shown that high levels of stress destroy neurons in the brain. A scientific paper in 2013 on major depression said:

> Enriched environment, exercise and learning for instance, are positive regulators while stress and age are major negative regulators. Stressful life events are not only shown to reduce adult neurogenesis levels but are also discussed to be a key element in the development of various neuropsychiatric disorders such as depression.... Additionally, disturbed adult neurogenesis, possibly resulting in a malfunctioning hippocampus, may contribute to the cognitive deficits and reduced hippocampal volumes observed in depressed patients.[1]

Chronic stress leads to impaired cognition and anhedonia (loss of interest in all activities), as a sign of major depression. God's prescriptions for chronic stress enhance neurogenesis, and can help prevent dementia and Alzheimer's disease, thus saving millions of lives. As you wait upon the Lord, meditating on the Word of God and His promises, you promote neurogenesis, creating new neurons. At the end of the twentieth century, scientists discovered that profound thinking, which I call meditation, causes the brain to create new neurons in our hippocampus.[2] This is the area where cortisol (the stress hormone) destroys neurons continuously during high levels of stress, affecting people's memory and mood. How exciting to know that our brains are programmed to make new neurons during meditation. The Bible says that meditating on the Word of God brings blessings. (See Psalm 1.)

In our brains we have about 86.1 billion neurons, but many of them are destroyed by unhealthy actions and behavior, especially when fear, worry, and anxiety cause cortisol to increase. Under high levels of stress, many people seek comfort from alcohol, smoking, and drugs, killing more neurons. For example, excessive alcohol or nicotine use will damage or kill neurons.[3] That is why alcohol, tobacco, drug use, gluttony, and sexual immorality are considered sins, because they will destroy the body, which is God's temple.

Now we know that new neurons are developed through healthy behavior and positive emotions such as joy and happiness, and hoping and meditating on God's promises. Isaiah 40:31 stated thousands of years ago: "They that wait upon the LORD shall renew their strength...they shall run, and not be weary; and they shall walk, and not faint" (KJV). Waiting upon the Lord is meditating on, hoping in, and believing His promises. It will even make you younger. Neurogenesis is the natural antiaging therapy!

MEDITATION BRINGS PROSPERITY AND SUCCESS

> Keep this Book of the Law always on your lips; meditate on it day and night, so that you may be careful to do everything written in it. Then you will be prosperous and successful.
> —JOSHUA 1:8

God even designed the benefits from meditation. He wants to give us an energized, healthy, prosperous, and successful life. Thousands of years later, scientists tell us, "Meditation is a complex process involving change in cognition, memory, and social and emotional control, and causes improvement in various cardiovascular, neurological, autoimmune, and renal pathologies."[4] Meditation is now recognized and used in medicine to treat physical and mental illnesses induced by stress from fear, worry, and anxiety. It is documented that meditation causes changes "in cerebral cortex, prefrontal area, cingulate gyrus, neurotransmitters, white matter, autonomic nervous system, limbic system, cytokines, endorphins, hormones, etc."[5]

Meditation prevents neurons from being destroyed by cortisol during high levels of stress. It is interesting that the hippocampus, where consolidation of memories takes place, is the place where cortisol receptors are predominantly present. Meditation will decrease the stress level and further decrease the level of cortisol. Researchers used PET scans to show that meditation will enhance the hippocampus region by preventing neurons from dying and by forming new neurons for memory and mood. More than 3,200 years ago God told man to meditate day and night on His law and His instructions.

THE BEST MEDICINE FOR STRESS

> For the word of God is alive and active. Sharper than any double-edged sword, it penetrates even to dividing soul and spirit, joints and marrow; it judges the thoughts and attitudes of the heart.
> —HEBREWS 4:12

As Hebrews 4:12 says, the Word of God is alive, active, and able to transform lives. Just as antioxidants, flavonoids, carotenoids and all the active enzymes from fresh fruits and vegetables are able to detoxify our cells,[6] the Word of God supernaturally performs "surgery in man's spirit and soul," dividing and judging thoughts and attitudes. God's Word performs spiritual surgery to clean all our filthy thinking. Verse 13 adds: "Nothing in all creation is hidden from God's sight."

The Word gives us directions, even in darkness. Darkness will wrap you in a cocoon and set limits on your life, but the Word of God goes beyond all limitations.

Continue to be washed by the Word of God and meditate on it day and night, and you will become wiser.

BE WISER THROUGH THE WORD

> Oh I love your law! I meditate on it all day long. Your commands are always with me and make me wiser than my enemies.
> —Psalm 119:97–98

Meditating on the Word of God gives you wisdom to make good decisions in stressful circumstances, which David acknowledged in Psalm 119:97–98. Wisdom will come when you ask God in prayer for more wisdom. The Word can move you out of a dark situation into the light. Are you ready to walk in the light, build a new life, and fulfill your God-given destiny?

Treasure the Word of God more than daily food. Value it, crave it, and hunger for it every day. It will give you vision in the dark. Don't let discouragement narrow your vision. Blind Bartimaeus, a roadside beggar, heard the Son of Light and cried out, "Son of David, have mercy on me!" (Mark 10:48). The crowd tried to shut him up, but he cried even more for his healing. Without spiritual vision, without light, people perish. Jesus is the Light of the world. Cry out to Him for spiritual vision.

Under communism we couldn't have Bibles. The communists wanted us to live in darkness, without vision or revelation from the Word of God. Intimidation and unworthiness demoralized people. I had to hide my Bible under my mattress or in a closet in my college dorm so I could read the Word when everyone else was sleeping. I often feared someone would see me and tell the communist supervisor. During those years I memorized powerful Scriptures that gave me wisdom and understanding. Secretly, I was able to read the New Testament five times during high school. The Word of God transformed my life.

Meditating on the Word will bring joy and gladness to your heart. "But let all who take refuge in you be glad; let them ever sing for joy. Spread your protection over them, that those who love your name may rejoice in You" (Ps. 5:11). Hope in the promises of God brings encouragement and joy.

THE WORD PRESERVES LIFE

> He has sent me to bind up the brokenhearted, to proclaim freedom for the captives and release from darkness for the prisoners, to proclaim the year of the Lord's favor and the day of vengeance of our God, to comfort all who mourn.
> —Isaiah 61:1–2

Hide the Word of God in your heart and memorize it to receive strength. It is such a rich and unimaginable treasure. I have seen people spend three or four hours in prayer, crying to God and reading the Word, who recovered their peace and found comfort.

Good news will always defeat anxiety and depressive thoughts. Jesus was anointed "to proclaim good news to the poor" and "to bind up the brokenhearted" (Isa. 61:1). When you are captive in your dark situation, do not isolate yourself. Seek godly people who bring good news, who speak words of encouragement and kindness that will bind your emotional wounds and bring you comfort through God's Word.

Acknowledge God everywhere. Nothing is more powerful than the Word of God. Did you know that in 1884 in Washington, DC, praise to God appeared on the city's highest tower?

The Washington Monument was complete, and it had surpassed the Cologne Cathedral to be the tallest building in the world at 555 feet, 5.125 inches. Inscribed on the aluminum cap, notable names and dates in the monument's construction are recalled, and on the east face, facing the rising sun, the Latin words "Laus Deo," which translate to, "Praise be to God."[7]

No one can touch those who praise the Lord. The Word of God preserves America. Where the Word of God is, there is power and connection with the supernatural. In our place of business my husband and I framed pictures with the promises of God in large print so people can read it and find hope in their emotional distress.

WISDOM THROUGH THE WORD

Everyone needs wisdom. Christian apologist Ravi Zacharias has stated that the leaders of the world are in desperate need of wisdom, and even their "cumulative wisdom" cannot meet the challenges of this age.[8] The leaders at the highest levels of society need divine wisdom. God will rescue you from fearful and stressful circumstances when you ask for wisdom without doubting in your heart. Be spiritually aware and willing to live a life of sacrifice, with an appetite for wisdom.

Make a stand for what is noble and God can reveal to you which direction to go. "This is what the LORD says—your Redeemer, the Holy One of Israel: 'I am the LORD your God, who teaches you what is the best for you, who directs you in the way you should go'" (Isa. 48:17). He will refine your desire and *reveal your dreams* to you through His wisdom. When you are desperate to know God more and to follow His prescriptions for an uncompromised life of victory, He will show you solutions for all the challenges in your life. God wants to transform you, and the entire world, through wisdom from His Word. "If any of you lacks wisdom, you should ask God, who gives generously to all without finding fault, and it will be given to you" (Jas. 1:5).

Wisdom for a Healthy Culture

People are trapped by so many poisonous elements in our modern, toxic culture. Years ago I read about a medical examiner who was dying. He had accidentally contracted HIV through a paper cut, while examining a dead body during an autopsy. The same thing can happen in the spiritual realm, when toxic sins enter your spirit, and then your body, through just a "paper cut" in your spirit. You are sentenced to die from an unnoticed small "paper cut" in your soul, where your spirit lives.

What you allow into your mind will affect your spirit and body. Walk away from bad thoughts and behaviors that can cause irrevocable devastation in your life. Change the way you think, the way you see things, the way you talk, and the way you process information. One of my friends, a physician, was diagnosed with cancer years ago. After surgery and all her treatments, she resumed her medical practice. She said she now looks at the patients in her practice much differently. Since her tragic experience, she sees "the face of God" in each patient. Her illness shaped her thinking. Shape your thinking and change your perceptions according to the Word of God, before tragedy happens.

What kind of "ammunition" will you store in your brain structures to prepare the atmosphere for the spiritual and physical "war" in your soul, spirit, and body? Refuse to stay in the danger zone with unhealthy thinking, and do not be afraid to make changes. Do not wait for a diagnosis to change the way you see things. One of my friends, a nurse manager for many years in a cardiac unit, lost a dear friend of hers to an incurable disease at a very young age. That was a devastating loss for my friend. Because of that experience, she decided to renew her mind before any diagnosis might affect her life. She began to pursue a healthier lifestyle, both physically and spiritually.

Ruth's Cultural Wisdom

> I've been told all about what you have done for your mother-in-law since the death of your husband—how you left your father and mother and your homeland and came to live with a people you did not know before. May the Lord repay you for what you have done.
> —Ruth 2:11–12

People will notice the Holy Spirit in you through your character. They will know that you have a healthy outlook. Ruth 2:11–12 summarizes how Boaz noticed Ruth's character and wisdom. People can tell that you have a different personality just by watching you interacting with others and studying your body language. From the Bible account, we know that people were watching Ruth, and noticed her character. She arrived in Bethlehem, widowed, with nothing to provide for Naomi, her mother-in-law; and herself. Ruth went into the fields to glean—to pick up the grain left behind by workers. By law the Israelites would leave some grain behind for the needy and poor so they could provide for themselves, as Ruth did.

Ruth wondered why Boaz was so kind toward her, a foreigner. By her attitude and actions, people in Bethlehem knew that Ruth was a loving, kind, and compassionate person. She was also faithful and hardworking. She gained a reputation that spread, so everyone knew about her. These character qualities gave her a reputation that positioned her to fulfill her destiny. God can use you in an amazing way to fulfill your destiny, even through the kind of tough times Ruth and Naomi suffered. Sometimes people may mock what God is doing in you, but the fear of the Lord leads you, and your godly character will prevail, promoting your spiritual and physical health.

Fear of the Lord Is a Treasure

> The fear of the Lord is the beginning of wisdom; all who follow his precepts have good understanding.
> —Psalm 111:10

> Oh, that their hearts would be inclined to fear me and keep all my commands always, so that it might go well with them and their children forever!
> —Deuteronomy 5:29

The fear of God keeps us close to the Lord and reminds us that nothing is hidden from God. This does not mean we should run away from God. It means we esteem and honor Him as our loving Father. As a teenager I was always trying to please my biological father, to honor his reputation as my father, and make him happy, because he worked hard to make a living for our large family. Our heavenly Father provided us with spiritual life by giving His only Son to die for our sins. The fear of the Lord causes people to keep His commandments, as evidenced by the above words from Psalm 111:10. The fear of the Lord will bring favor and benefits to the next generations who keep God's commandments; Deuteronomy 5:29 says doing so means things will go well with our children and succeeding ancestors. This supports the science of epigenetics, through which blessings can be passed on from one generation to the next.

The fear of the Lord is the foundation of wisdom and helps us make the right choice when opportunity comes. Through wisdom a house is built (Prov. 24:3). When I need to make a decision in my business or profession, I ask God for wisdom. I know that on my own I could make a poor one.

I do not know the future, so I fast and pray for God's wisdom and inspiration through the power of the Holy Spirit. A few years ago I had an impossible situation in my business. It needed heaven's attention. I called on God with all my strength, even fasting for an extended period of time as Daniel did (with fruits and vegetables only) for wisdom. I needed wisdom only God could give to make that business decision. The answer came several months later, when I needed it the most.

What was impossible became possible through God's supernatural intervention, activated by obedience. He gives us wisdom and favor with the right people. At that time more than ever, I understood the admonition not to lean on my own understanding. I literally followed the Word, "Trust in the Lord with all your heart and lean not on your own understanding; in all your ways submit to him and he will make your paths straight" (Prov. 3:5–6).

The fear of the Lord keeps us from sin, and it keeps us and our children from departing from God. Many people think the Lord does not see, but He declared, "I am the Lord of all mankind. Is anything too hard for me?" (Jer. 32:27). Obey Him instantly and fear Him, even if it hurts or you do not see the benefit. Many times in my struggles I had to choose to either fear the Lord and obey, or live my own way, to escape a hard situation. But now, looking back, if I had not obeyed God, where would I be today?

I have no regrets. My heart was completely His and I followed Him with my whole heart. I enjoy my family now, with many blessings, as the result of obeying God in spite of many difficulties. We have great satisfaction from taking care of the elderly with multiple chronic conditions, and dealing with challenging behaviors of marginalized people. The community is our family.

The fear of the Lord changed my life. It will change you, and the world, one person at a time. That is because, "The precepts of the Lord are right, giving joy to the heart. The commands of the Lord are radiant, giving light to the eyes. The fear of the Lord is pure, enduring forever" (Ps. 19:8–9). People who do not fear God do not endure forever. For example, after seventy-four years of ignoring God completely, the Communist system in the Soviet Union—and its shorter-lasting counterparts in Eastern Europe—collapsed. Who dreamt of this sudden collapse of communist power in the Soviet Union and surrounding countries after so many years? They did not fear the Lord at all, teaching children for decades that there is no God. For decades those children were deprived of blessings, and their futures were destroyed. They lived under a curse. Now the generations after them are completely disoriented and have no knowledge of the Word of God, the Creator of the universe. They still continue to suffer the consequences of disobedience.

Communism brought curses upon generations through atheistic teaching and the evolutionists' deception that the universe was created by chance. If life was formed by chance, there would be no life on earth today, because mutation in human genes—if left to chance—would cause uncontrolled, abnormal cell division and proliferation, leading to cancer and death. Cancer of any kind is an accidental gene mutation with uncontrolled and abnormal division of cells in the body.[9] People who have uncontrolled gene mutations undergo radiation or chemotherapy to eradicate those abnormal cells. To have a healthy body, all cells must function in the perfection created by God, the supernatural designer. In order for life to exist on this planet, cells must divide according to the divine programming and precise instructions built into our human DNA by the King of the universe.

When the structure of DNA, with a double helix, was discovered in 1953 by James Watson and Francis Crick, it was the highest accomplishment and a great scientific revolution, proving we have a Creator and life is not by chance. We now know more about DNA and cell function and cannot believe the lie that life appeared on earth spontaneously, by accident. The communists took advantage of the lack of knowledge and lack of scientific proof, and deceived huge masses of people by forcing them through a controlling dictatorship, depriving them of the blessings of knowing God and the treasure of fearing the Lord.

Chapter 16

FAVOR

These are the ones I look on with favor: those who are humbled and contrite in spirit, and who tremble at my word.
—Isaiah 66:2

I first mentioned Mephibosheth in chapter 12. This Old Testament story is relevant for you and me. After King David's friend Jonathan passed away, God moved on David's heart to show kindness to Jonathan's house, so David brought Mephibosheth to his home because of his covenant with Jonathan. David wanted to restore his best friend's son's joy and relationship with the royal family (without him even knowing it). Your Father in heaven wants to restore the covenant relationship between Himself and His family on earth. Christ wants to restore your relationship with His royal family by forgiving your sins to bring you joy. Joy is the key to calming and reprogramming your brain. Joy stimulates healthy amounts of neurotransmitters, restoring your memory and mood in your brain's structures.

Saul's disobedience to God and sin brought famine to the land. But Saul's grandson, Mephibosheth, received protection when his relationship with the royal family was restored. There is a worldwide famine today—a desperate hunger for relationship restoration. Jesus is our Advocate for such a miracle, but He is waiting for us to decide to come to the King's table. He took away your iniquity and spiritual infirmities and covered you with His blood. That is the kindness of God, which leads you to repentance. He took away your sin and its consequences, so you are called to repent, because "God's kindness is intended to lead you to repentance" (Rom. 2:4). Mephibosheth was the victim of a fall; King David had never met him because of his resulting disability. But the king's kindness brought Mephibosheth from anonymity to the king's table.

God, the King of the universe, made man in His own image. You descend from a royal family. You carry the image of the King of kings. You are His child. God cares about you, and His heart is touched by your problems. God wants to raise you up and give you an unending feast at His banquet table. Mephibosheth was elevated from obscurity to the king's table, for life (2 Sam. 4:4).

Your soul is more precious to God than all the wealth of the world. Let the Holy Spirit guide you, even in the lowest moments of your life. Seek His advice. You are also a victim of a fall, but God wants to put "holy oil" on your wounds. Jesus did the same with the woman caught in adultery. He lifted her up from the calamities of her sins and told her to "go and sin no more." God wants to lift you up from all your circumstances by cleansing away your sin. The blood of Jesus has the power to wash your sins away. You need to obey Him, follow His powerful prescription to "go, and sin no more" (John 8:11, KJV) and have fellowship with the Lord. You will not be a victim anymore; you are the temple of God, and His favorite.

THE FAVOR OF GOD

In 2006 I was invited to speak to a national women's conference in Bucharest, Romania. My husband remained in Portland to manage our business and to be home with our daughter, who was in high school at that time. We were also running the business of a friend who had passed away and left behind her children with many needs. We took on the responsibility of managing her business for one year after her death so her children would have their needs met. During the conference, my husband called to say that the live-in caregiver of my friend's business was waiting with her luggage, ready to leave upon my return to Portland. That news struck me so hard I couldn't even talk. My stress level suddenly skyrocketed from that bad news. All I could do was get on my knees and cry out to God with my entire being. If the live-in caregiver left, the business would be lost, leaving my friend's children homeless. My heart was broken for these children who had lost their mom, and now their resources. After that fervent prayer I received a peace deep in my heart, knowing that God would provide.

Three days after I got home from that mission trip, a nice young woman knocked at the door, desperate for a job. She was well-educated, willing to be trained, and ready to take that vacant live-in caregiver position. I knew that was God's favor, and the answer to my prayer in Bucharest for provisions in Portland. We read in the Book of Isaiah that "these are the ones I look on with favor: those who are humble and contrite in spirit, and who tremble at my word" (Isa. 66:2). I had humbled myself and cried out to God, and He demonstrated His divine favor. In order to have favors from God we must follow His standards. God will move in people's hearts to work in our favor when we are under the burden of an increased level of stress from worry.

Chapter 17

KEEP A BIBLICAL ATTITUDE

*See, darkness is over the earth and thick darkness is over the people, but the L*ORD *rises upon you and His glory appears over you. Nations will come to your light.*
—ISAIAH 60:2–3

You are designed to win, but only when you abandon the world's ways and choose God's way. The world lives in the dark, but God wants His glory to shine on the earth over His people. God's divine prescriptions are for you to win and have an excellent life. Follow His directions, listen to His instructions, and respect His guidelines. This will provide a therapy for your divine restoration from sin—mentally, emotionally, and physically. Do not miss the opportunity. You need power and energy from the Holy Spirit, as outlined in Isaiah 60:2–3. God endowed you on earth with wisdom to live in the light and in health. You have a destiny to fulfill, so be faithful in everything you do, and let your light shine around you. God has an open door for you, but you must have an appropriate attitude and "contend for the faith that was once for all entrusted to God's holy people" (Jude 3).

Changing your attitude is necessary for reducing the stress levels in your life and improving your physical and spiritual health. Your attitude should reflect love, honesty, integrity, and unity. Maintain high standards in your life, because darkness covers the earth. Isaiah prophesied thousands of years ago about the Lord's glory bringing nations to your light. You are called to live with a tender heart, live in the light, and forgive and help others. You must be like Christ for His glory to appear over you.

POWER TO CHANGE YOUR ATTITUDE

> Now to him who is able to do immeasurably more then all we ask or imagine, according to his power that is at work within us.
> —Ephesians 3:20

In his book, *Reposition Yourself*, Bishop Jakes challenges us to stop procrastinating or blaming the past. He says we should not embrace the role of a loser, but be the "make-it-happen person." He describes a person who is willing to change their attitude: "These are the people who see what is coming and they make it happen rather than hope it happens or react to what happens." Jakes emphasizes that the power to change your attitude is in you.[1] We should embrace the message of Ephesians 3:20 because God built certain features in us that, if activated by our will and desire to change, will give us divine power to make it happen.

Bad attitudes generate from bad thoughts. Such negative thinking damages our bodies by releasing abnormal amounts of neurochemicals and hormones, and redirecting the blood flow in different parts of the body, resulting in sickness and disease. Worthless secular pleasures that contradict godly standards will enslave you, creating addictions. Addiction is a symptom of spiritual disease, and calls for effective intervention. If you are trapped, pray an emergency prayer to deepen your relationship with God and free you from all bondage. Fasting will improve your self-discipline and help free you from destructive behaviors. You will regain your willpower and refocus your attitude. It will impact your thinking and renew your mind. Turn away from useless things, break your addictions, and focus on what matters the most. Time is a precious gift from God, and you need to act now.

An attitude of forgiveness brings healing. Your body delivers natural chemicals for healing, including endorphins (acting as a natural antidepressant) when you change your attitude toward others, forgiving them for offending you or hurting you. Forgiving brings joy. I love this ancient truth: "The joy of the Lord is your strength" (Neh. 8:10). Joy is necessary. It strengthens by releasing healthy amounts of neurotransmitters to restore the body, soul, and spirit—beyond science.

You cannot control what other people say, but you can control what you believe and how you react and interact. You cannot control the circumstances and events of life, but you can control how you react in any situation. Your constant meditation on the living Word of God will increase your faith. Act according to your faith and your attitude will change. It is a divine exchange. Decide to walk in the light, and receive the rewards of light. You have been chosen by Jesus to bring the fruit of joy, peace, kindness, goodness, patience, endurance, and self-control, and to walk in the light with a great attitude. (See 1 John 1:7.) People will admire your attitude in the light.

Awaken Your Mind Through Wisdom

> The Sovereign Lord has given me his words of wisdom, so that I know how to comfort the weary. Morning by morning he wakens me and opens my understanding to his will.
> —Isaiah 50:4, NLT

The Spirit of God can awaken a person's heart through a transformed mind, renewed thoughts for the right perceptions of an unhealthy environment, and a changed character. Your character is encoded in your unique DNA, designed by God, the superintelligent designer. In your DNA lies God's plan for your life, your destiny, and your purpose on earth. All God's plans for you are in your DNA, encoded from creation. The Bible says incorruptible seed is in you, and thoughts of eternity (Eccles. 3:11). God wrote your destiny before you were born (Ps. 139:16). Activate that touch of eternity in you.

You have precise instructions, inside you since you were in your mother's womb; "from my mother's womb he has spoken my name" (Isa. 49:1). Read God's Word to learn what God intended you to be. You are created by God's hands and programmed to be who God wants you to be. You just need to let Him open your "understanding to His will" when He wakes you morning by morning, as Isaiah 50:4 says.

The world is trying to reprogram your mind with unhealthy thoughts that are toxic, as well as unbiblical. The customs and attitudes of the world do not follow God's prescriptions. Knowing the Word of God awakens you through wisdom and revelation, to transform you into a person more like God's Son, Jesus Christ. You can reprogram your brain and become who God created you to be from the beginning. You need power, energy from the Holy Spirit, and infilling through prayer. Trust that He who began the good work in you will help you to accomplish it when you follow His prescriptions and instructions. Study His excellent words of wisdom that excel far beyond the science of this world. (See Philippians 1:6.)

The heroes of the Bible were men and women whose spirits were awakened and touched by the Holy Spirit. Daniel and his three compatriots decided not to defile themselves with the food from the king's table. They drew the line and made it known to the people surrounding them. (See the Book of Daniel.) They had an awakening in their spirits, and their appetites were changed. In addition to their healthy physical appetite, they had a "spiritual appetite" in their heart—a hunger for God. We need to train our spiritual appetite, be willing to change our souls' diets, and receive nourishment from the Word of God. His prescriptions contain the power, wisdom, revelation, and knowledge to change our character and transform our minds and our personality. This is the only way to overcome fear, worry, anxiety, and depression, and enjoy a healthy life.

Changing Your Mind Changes Your Attitude

> I have set before you life and death, blessings and curses. Now choose life, so that you and your children may live and that you may love the Lord your God, listen to his voice and hold fast to him. For the Lord is your life.
> —Deuteronomy 30:19–20

> You were taught...to put off your old self...(and) to be made new in the attitude of your minds; and to put on the new self, created to be like God in true righteousness and holiness.
> —Ephesians 4:22–24

People get stuck in their human thinking. They spread bad reports of their negative mentality. I had to meditate on this verse many times until it became a part of me: "I can do all things through Christ who strengthens me" (Phil. 4:13, NKJV). Thinking differently today will change your tomorrows. The mind is powerful. God is waiting for you to make choices. Don't let your mind be programmed by worldly things. Take responsibility for your life. We are directed to choose life, as Moses wrote to the children of Israel in Deuteronomy 30:19–20. The Word of God has the power to change your attitude. Watch what you choose in your life and what you are thinking. The Spirit of God renews your thoughts and attitudes so you can "be made new in the attitude of your minds" (Eph. 4:23).

I allowed the Spirit to renew my thoughts during the communist regime, when the communists declared there was no God. I allowed the Word of God to reprogram my mind, thinking, attitudes, and speech, as it is written: "May these words of my mouth and this meditation of my heart be pleasing in your sight, my Rock my Redeemer" (Ps. 19:14). I worked on reprogramming my mind by repeating new thoughts out loud. I would recite verses from the Bible throughout the day. In this way I received new thoughts and new directions. "For out of the abundance of the heart the mouth speaks" (Matt. 12:34, ESV). I was memorizing verses and poems inspired from stories of biblical characters who achieved great victories. They are stored in my brain structures, and I can easily activate them and bring them into my conscious mind anytime I need them. Those stories are written in the Bible to encourage us and to build our faith in the Almighty God who can do anything, anytime. He has done great things in the past, and He will do more today for you, because "Jesus Christ is the same yesterday and today and forever" (Heb. 13:8).

God gives us a *new life* through the Holy Spirit. If your heart is overflowing with promises from God's Word, you will share them. People around you will be encouraged, thus their minds can be transformed and reprogrammed. It takes effort and work to change and reprogram your thoughts and help those around you.

I cannot stop thinking about Ruth's attitude. She reprogrammed her thinking to accompany her mother-in-law to Bethlehem, demonstrating a "do-whatever-it-takes" attitude to help Naomi. Through her positive, overcoming attitude Ruth positioned herself for blessings for the rest of her life, and for eternity. Ruth was overwhelmed by the favor God gave her with Boaz. Ruth's life exhibited admirable qualities. She was hardworking, loving, kind, and faithful. She had gained a reputation for these qualities and for her amazing attitude. Ruth's character remained unchanged, even when the circumstances changed.

Learn God's language and do not be afraid to live it out and speak it out loud. God's language remains unique through the ages. People will notice that your language is different. Position yourself for the blessings of God through your attitude and character. Consider your actions too. What do your actions say about your reputation? Remember, a good reputation is something we earn when we live according to our values and beliefs, in line with biblical standards.

Ruth activated the potential that God had placed in her DNA, even though she was a stranger in a foreign country. I love Ruth's story because I was a foreigner on foreign ground, but God was watching over me the entire time to fulfill His promises in my life. He gave me power to consistently work toward my goals and His plans. Today is the result of yesterday's decisions and actions. Your health problems today are the results of yesterday's bad habits. Learn from your past situation (like the prodigal son) and correct your present to be blessed in the future.

Fruits of Your Attitude

> Stand at the crossroads and look; ask for the ancient paths, ask where the good way is, and walk in it, and you will find rest for your souls.
> —Jeremiah 6:16

> May God himself, the God of peace, sanctify you through and through. May your whole spirit, soul and body be kept blameless at the coming of our Lord Jesus Christ.
> —1 Thessalonians 5:23

We have learned that the brain structures (including the thalamus, amygdala, hippocampus, and hypothalamus) are associated with memories, emotions, and processing and storing information. The amygdala is linked to emotions and behaviors relating to fear and pleasure. The Creator gave us a desire for happiness and socialization, aided by serotonin, endorphin, oxytocin, testosterone, and other neurochemicals. For example, if the serotonin level is too low for an extended time, fear, depression, eating disorders, and other diseases can invade our bodies, affecting the soul and the spirit.[2] The link between the amygdala, hippocampus, hypothalamus, septal area, and prefrontal cortex helps us decide what is right or wrong.[3] The GABA neurotransmitter prevents us from harmful bad behavior and calms down the brain.[4] We are divinely equipped to be able to produce the fruit of the Spirit: joy, love, peace, goodness, kindness, gentleness, patience, faithfulness, and self-control. These qualities will create an atmosphere in our brains for healthy amounts of neurotransmitters to store healthy thoughts and emotions. They will affect all our attitudes, everywhere we go.

The entire Bible is a Book of restoration and attitude change. From the Book of Genesis we know that Jacob met God in a dream. After his attitude changed and his character transformed, he was able to look at those around him differently. After your attitude changes, a heavenly atmosphere descends on you. In Jacob's situation angels were ascending and descending from heaven as they changed the atmosphere around him. (See Genesis 28:16–22.) The window of heaven opens when your attitude is changed through prayer. Your obedience moves the heart of God. When Jacob's heart and attitude changed, his future changed. Jacob prayed, and after that his heart was transformed. As a foreigner, I had to maintain an attitude of prayer. I vowed to share my blessings with the poor and needy if God would bless me. And He did.

God changes our attitude so we can love the people around us. When you experience the power of the Holy Spirit, you want to share with others right away. When you have an authentic experience with God, people will notice. In the presence of God is joy and rest, as was written thousands of years ago: "My Presence will go with you, and I will give you rest" (Exod. 33:14). To find rest for your soul, choose to walk in a godly way. Change your attitude, to choose the better way when at a crossroads, as Jeremiah 6:16 (above) assures us.

If you choose to follow the ways of the world, you open yourself up to experiencing catastrophic things. As 1 Thessalonians 5:23 says, only God can keep your whole spirit, soul, and body blameless. The fruit of the flesh (such as envy, jealousy, anger, unforgiveness, and bitterness) increase stress levels, and cause the stress hormone cortisol to go up, lowering the T-cell level and compromising your immune system.[5] Prolonged high levels of cortisol due to increased stress levels will cause heart disease, sleep disturbances, depression, and many other complications.

CHOOSE TO HAVE A DIFFERENT SPIRIT

> But because my servant Caleb has a different spirit and follows me wholeheartedly, I will bring him into the land he went to, and his descendants will inherit it.
>
> —NUMBERS 14:24

Repeated actions become habits. Let the Spirit renew your thoughts "to be made new in the attitude of your minds" (Eph. 4:23). Many times I have chosen to refuse thoughts of fear and anxiety. Like many successful people, I choose to have a different attitude and a different spirit. God's blueprint is in your spirit. He put His promises in you, but you need to *activate* what God put in you and *decide* to have a different spirit. Develop a spirit of excellence through obedience. A right spirit will give you right attitudes to sustain your relationships in marriage, family, business, and society.

A gentle and quiet spirit is precious in the sight of God. We read in the Book of Joshua that Joshua and Caleb received the promises of God because they had a right spirit. Bible characters who followed God's prescriptions disciplined themselves. They are examples for us, so we may consider their character as a model. Discipline can be painful, As Hebrews 12:11 points out: "No discipline seems pleasant at the time, but painful. Later on, however, it produces a harvest of righteousness and peace for those who have been trained by it." God chose to give the promised land to the sons of Israel, but they had to discipline themselves and faithfully follow God's prescriptions and instructions. God gave us promises for health, family, success, prosperity, etc., but we must follow His advice and recommendations. Choose God's perspective to wake up your spirit.

We learn in the Book of Joshua that during Joshua and Caleb's time, the ten spies missed the true perspective, and lost the blessing. People miss blessings because they lack self-discipline, refuse God's prescriptions, and lose their way. You can develop a right spirit through prayer. Be willing to learn. You are well able to overcome difficulties through an obedient spirit.

Choose a lifestyle of forgiveness, kindness, and faith to prevent adverse effects. Disobedience will separate you from God's promises and from arriving at your God-given destination. We must become the people God wants us to be. God wants people like Caleb, whom He praised in Numbers 14:24.

A different (right) spirit will bring blessings over you and your descendants through the blessings of God, activated by the epigenetics mechanism that facilitates the "good" gene expression for the next generation. You must encourage yourself, even in tough situations. A different spirit was needed in the promised land. The other spies had ignorant and contemptuous spirits. You need the right spirit to benefit from God's blessings in your daily life. Cultivate a spirit that follows God's prescriptions and obeys His Word.

You can overcome any circumstances through the power of God. Nothing is impossible for those who believe God's Word and His promises. He promised, "Never will I leave you; never will I forsake you" (Heb. 13:6). He promised to be with us always, if we seek Him and His presence. If you do not stay in the presence of God, you will end up in the presence of demons. Leave aside compulsive behavior that you cannot control: cigarettes, alcohol, drugs, lies, cheating, stealing, pornography, adultery, or fornication, which debilitate your life. The enemy tells you it is "only one time," and then again, "only one time." You must say, *"No more."* Do a U-turn from everything that is ungodly.

Protect your eye gates and your ear gates. TV steals your time, and video games are an addictive stronghold. Addictions start with "one time only," but that time never ends. Do not let addictions deplete your body of dopamine. I have seen people crying, trying to get delivered, then experiencing withdrawal symptoms and going back into the same destructive behavior. They cannot break the bondage of addiction. Those are strongholds that must be broken by choosing to have a different spirit.

Deliverance can be slow, because of the receptors that were developed during the addiction. However, deliverance can be quick when a supernatural intervention from the Spirit of God touches you. Many people cannot feel the touch of God because they are numbed by their addiction. I do not leave room for addictions. The only time I watch TV is when I need to know the news, or watch a Christian channel that builds up my faith. You must pursue knowledge and wisdom to develop a healthy conscious mind, one that is willing to make the right decisions and listen to God's spirit.

Other people will see your changed attitude and your unconditional love for people in distress. They will follow your example when you are transformed according to the Word of God. It takes only one minute to pray the prayer that Jesus taught His disciples to pray, the Lord's Prayer (Matt. 6:9–13). Why don't you pray that prayer now? God wants to polish you, and change your attitude and your reputation. You need to become the person God wants you to be. Look at life through your spiritual lenses. Think about what Jesus would do when temptations came. He fasted and prayed and refused to be enticed by the devil's snare.

COMMUNICATING OUR ATTITUDE

> The soothing tongue is a tree of life, but a perverse tongue crushes the spirit.
>
> —Proverbs 15:4

Mirroring activity helps people communicate with each other. Science shows us that "mirroring, besides being a tool for communication between individuals, also corresponds to the basic function of developing knowledge and connection between people. Recent findings in the field of neuroscience have shown the presence of 'mirror neurons' in the neural system of primates and humans. These neurons make possible exchanges between people, the development of the psyche and the inter-subjective processes that are a basic condition for knowledge acquisition from others and for development of relational life."[6] Through the mirror neurons we learn from each other. Who controls your mirror neurons?

> Then those who feared the Lord talked with each other, and the Lord listened and heard. A scroll of remembrance was written in His presence concerning those who feared the Lord and honored His name. "On the day when I act," says the Lord Almighty, "they will be my treasured possession. I will spare them, just as a father has compassion and spares his son who serves him. And you will again see the distinction

between the righteous and the wicked, between those who serve God and those who do not."

—Malachi 3:16–18

Communication prevents isolation and further depression and pain. God intentionally created mirror neurons in us with the ability to communicate, develop good relationships, and love one another. God gave us the powerful prescription to "love one another," and He gave us the ability to love by using our mirror neurons. That will also reduce our stress level.

Our health flourishes when we communicate with a soothing tongue. Words have the power to either destroy someone's future, or build and transform a life for eternity. "The tongue has the power of life and death" (Prov. 18:21). What you speak has the power to bring life. God brought all of creation into existence by the power of His Word. He used the Word to create the universe. We who bear God's image have the ability to create through our words. Words can create or destroy. Words have emotions attached to them, based on our perception. As soon as they touch the ears, they are processed and stored as a memory in your brain structures, ready to be accessed for healing or destruction. Proverbs 15:4 (above) contrasts the difference between a tongue that praises and one that destroys.

Words arrive as a "breeze" (electrical impulses) in your brain cortex, with the neurons as "a forest of trees containing ten thousand trees per square mile."[7] If those words are kind and pleasant, they will bring fruits of their kind and healing to a bruised soul. But the tongue can also crush the spirit. Harsh and derogatory words spoken to you will crush you—words like: "You are ugly," "You are worthless," or, "You're not so smart." You cannot handle those words. But if somebody speaks uplifting words, such as: "You look good," "You can do that," "You are so smart," or, "You are strong," they have the power to build you up, shape your outlook, and improve your attitude. Remember to declare the promises of God that bring encouragement, faith, hope, and restoration.

There is power in your words. Your words can heal or hurt, regardless of your culture or nationality. Words become thoughts that are stored in your unconscious mind, and they can stay in your unconscious mind your entire life.[8] If unhealthy words caused unhealthy emotions, even those memories can be changed with healthy words (with healthy emotions attached to them) to build new, healthy memories for a healthier future. Mental health specialists deal with people whose episodes of angry outbursts are triggered by unhealthy words spoken to them even forty or fifty years ago, resulting in unhealthy emotions and hurtful memories.[9] You must select which words you allow to grow in your neurons.

When I was a child, if Mom gave me an assignment, I did everything I could to accomplish the task. One time I heard Mom say to another woman, "She could penetrate even a hard rock if needed, to do what I tell her to do." That comment remains with me today. No matter what is happening and how hard it is, I am determined to complete my assignments. The Bible says it is important to successfully finish everything we start. Do not give up easily or leave your tasks unfinished.

The Book of 1 Samuel tells us about David and Goliath's epic battle. David saw that Goliath was a giant, but declared, "I come against you in the name of the LORD Almighty" (1 Sam. 17:45). He knew God was (and still is) bigger than Goliath. Goliath tried to intimidate David with derogatory words, but David knew that Jehovah Jireh would provide victory, just as He had protected him many times when he fought lions and bears. David knew God as His rock of salvation, full of power and victory.

Do not talk against your destiny. Joshua 6:10–11 says, "Joshua commanded the army: 'Do not give a war cry, do not raise your voices, do not say a word until the day I tell you to shout. Then shout!'" When they followed Joshua's instructions, the impossible became possible because of their obedience. God's promises for victory became real to them. They were commanded not to talk, because the risk and temptation for negative words would bring discouragement and destruction. They could never have been victorious if they had not obeyed and remained silent until the day of victory.

> Do not let any unwholesome talk come out of your mouth, but only what is helpful for building others up according to their needs, that it may benefit those who listen.
> —EPHESIANS 4:29

Ephesians 4:29 advises us to be conscious about what kinds of words are coming out of our mouths concerning God's prescriptions. When you carefully choose your words, you increase people's faith because faith comes by hearing the Word of God (Rom. 10:14). Good words will be deposited in their unconscious mind, and available when needed. Your testimony is a powerful weapon. Your message, your worship, your prayers, and your walk with Jesus can influence those around you. The power of God's prescriptions, His Word, and your testimony about what God has done in your life will change other people's lives.

Sometimes we hear about a good medical specialist, and highly recommend him or her to our patients. But we all have the specialist of the universe giving free prescriptions for life, for us here on earth and for eternity, which I highly recommend. Run to Him and benefit from His presence, wisdom, revelation, healing, and restoration.

When Jesus lives through us, others will want to have the same power to change their attitude. So, go public with your testimony. "For we are God's handiwork, created in Christ Jesus to do good works, which God prepared in advance for us to do" (Eph. 2:10). Continue to do good to people around you. Speak life into other people's lives every chance you get. Be confident that you are who God said you are: a child of God, His creation, saved by grace. Do not hide your identity. If I had ignored the Word of God, I could have missed my destiny and my calling in life.

Chapter 18

THOUGHTS

*The mind governed by the flesh is death, but
the mind governed by the Spirit is life and peace.*
—Romans 8:6

We take captive every thought to make it obedient to Christ.
—2 Corinthians 10:5

Wholesome thoughts bring life and peace, promote health, and bring glory to God. Refresh your thoughts, your memory, and your heart by meditating on the Word of God and reflecting on its transforming power. Filter your thoughts, selecting only the constructive, healthy ones. God wants you to enjoy a healthy body, soul, and mind. He wants to preserve you until the coming of the Lord Jesus Christ. "May my meditation be pleasing to him, as I rejoice in the Lord" (Ps 104:34). Your thoughts influence your destiny. If your thinking is controlled by the flesh and unwholesome things, it will lead to death from incurable diseases. Let the Holy Spirit control your thoughts, because "the mind governed by the Spirit is life and peace" (Rom. 8:6).

Your thoughts actually do run your life—so be careful what you think. Examine and evaluate your thoughts. You can hide your thoughts from people, but God knows every one of them. When you have better thoughts, your world is better. Thoughts dictate your attitudes and how you walk in daily life. God's thoughts are not like yours: "For my thoughts are not your thoughts, neither are your ways my ways," declares the Lord (Isa. 55:8). As a result, your thoughts dictate your ways, which must follow God's ways. "As the heavens are higher than earth, so are my ways higher than your ways and my thoughts than your thoughts" (v. 9). Would you like to know God's thoughts? Read His Word and pray for revelation through the power of the Holy Spirit.

Your attitudes and behavior reveal what kind of thoughts you have been focusing on. Jesus said, "What comes out of a person is what defiles them…sexual immorality, theft, murder, adultery, greed, malice, deceit, lewdness, envy, slander, arrogance and folly" (Mark 7:20–22). Those attitudes lead to destruction, and "all sinners will be destroyed" (Ps. 37:38). You can make every thought obedient to Christ, as written in Scripture: "We take captive every thought to make it obedient to Christ" (2 Cor. 10:5). Christ's thoughts are pure thoughts.

PURE THOUGHTS

> Finally, brothers and sisters, whatever is true, whatever is noble, whatever is right, whatever is pure, whatever is lovely, whatever is admirable—if anything is excellent or praiseworthy—think about such things.
> —PHILIPPIANS 4:8

Pure thoughts are the pathway to a right attitude. "Blessed are the pure in heart, for they will see God" (Matt. 5:8). Follow God's prescription from Philippians 4:8 and focus your thoughts on what is honorable, true, pure, lovely, and admirable. Think about things that are excellent and worthy of praise. If you put your thoughts on God and His Word, it will be well with you physically and spiritually; as Isaiah 26:3 says, "You will keep him in perfect peace whose mind is stayed on You because he trusts in You" (NKJV).

REJOICE EVEN IN DIFFICULT TIMES

> Not only so, but we also glory in our sufferings, because we know that suffering produces perseverance; perseverance character, and character, hope, and hope does not put us to shame.
> —ROMANS 5:3–4

Choose to rejoice, even in unfavorable situations, as Paul advised in Romans 5:3–4. God is always working in your life, building your character into who God wants you to be. Character is important. When you go through fiery trials and discouraging situations, God is there with you to show His glory, just as He is always watching you: "For the eyes of the LORD run to and fro throughout the whole earth, to show Himself strong on behalf of those whose heart is loyal to Him" (2 Chron. 16:9, NKJV). Our eyes are focused on the trial, but a supernatural intervention will bring joy and accomplishment. Judy Squier, a speech pathologist born with underdeveloped legs and a deformed hand—but now the mother of three healthy girls—wrote in her book, *His Majesty in Brokenness: Finding God's Masterpiece in Your Missing Piece*:

> Our seeming catastrophe can become a blessing in disguise when our last breath gasps, *For this I have Jesus!* The minute we welcome Jesus on the scene, His Majesty transcends our lowest point so that we Much Afraids are seen as pillars of strength, not because we have courage, but because we have Him.[1]

Though her life was not free of difficulties, Judy she saw herself strong in her brokenness because she received Jesus in her heart.

HOLY SPIRIT THINKING

> The fruit of the Spirit is love, joy, peace, forbearance, kindness, goodness, faithfulness, gentleness and self-control. Against such there is no law.
> —GALATIANS 5:22–23

Negative, unhealthy thinking (from lack of knowledge of the Word of God) brings confusion, fear, anxiety, depression, isolation, suicidal thoughts, multiple chronic conditions, complications, and premature death. To avoid and prevent all those conditions, you need to clean negativism from your thoughts. Scientists are more interested than ever in studying the effects of optimism on the brain, to develop new interventions and methods to treat depression and anxiety disorder.[2] Have the mind of Christ. Only Jesus can bring maximum hope and optimism. He brought abundant life for those willing to renew their minds. Your thoughts improve when you seek God's thoughts for your life and grow in God's thoughts. "Now I commit you to God and to the word of his grace, which can build you up" (Acts 20:32). The Word of God is necessary for spiritual growth and healthy thoughts. The Word has the power to build you up and change your thinking by bringing you revelation, knowledge, wisdom, and understanding—the mind of Christ. Devour the Word of God to develop positive ways of thinking and an optimistic point of view—beyond science.

The Holy Spirit's presence in your life is shown by the fruit of the Spirit, listed in Galatians 5:22–23. Choosing behaviors and thoughts that reflect the fruit of the Spirit can reprogram your mind. If you want your brain to have the right atmosphere for a healthy neurochemical balance and healthy amounts of neurotransmitters (endorphins, serotonin, oxytocin, dopamine, and others) and to promote healing in your entire body and restore your spirit and soul, then make the fruit of the Spirit your own. The Holy Spirit offers a life full of optimism.

The Holy Spirit wants to live in us, but He can be grieved by our negativism and harmful thoughts. The Spirit gives gifts of wisdom, knowledge, faith, healing, miracles, prophecy, discernment, and speaking in heavenly languages, according to His will. (See 1 Corinthians 12:7–11.) Through the power of the Holy Spirit you can speak directly to God. The Holy Spirit will build your faith in Jesus. "But you, dear friends, by building yourself up in your most holy faith and praying in the Holy Spirit, keep yourselves in God's love as you wait for the mercy of our Lord Jesus Christ to bring you to eternal life" (Jude 20–21).

When the Holy Spirit comes over you and resides in you, you will change your thinking completely. Fear, worry, anxiety, depression, and discouragement are gone—replaced by love, joy, peace, forbearance, kindness, goodness, faithfulness, gentleness, and self-control. You need to encounter the power of God through the power of Holy Spirit, for "you will receive power when the Holy Spirit comes on you" (Acts 1:8).

Ruth changed her mind when her father-in-law and her husband both died. She did not allow depression to take over her life. She did not let bitter thoughts and pessimism ruin her life. She made the decision to let the Spirit of God reside in her, to guide and lead her. She cared for Naomi with a changed mind. Ruth was loving, kind, and compassionate to her mother-in-law, now an old widow suffering from loneliness.

Ruth, choosing to be possessed by the Spirit of God, positioned herself for future blessings and prompted admiration from people around her, because she had changed her thinking. Instead of going back to her own people—her country, her culture, her old habits—she chose to follow her mother-in-law's God. She was faithful, positive, and hardworking, day in and day out. God gave her an amazing reward. The changes she made in her mind changed her future and brought her an eternal reward. She activated the character in her DNA to its maximum potential. She was willing to activate—by God's Spirit—what already existed within her.

CHANGE YOUR THINKING—CHANGE YOUR BRAIN

You can change your brain by changing your thought process. Leading neuroscientists report breakthrough findings of how our brains are wired biologically to be changed by God through healthy thinking.[3] People resist changing their thinking. They think they are in control of their lives, are independent from God, and can live without responsibilities or consequences. Delaying acceptance of the need for God in our lives will sooner or later bring the consequences of disobedience. Denial of a need for divine intervention in our lives does not change God one bit but can prevent us from living lives according to God's will and His divine purpose for creating us. Acceptance that our brief lives on earth are temporary may change our perspective. Our attitude might need a makeover, and our brains need to be reprogrammed to coincide with reality. People need to deal with changes all the time—such as new cultures, new technologies, new generations, or new approaches to manage stress. When you change your thinking you "change your brain."

People often feel vulnerable and insecure from all the rapid changes in the world. Acknowledging and admitting that we must adapt our thinking for the changes in technology, and in many other areas of life, does not exonerate us from the responsibility that one day we will leave this planet. We will need to face the day of judgment for our lives on earth. That is the main reason we need to change our thinking.

Making the change in your mind is crucial. Seek help in the Word of God, and from others who already obey and serve their divine Creator. From birth to adulthood we must navigate our way through various life stages and changing circumstances that affect our minds. Changes are needed to reshape our thinking and mind. Sometimes we do not like these changes, but we must acknowledge and accept them. God is ready to intervene and help us change our thinking. Identifying the need for change, and responding appropriately, is the key to a healthy life.

Listen to God's instructions and guidance; stay connected with all the great giants of faith to preserve your life here on earth and to secure your place in heaven so you can spend your eternal life with Jesus and His followers. Your miracles are in your thoughts and your faith. When I see people suffering because of bad choices and wrong thinking in the past, such as drugs or alcohol-related dementia, I feel like writing the instructions from the Word of God on the prescription pad: "Urgent: read ten chapters daily from the Word of God and meditate on it day and night to preserve your neurons from dying prematurely. Take the Word with prayers and meditation to restore your health. The Word is life for your soul and for your spirit." As a primary care provider, actually I do pray with my patients and encourage them to read the Word of God for their benefit. Medication alone cannot solve all our problems.

Captive Thoughts

The Holy Spirit searches your mind, your thoughts, your emotions. He knows your brokenness. Every thought must be captive and obedient to Christ's teaching (2 Cor. 10:5). We must embrace the mind of Christ (1 Cor. 2:16) because God has good thoughts for our future (Jer. 29:11). The devil has evil plans for you. He is the one who is looking for ways to steal your joy, kill your passion and enthusiasm for God's promises, and destroy your health by bringing unhealthy thoughts into your mind. Our shortcoming in medicine is failing to address the fact that so many people are suffering from anxiety, worry, and depression because of wrong thoughts, poor attitudes, and bad habits. We can reverse those epidemics created by destructive thoughts, replacing them with God's promises that bring healing and restoration. The forces of darkness that bring addiction, sickness, and poverty can be overcome with healthy thoughts from the Word of God. Fight the forces of darkness by declaring the promises in God's Word over your life, again and again.

Chapter 19

THE WILL OF GOD

In all things we are more than conquerors through Him who loved us.
—Romans 8:37

Outside the will of God there is never complete success in managing stress. People attend stress-management classes, receive pharmacological and non-pharmacological interventions, and try many kinds of therapy classes with different kinds of advice, procedures, and treatments with different medications. But they still only bring temporary results; we see relapses all the time. It is an endless battle. Besides all those interventions people need permanent hope—beyond science—to stay strong and firm to overcome stressful situations, especially during a crisis. In order to manage stress, you need to have an open mind to the will of God, beyond science, and become the person God created you to be for His glory.

We can see the will of God for mankind in Jeremiah 29:11: "'For I know the plans I have for you,' declares the Lord, 'plans to prosper you and not to harm you, plans to give you hope and a future.'" The will of God gives hope and a future to a broken heart in a broken world. You need to know God's will for your life and dwell in Him. If you do not know His will you can keep fighting, yet feel that you have lost, because you are on the wrong path. The will of God is built in, inside of you, in your DNA. He has written His will into your physical DNA (deoxyribonucleic acid). You have the blueprint of God and His language, with all the characteristics that you were created to be. You need to discover His will and learn to know and accept it. His plan may be different than you expect, but His will is the best for you. You know that is God's plan for your life, when you ask something according to His will and He gives you what you ask. Everything that is impossible with men is possible with God. When you pray God's will in faith, you will find solutions for your problems and circumstances.

Being a stable person of faith will bring victory in your life. My husband and I had to believe that God wanted to bring victory in our lives. David confessed the same in Psalm 66:17: "I cried out to him with my mouth; his praise was on my tongue." God has done great things for us when we focused our attention on His will. We had to believe and follow His prescription to stay still, until He intervened on our behalf.

You cannot know someone else's thoughts, except through their spoken words and their actions. It is written that the Lord knows your thoughts. "You have searched me, Lord, and You know me. You know when I sit and when I rise; you perceive my thoughts from afar" (Ps. 139:1–2). People can think lawless and miserable thoughts that contaminate their souls. Dirty, filthy thoughts can enter in your mind through different sources: bad friends with wrong influences, media outlets (internet, magazines, movies), and books that are contrary to God's character. All of those will cause you to feel far from God and in much distress.

Be careful and pay attention to what you hear, what you read, what you see, and what you say so that you are in God's will. This will reduce the stress in your life. People with unclean thoughts depart from God and end up destroying their future and their family. Those tragedies create ripple effects in their community, city, and nation. Two cities, Sodom and Gomorrah, were destroyed completely because of the people's wickedness. (See Genesis 19.)

A good friend's family was destroyed because her husband opened the door to another woman in his life after many years of marriage. Her husband's actions destroyed her life and her children's future. The children lived under terrible stress caused by their parents' divorce, which led to anxiety, depression, and their consequences. My friend's immune system was compromised and she developed a terminal illness very soon after the shock—caused by a disastrous, unexpected divorce, which created overwhelming stress.

Jesus gave instructions to His disciples and to us all to watch in prayer so we do not fall into temptations. In this postmodern era we face multiple temptations, but we can watch vigilantly over our lives and stay in God's will. Many families are destroyed because of a lack of knowledge of the Word of God and His will. They lack faith in God, do not fast and pray, and never know God's will. People who don't know God's Word lack wisdom from heaven regarding their families.

Where there is peace, joy, and unity there is victory. Seek peace with your wife or your husband, your children, and everyone around you, giving priority to God's will. It is up to you to live in peace. If you provoke and create pain in somebody else's life, start a dialogue and ask for forgiveness to prevent further emotional distress and damage. You must pursue peace and love in any relationship. "And now these three remain: faith, hope and love" (1 Cor. 13:13). These three virtues—faith, hope, and love—will last forever. God's will for you is to have faith, hope, and love, but love is greatest. When you have love, you can live in peace with everyone, because God is love and He loves all His creation.

The Will of God

The will of God is included in all the promises written in the Word of God, which is good news for those who believe. Good news brings joy. Physical joy triggers thoughts of happiness that result in healthy amounts of neurotransmitters being released in your body. This repairs the cells affected by thoughts of fear, anxiety, depression, doubt, and unbelief. Healthy neurotransmitters will promote a good attitude.[1] Proclaiming the good news to those around you will cause them to be happy, thus promoting health in their body and building a healthier community.

I had unbelieving colleagues under the communist regime who wanted to spend time secretly talking to me and listening to my testimonies, because they sensed the good news would bring joy to their heart. They were hungry for it, but sharing it was illegal during the communist regime.

Good news can be mysterious and unexpected. For example, one day in Romania, I was in the office when the telephone rang. A colleague who picked up the phone said the call was for me. I was surprised because I did not expect anybody to call me at work. When I heard a voice with an accent, I asked her identity; the caller told me and reminded me we met at an all-night, underground prayer meeting at her grandparents' house in 1977. Of course, I had to search my memory to find and activate that information from ten years earlier. I remembered very well that night of prayer and the people who attended. But I was astonished to hear from her after so long. She told me she had moved to the United States because the communists had forced her to leave the country, but was back on a visit and wanted to see me. That was such good news and brought so much joy to my heart. I had reconnected with a close friend! But God had a mysterious plan for me. After our meeting the Lord started to work in my heart, convincing me that I must leave Romania too. I was sure that God had a plan for my future, even though everything seemed contradictory to my circumstances.

After this call, the communists started secretly following me, to stop me from pursuing a visa to leave the country. It was very intimidating. They could do anything they wanted to me or my family, to hinder God's plan for my future. Once I had applied for a visa to leave the country, my future was not secure in Romania. I had become a problem for them. So, I had to trust God in every situation. I knew my future was in God's hands. I felt like Nehemiah facing opposition: "They were all trying to frighten us, thinking, 'Their hands will get too weak for work, and it will not be completed'" (Neh. 6:9). This was what happened to me and my husband. They were trying to intimidate us and stop us from planning for our future. But I prayed: "Now strengthen my hands" (v. 10).

We continued to pursue the exit visa with even greater determination, knowing that the communists could still stop us from leaving the country. So we continued to pray and believe God for miracles, because the barriers were so great. I prayed continuously for strength in that difficult time. If you feel intimidated, or it seems impossible to find a solution for your situation, you must allow God into your life now to strengthen your soul, and declare, "In all things we are more than conquerors through him who loved us" (Rom. 8:37).

Did you know that when you are in God's will, you will fulfill your destiny? To find your destiny, you must know God's expectations for you. God has a vision for your future and your destiny. Many people ask, "What am I created for?" "Why I am here on earth?" "Why I was born?" or "What is the purpose of my existence?" In my profession, and in my business, I spend time at the bedside of many dying patients—people like you and me. They were born, then grew up, and in their childhood and adulthood they often had the same questions about their reason for being on this earth. I am sure that God had a plan for each one of their lives, until they arrived in our facility, on their deathbed. God planned a precise destiny for each of us. Life is a mystery, but you need to know what you are here for.

You must discern what is best for your life. As Philippians instructs: "This is my prayer: that…you may be able to discern what is best and may be pure and blameless for the day of Christ, filled with the fruit of righteousness that comes through Jesus Christ—to the glory and praise of God" (Phil. 1:9–11). Many people are miserable because they do not know their destiny, or they are apathetic. They are lukewarm and have no passion, living a life that will have discouraging consequences. God wants us to live a life with passion for Him.

God tests us to see if we are hungry to know Him more and find out His will for our lives. God is working at the level of your desire. If you are hungry and thirsty for more, He will help you achieve more. The spiritual realm is the same as the natural realm. For example, after I arrived in the United States, I started cleaning toilets in a nursing home, but my desire was to know more about how to care for the aging population. Slowly I proceeded to take classes, to learn more, and was accepted into different programs for education—up to the highest levels. It is the same in the spiritual realm. You can have as much of God as you want. Are you thirsty for more of Jesus? When you desire to work more for Him, God will bless you more in everything you do. God gives approval to those who seek His will on earth and who have faith. (See Matthew 5:45.)

SURRENDER TO GOD

When you surrender to God, the will of God and His presence brings happiness. Turning bitterness into joy will reduce your level of stress. Joy will bring health to your body. He will bless you and help you impact other people. When we surrendered to His will, He changed our years of bitterness into blessings, so we now can bless others and bring joy into our lives and their lives. Surrender to God in every situation because God wants to give you peace in the storm. He wants to restore your relationships with your loved ones, reconnect you with them, restore your health in body and spirit, refresh your spirit, and renew your heart. You may face storms in your life, but you must look to Jesus and pray. Jesus' storm was bigger than ours, and all He did was pray every day early in the morning, or sometimes all night long. Your help comes from the Lord. I have had many storms and tough times, and always when I prayed to the Lord, He rescued me. (See Psalms 91 and 121.)

Remember what God has already done for you. Keep your conscious mind clear before God and man. God is a lover of those who messed up, but wants each person on earth to surrender and live in truth and in righteousness (Acts 24:16). God provided everything for us. Everything comes from Him. Yield your heart to the Lord and you will be blessed by Him. There are consequences if you do not pay attention. (See Joshua 24:22–24.) Many people are not willing to yield to the Lord, and then they must "reap what they sow."

Many people grieve and experience bitterness, because they do not want to surrender to God and repent. Yet true peace is only obtained through yielding and repentance. Selfishness brings bitterness, because you do not get what you want for yourself. You set unrealistic, high expectations, which you are never able to achieve. When you surrender, you will develop a selfless life and a heart of gratitude. Through joy and love you will have a charitable heart that will bring you great rewards. Train yourself to be joyful, even through difficult situations. Get rid of bitterness in your soul with the joy and love of the Lord, who gives you strength.

True joy in your life happens when you are connected with Jesus' love. Nothing can bring more joy than Jesus the Prince of Peace, the Bright and Morning Star, the Sun of Righteousness. There is power in the name of Jesus. In His name you are able to love people who do not love you back—even people who hurt you. You will be able to forgive them as the Father forgave you, and that will bring healing to your soul and body. Do not blame the church, or God, or other people for their mistakes. Surrender to God's will and seek God's mercy, grace, and love. When you have a surrendered heart, you rejoice with those who rejoice and weep with those who weep.

People Are Lost Without Direction

> As for you, if you redirect your heart and spread out your hands to Him in prayer...then you will hold your head high, free from fault.
> —Job 11:13, 15, csb

Knowing God's will for your life and following it is literally a matter of life and death. Those whose lifestyles run contrary to the Word of God put themselves in very dangerous situations. I see ignorance of the Word and good health practices in my medical office all the time. I give instructions to patients for lifestyle changes, and they ignore them completely. One time I instructed a patient with a serious heart condition to follow up with me for her treatment, and with her cardiologist for further cardiac investigations and interventions, to prevent a fatal event. She ignored my clinical advice, did not follow my strict instructions, and a few weeks later collapsed on the street. She was taken to the ER and resuscitated there for several minutes, then spent weeks in intensive care and in the hospital—all at great cost.

People can end up in terrible situations by ignoring God's instructions. Having no direction in life, their careless behavior often results in tragic consequences. We are known by our character, personality, and lifestyle. The Bible warns about the falling away before the coming of Christ. "Don't let anyone deceive you in any way, for that day will not come until the rebellion occurs and the man of lawlessness is revealed, the man doomed to destruction" (2 Thess. 2:3). Only the Holy Spirit can draw us back to Jesus.

People who depart from faith and truth are on a path to death. "Whoever strays from the path of prudence comes to rest in the company of the dead" (Prov. 21:16). People need to know about Jesus so their lives may be written in the Lamb's Book of Life. If their name is not in this book, they will be cast into the lake of fire. (See Revelation 20:14–15.) Many people's names will be missing from the Book of Life, due their ignorance of God's prescriptions. (See Revelation 3:3.)

Chapter 20

GENDER DIFFERENCES

*That is why a man leaves his father and mother
and is united to his wife, and they become one flesh.*
—Genesis 2:24

Be fruitful and increase in number; fill the earth and subdue it.
—Genesis 1:28

Therefore what God has joined together, let no one separate.
—Mark 10:9

One major relationship area that can trigger high levels of stress, worry, fear, and anxiety is marriage. Marital partners share a physical, emotional, and spiritual union, creating an eternal bond together. You desire and expect a safe relationship for life with your spouse, but if one of you gives in to disobedience or unfaithfulness, the marriage bond quickly fizzles and breaks down. What should have been a blessing can become twisted, putting the marriage and even lives in danger.

God's prescription for marriage establishes wholesome standards for a successful, loving union. Two unique souls become united through intimacy. Sex was created to be a central, holy element in the marriage covenant, yet marriage is not only for having sex. It was God's idea—not man's—that a man and a woman should become one in love, bonding together physically, emotionally, and spiritually for a divine purpose. They need to be as one emotionally and spiritually to be overcomers in spiritual warfare. Husband and wife must be committed to one other. Separation in marriage is not healthy—physically, emotionally, or spiritually—because of the overwhelming emotional pain that can result. In cases of divorce, each person experiences the unbearable pain of separation, similar to death. Because man and woman were not designed to bear the pain of divorce, the stress level created by divorce and separation is extremely high, causing real damage to the spirit, soul, and body. Divorce is one of the reasons for "broken heart syndrome."

In marriage relationships, poor communication is the usual culprit leading to divorce, because your words reflect what's inside your heart, mind, and soul. Words reveal your internal condition. Words have meaning and power in the spiritual realm. They can bring people closer or produce distance and separation. The power to become closer is in you. You just need to activate it through the power of the Holy Spirit to create the atmosphere in your mind that promotes love, joy, peace, and happiness. That is how you strengthen a marriage. One main ingredient in the divine marriage prescription for a lifelong healthy relationship is for both husband and wife to be filled with the Holy Spirit.

Abstinence

> Flee the evil desires of youth and pursue righteousness, faith, love, and peace, along with those who call on the Lord out of a pure heart.
> —2 Timothy 2:22

> Do not be deceived: Neither the sexually immoral nor idolaters nor adulterers nor men who have sex with men nor thieves nor the greedy nor drunkards nor slanderers nor swindlers will inherit the kingdom of God.
> —1 Corinthians 6:9–10

Medically, we know that adultery opens the door to sexually transmitted diseases—among them chlamydia, gonorrhea, genital herpes, HPV, hepatitis, syphilis, HIV, and AIDS. Thus, God gave us prescriptions for how to prevent those diseases: abstinence and self-control. Abstinence before marriage was commanded by God to help people avoid disaster. (See Genesis 2.) It is one of His instructions for a healthy lifestyle. Marry at the right time with the right person, and stay married for life. God hates divorce (Mal. 2:16). It is important for young men and women to be extremely careful about whom they marry, and to discern the right time. If you are not married yet, look for a godly person, because marriage is for life. When teaching about marriage we must lay out the foundations for future generations. Disastrous ideas pervade the educational system and the media. The constant stream of movies and video games promoting violence, immorality, and pornography seems unending. What principles do we want to promote? Do not lose the battle for lack of wisdom.

Due to rapidly changing technologies, our culture is constantly changing all around us. We are bombarded with chaotic and conflicting messages on every level. Contrary to God's instructions, worldly attitudes promote countless unhealthy behaviors that lead to chronic physical and mental diseases. Society is becoming sicker and sicker, with many dying a premature death due to corruption and man-made diseases. First Corinthians 6:9–10 spells out some of the behavior that can keep us out of God's kingdom. None of those have a place there. That is why Jesus Christ paid for our sins with His blood, and He is calling us to repent and be forgiven of all those sins.

A multinational study conducted in 2011 showed the number of young people having unprotected sex with new partners had increased 39 percent in the US, 19 percent in the UK and 111 percent in France over a three-year period.[1] Millions are being spent on medical research to discover cures and vaccinations for devastating sexually transmitted diseases, when simple prevention through abstinence has superior results.

The Centers for Disease Control reported in 2017 that cases of chlamydia totaled 1,708,569—the highest recorded for any condition.[2] These sexually transmitted diseases are due to sex outside marriage with multiple partners. Even young teens, students in grades seven to twelve, are engaged in destructive behaviors, such as gambling, substance abuse, sex, pornography, and attempted suicide. "Approximately 1 in 5 adults in the U.S. (46.6 million) experiences mental illness in a given year."[3] The costs for their care tremendously increase stress throughout society. When I look at these numbers something screams inside of me, "We must wake up!"

UNDERSTANDING OUR DIFFERENCES

> So God created mankind in his own image, in the image of God he created them; male and female he created them.
> —GENESIS 1:27

To manage stress in marriage you need to understand that God, our super-intelligent designer, created men and women differently. No one should doubt that. Physically we have obvious differences in our reproductive systems and their functions. We do not need somebody else to tell us who is a woman or who is a man. There is no confusion in God's creation of a man and a woman. What we cannot see is the hidden physiology in the circulatory system or in the brain. For example, women's arteries are smaller than men's arteries, putting women at higher risk for heart disease, and different circulatory symptoms have different complications.[4] Cardiology studies show differences in women's and men's hearts, and how they are differently affected by stressors.[5]

Because women's arteries are narrower, they carry an increased risk for atherosclerosis and its complications later in life.[6] Also, in women and men the brain is designed differently and uniquely programmed by God. Female and male brain structures and neurons also have physiological differences.[7]

Our gender differences remain as long as we live. Many women complain about their husband's behavior and make huge efforts to change him after they get married. They often use manipulation, humiliation, complaints, disrespect, cheating, and flirting with other men or women, jeopardizing their relationship. The same is true of men toward their wives.

Misunderstandings about the differences create further stress. God created men and women with physiological and psychological differences. Not understanding the differences in our brain structures can be extremely stressful for a married couple. The majority of us learn from our mistakes, and only by God's grace are we able to manage the stress in our marriage. Marriage should bring comfort, not worry, fear, and anxiety. Looking for comfort from immediate gratification, and entering into marriage primarily for sex, results in bitterness. Not waiting upon the Lord will have repercussions later in life.

My husband and I grew up subscribing to biblical standards about marriage. When our daughter Andreea was in high school, she prepared a list of thirty-five points and conditions to be met by her future husband. Our daughter knew she would want to get married according to God's instructions and prescriptions and His will for her life. She did not want to "play" marriage. She knew that marriage is for life. I really wondered where she would find a guy to meet all of her conditions! I started praying for a miracle, because these days it would take a miracle to find such a young man with a pure heart. Then God brought Jeff into her life, and she quickly checked off each point on her list. I told myself, "He must be the one." God had prepared the one who was to be her husband for life. She had trusted His promises; as Psalm 46:10 says: "Be still and know that I am God."

Obedience to the Word of God in marriage is not optional. With God all things are possible—when you wait for His divine intervention. God knows everything. You must have faith that He will provide the right person for you. Jesus sees your tears when you cry out to Him for the right one. Do not despair. Prayer and fasting is a key element in this. If we fear God and do His will, He will hear us. Unbelief will only produce fear and cripple your future. Renew your mind and meditate on the Bible's clear instructions about marriage.

We need to enjoy the mystery of God's creation in marriage. Marriage is a lifelong commitment and should be full of love, joy, happiness, peace, and all the fruit of the Spirit. The brain's various structures release neurotransmitters in different ways in men and women.[8] Neurotransmitters (serotonin, epinephrine, norepinephrine, oxytocin, dopamine, endorphin, and other neurochemicals and hormones) are released in different amounts in each man or woman, based on what kind of thoughts you dwell on. Your thoughts influence your attitude and behavior in your marriage. Dr. Caroline Leaf, in her book *Who Switched Off Your Brain?: Solving* the Mystery of He Said/She Said, stated, "When the weight of stress and pressure becomes toxic and unhealthy, woman will talk without thinking and man will act without thinking."[9] Male and female thought processes are different and they do affect relationships in marriage.

You can read Dr. Leaf's book for a clearer scientific picture, and a fuller understanding—beyond science—of the difference between male and female brain anatomy, physiology, and functions. You will gain more insights about gender differences and a different perspective about relationships in marriage.

THE WISE WOMAN

> The wise woman builds her house, but with her own hands the foolish one tears hers down.
> —PROVERBS 14:1

Oxytocin is the neurotransmitter with a clear assignment to keep the family together. To prevent and avoid divorce in your family, keep the oxytocin level high, giving you the comfort and assurance of well-being in your marriage.[10] The release of oxytocin gives you confidence and comfort in your marriage, so you will not look for the "D" word when things get tough. God is against separation and divorce. Keep love alive in your heart and brain so your relationship in your marriage will last, just as God intended. You are equipped by your Creator for marriage to last your entire life.

To keep her family together and to please God, a woman needs the virtues of the Proverbs 31 woman (found in Proverbs 31:10–31.) By enriching your knowledge and acting more like this woman, you will have a life full of victory and success.

We need the Word of God in our heart at all times. Study the Bible and memorize the Scriptures. This is good not only for spiritual discipline; it can physically create new neurons and restore your emotions and relationships in your marriage. Your brain will produce more healthy neurotransmitters if your attitude is right. Love will never fail because God, the source of love, is infinite. Neuroscientists have discovered that oxytocin is created in the hypothalamus and secreted by the pituitary gland, when triggered by love.[11] Living by the power of the Holy Spirit, you will have what lasts forever: love.

Love will cause more joy, peace, goodness, kindness, gentleness, patience, faithfulness, and self-control, and—if troubled—heal your marriage. When you create a healthy atmosphere for the brain to release the right chemicals, as God intended in His intelligent design, it draws husband and wife together again and again.

Oxytocin, the "love hormone," facilitates attachment. God's prescription for man is to love his wife. Oxytocin, released when you love, is important for reproduction and survival of the species. It helps develop lifelong bonds for a family to produce offspring in a covenant of marriage. Oxytocin has been important in monogamy since creation.[12] God wrote prescriptions and instructions for marriage between a man and a woman, who were complete strangers in Genesis. "That is why a man leaves his father and mother and is united to his wife, and they become one flesh" (Gen. 2:24). God also gave the command to "be fruitful and increase in number; fill the earth and subdue it" (Gen. 1:28). Then, in Mark 10:9 we read, "Therefore what God has joined together, let no one separate."

Oxytocin, released through love, keeps man and woman "glued" together. Since creation—beyond science—what God united, man should not separate. Scientists marvel at the biological mystery of monogamy, enabled through this hormone oxytocin and released through love.[13] Reprogram your brain to love and to increase oxytocin levels through the "power of touch" through hugs, kisses, holding hands, and an intimate relationship.[14] All these expressions will cause the release of oxytocin to improve your relationship with longer, stronger bonds.

Oxytocin also helps bond a mother to her baby.[15] Isaiah wrote, "Can a mother forget the baby at her breast and have no compassion on the child she has borne?" (Isa. 49:15). Oxytocin is released when triggered by love and is involved in nurturing, helping strangers marry for life, and in empathy and compassion.[16] Oxytocin involved in overcoming fear and anxiety can be beneficial for an individual's survival.[17] As Paul warned Timothy: "Flee the evil desires of youth and pursue righteousness, faith, love, and peace, along with those who call on the Lord out of a pure heart" (2 Tim. 2:22).

Oxytocin reduces stress. It helps you forgive others, helps with social skills, and lifts the burden of bitterness from your heart. God's love has been poured out in our hearts. But separated from God, you deprive your body of these amazing resources. Read 1 Corinthians 13, the "love chapter," which assures us that love never fails. "Now these three remain: faith, hope and love. But the greatest of these is love" (v. 13). Love will remain forever. Use the "power of touch" to release oxytocin in the brain. This is what touch does for us in our family life. Love is the fruit of the Spirit; it is what God desired from the beginning, both for and from His creation. Only through the power of the Holy Spirit, given by Christ Jesus, can we have true love. God is love.

LOVE

> Let love and faithfulness never leave you; bind them around your neck, write them on the tablet of your heart.
>
> —Proverbs 3:3

According to neuroscientists, healthy amounts of neurotransmitters are released in your body through love as endorphin, the natural antidepressant, and oxytocin, "the love hormone," for nurturing.[18] Together, they influence your physical health in a positive way. Love will calm your brain. Your anxiety level will decrease, your heart rate will decrease, and your heart can relax, improving circulation, breathing, and the oxygenation of all your cells. It will enhance the immune system's ability to fight infections, viruses, and cancer when you follow the high potency prescription in Proverbs 3:3.

Stress can be managed through love. Love is a feeling that will trigger a healthy amount of chemicals to be released in your body, reprogramming your thinking. All is based on love. Jesus gave us the fundamental commandment for the human race: "Love one another" (John 15:17). Jesus was driven by love; everything He did was loving. We must be driven by love too. Love is crucial. Living without love means we are like a brass cymbal—nothing but noise. If you do not love, you accomplish nothing. (See 1 Corinthians 13:1–3.) Your influence on the job, at school, and in society is driven by love. We must prove our love. Love is a force, a power, an effort, an exertion. Love makes an impact, because God is love. He supernaturally pours His love into our hearts.

Use your imagination. Imagine that God's love from the invisible world, "the spiritual realm," hits the threshold of our cerebral cortex. There it is transformed into electrical impulses flowing through "the forest of neurons" rushing to the amygdala, casting out all thoughts, emotions, and feelings of fear and anxiety. Another neurotransmitter associated with love is dopamine, with its excitatory function.[19] It is amazing how Jesus gave us instructions about loving one another. He did not explain why, but from creation—beyond science—our heart and brain and spirit were created with the capacity to love. We were created for relationship, and given all the necessary equipment to love. We just need to follow God's prescription. Selfishness is the opposite of love.

Love becomes real when someone touches Jesus, who was consumed with love for us. Love is serving others. (See Matthew 20:29–34 and Galatians 5:13.) Jesus served people. In response to His great love you need to be full of holiness, pray for others, and live your life for others. You carry the "living water." Day in and day out you can bring "living water" to the lost. Love-deprived people need our compassion and love.

In our business, we have the opportunity to serve homeless people. We know how deprived of love they have been for many years. When they come to our place, we show them love through our services, but we also give them hugs and tell them verbally that we love them. We can see joy and happiness in their eyes, from love they had not felt for years. To receive, you must give, and to have harvest, you must sow. These are the signs that point the way to God. God gave His only begotten Son, to leave the glory of heaven, to be born in the lowest place on earth, and be wrapped in swaddling clothes, lying in a humble manger. He grew in God's wisdom and power, ministered to others, and died on the cross for the entire world. Then He was raised from the dead and ascended to our heavenly Father to intercede on our behalf, even now, in this moment.

This is how God loved and continues to love us, no matter what. In return we must have a humble spirit. Jesus is now in glory because He humbled Himself on earth. If you want God to give you glory, you must humble yourself. We need to be like Christ. He came to break the chain, to cleanse us from our sins. We must become like Him. Through love, you win favor with people and with God, as well as promote health and prevent diseases. Through love He will show you His will in everything you do, and He will show you which path to take.

I did not know what to expect when I arrived in the United States, but through His love and through fasting and prayer, God showed us what to do every single day. Even though I often felt tired and discouraged, I felt God's love. He gave me strength through His Word, and by the power of the Holy Spirit. I felt His love through His presence in my lowest moments of loneliness. I kept the Bible open on the table so I could read it each time I had a chance throughout the day, to stay connected with God's love. I memorized the Word of God during my adolescence and adulthood in Romania, and here in the United States I recited it to myself to remind me of His promise that He loves me.

You must renew and guard your heart with God's love. Through fasting and praying, we become stronger in the Lord and closer to Him. He promised, "Those who hope in the LORD will renew their strength. They will soar on wings like eagles; they will run and not grow weary, they will walk and not be faint" (Isa. 40:31). When you hope in the Lord and recognize His love for you, your strength will be renewed.

So hoping in the Lord will give you more energy to function well. It is the hope in His love for you that your brain is programmed to produce healthy neurotransmitters that will increase your energy. I was working two jobs full time, with no days off, for almost two years after I arrived in the United States. At the same time, I also studied English daily, late into the night. I was able to run and not grow weary, to work and not be faint, because God's love gave me strength. God will do a new thing in your heart too, if you are sensitive to God's love every day and find your hope for a blessed future.

Focus on the good news that God loves you, and feed your soul with joy. Always look for the good news in the Word of God, which brings joy and excitement to your heart. Beni Johnson—who with her husband, Bill, pastors Bethel Church—stated in her book, *The Happy Intercessor*: "When you carry the joy of the Lord with you, all kinds of things happen. Joy brings excitement to the air, and it releases life."[20] Joy comes after you find the good news. Good news can be unexpected and mysterious, as when God sent Jesus Christ, His Son, in the form of a man, to planet Earth. Nothing brings more joy than knowing God loves you.

As a young girl under the communist system I was so hungry for God's love, I would wake up at 3:00 or 4:00 a.m. to go to a prayer meeting. We did not have electricity in my village, so our path was lit by the light of the moon in the early morning. My heart was filled with the joy of God's presence. Where God is present, His love is felt. I could sing all day long, working tirelessly, because of His love in my heart. My work was efficient and time passed quickly, even though the work was so hard.

When you love with the love of God, fears will disappear. Love is powerful. God's love gives confidence and encouragement that is fearless. The love of God can change the culture of every nation. People develop their own code of living and call it good, unwilling to recognize the love of God in their lives. During a certain time in the Old Testament, it is written that "everyone did what was right in their own eyes" (Judg. 17:6), where people were not seeking God's advice, nor recognizing His authority. When they acted this way and followed their own fleshly desires with destructive behaviors, they put themselves in the position to be destroyed because of their lack of obedience. God always punishes disobedience, but He gives blessings beyond imagination to those with a heart after His own heart and to those who surrender to Him through love.

Chapter 21

MEDITATION AND ANTIAGING

May these words of my mouth and this meditation of my heart be pleasing in your sight, Lord, my Rock and my Redeemer.
—Psalm 19:14

MEDITATION IS A proven antiaging therapy that produces new neurons in your brain through neurogenesis. New neurons preserve cognition and prevent dementia and Alzheimer's later in life. Turn everything over to God, and meditate day and night on His Word, and you will renew your mind. The Queen of England declared in one of her speeches, "Reflection, meditation and prayer help us to renew ourselves in God's love."[1]

Spiritual heart disease—sin—brings futility and emptiness. Replace sin in your heart with meditation and the Word of God, and heed the warning of Solomon: "God created mankind upright, but they have gone in search of many schemes" (Eccles. 7:29). We live in a dark world where sin is accepted as normal and rationalized with the theory of relativism. Those who live in the light are often despised or persecuted, as I was under communism. But there is nothing too dark or too dirty to be redeemed by the grace of God. God wants to restore your relationships, renew your spirit, and change your heart. Begin to seek a fresh revelation of Jesus Christ and what He is doing right now in your life and in the world.

We need fresh spiritual eyes to see who Jesus is and so the Holy Spirit can reveal Jesus to us in our daily lives. Jesus is the answer for a broken world, broken nations, broken cities, broken families, and broken people. People are drowning in sin, and Jesus is the rescuer. Where we see Jesus, we see love and grace, and people transformed by His love and power. We don't need clinical trials to demonstrate the power of Jesus Christ transforming people. The best evidence since Jesus died on that cross almost two thousand years ago has been witnessed over and over. People are healed in the presence of His power. Victory is in Jesus' name. Surrender to God, ask Him to intervene, and let His Spirit rule again.

The world perverts everything: music, science, creativity in the arts, education, economics, technology, sex, and family life. Only God can restore everything back to its original form and give vision, dreams, revelation, and supernatural signs. Our society needs to return to a godly life to receive the provisions of unmerited grace. Grace can transform everyone and everything.

Meditate on God's Word

God is pleased when we humble ourselves. We need to meditate on His precepts so we can hear God's voice when Jesus knocks at the door. "Apart from me you can do nothing" (John 15:5). When you meditate day and night on God's Word, you hear His voice, because you create an atmosphere in your brain to allow the Holy Spirit to come into your mind and speak to you. In one of his past daily devotionals, Pastor Joel Osteen observed:

> When you constantly focus on external things: distractions, worry, and cares of the world, they become bigger in your mind's eye. But when you focus on what God has given you: peace, freedom, and abundant life, those are the things that you will see manifest in your life.... Remember, where the Spirit of the Lord is, there is liberty. So focus on Him and focus on freedom![2]

"Now the Lord is the Spirit, and where the Spirit of the Lord is, there is freedom" (2 Cor. 3:17). When you meditate on the work of the Spirit through the Word of God, you grow new neurons in your brain's structure and receive healing—physically and spiritually.

Because our brain structures produce neurotransmitters (like GABA with inhibitory action), we can avoid unsafe actions (protecting us from bad habits and bad consequences). But GABA needs to be activated to calm your brain; one way to do this is through meditation.[3] Meditate on the Word of God, because all Scripture is profitable and is inspired by God. Solomon was wiser than everyone else. He "spoke 3,000 proverbs, and his songs were 1,005" (1 Kings 4:32, ESV). Solomon experienced the power of God's presence, but in spite of his wisdom, he concluded that everything in life is meaningless. (Read the Book of Ecclesiastes.) He became pessimistic, departed from the truth, and stopped meditating on God's Word. He could no longer discern the voice of God.

Discerning and being sensitive to the voice of God is the most important thing in life. Solomon, looking for meaning in life, said, "Fear God and keep his commandments" (Eccles. 12:13). Make life count and keep His commandments, meditating on His Word. Solomon talks about how to make life meaningful, with skills that bring success. Solomon is telling us—thousands of years later—to stop and analyze what we are doing. Take time to meditate on the Word of God.

When we do not meditate on the Word of God, we can become exhausted. When you lose your passion, you work harder, but with little progress, becoming emotionless and spiritually hollow. Authentic meaning is found only in God. Solomon became addicted to things, but he missed out on meeting with God, who had blessed Him. Concentrating on material things, wanting more, and shifting our focus from God only brings depression. Ask yourself what really matters. People often sacrifice faith, family, friends, morals, and values for meaningless things. Tragically, as they reflect at the end of their lives, they acknowledge reality. Then it is too late.

Chapter 22

HELPING OTHERS

For we are God's handiwork, created in Christ Jesus to do good works, which God prepared in advance for us to do.
—Ephesians 2:10

H ELPING OTHERS HELPS us manage our stress. Follow Jesus' example: "Because Christ suffered for you, leaving an example, that you should follow in his steps" (1 Pet. 2:21), and walk as He walked, sacrificing for others. "Whoever claims to live in him must live as Jesus did" (1 John 2:6). Walk in love, have the heart of a servant, humble yourself and be obedient. "Have the same mindset as Christ Jesus: Who, being in the nature of God, did not consider equality with God something to be used to his own advantage; rather, he made himself nothing by taking the very nature of a servant, being made in human likeness and being found in appearance as a man, he humbled himself by becoming obedient to death—even death on a cross!" (Phil. 2:5–8). In her book *Having a Mary Heart in a Martha World: Finding Intimacy With God in the Busyness of Life*, best-selling author and Bible teacher Joanna Weaver wrote: "The Lord has gone out of his way to make us his own. Yes, he died and rose again. He sent the Holy Spirit to teach and guide us. He's invested his own life to make us holy, and he'll take what we offer him and make it into something good. But we're still expected to partner in the process."[1]

Trying to do everything in your own power will produce stress. Bring your cares and worries to Him. The best prescription, with no expiration date, says, "Come, follow me" (Matt. 4:19). Find the direction God is leading you, and follow Him. When you are disoriented, discouraged, or depressed, and at a crossroads in life, just remember His instruction—follow Him.

We must also practice servanthood. To see the power of God working in your life you must humble yourself and feed on God's faithfulness. Follow Jesus' example and start helping others. Jesus wants to provide a fresh start for everyone, and through His Spirit new "spiritual DNA" is available for all. Find out His purpose for you, and you will have a new passion for this life, and a purpose to prepare for eternal life. Jesus came to give life more abundantly, and eternal life to those who believe in Him. He wants no one to perish. He gave selflessly, and so must we. Help others break free from bondage. You must put your life on the line by helping others. Help somebody who is broken and hurting; God's heart breaks for the needy and the lost. Sacrifice for others, help others, and let your light shine. People will see your light in your good works. You have a treasure in you, given by the Lord Jesus—His seed of love and compassion.

As you help others on your journey to your own destiny, people can be transformed by your acts of kindness. They will admire you and follow your example when you are doing good deeds, and God will be glorified. So many people have a broken spirit, and there is a crying need everywhere for kindness.

Give God the first place in your heart. He rules the universe, but He will not force His way in your heart. David, when devastated by sin, prayed, "Renew a steadfast spirit within me" (Ps. 51:10). With a renewed spirit your heart will break for others. Caring for others is the most wonderful thing. We provide the care, but Jesus heals the soul and the body. By helping others we can build a bridge for people who are seeking God.

Serving Others by Grace

> Rejoice with those who rejoice; mourn with those who mourn.
> —Romans 12:15

> Each one of you should use whatever gift you have received to serve others.
> —1 Peter 4:10

> His word burns in my heart like a fire.
> —Jeremiah 20:9, nlt

The Mirror Neurons

Joel Osteen, senior pastor of Lakewood Church in Houston—the nation's largest in weekly attendance—stated in his book *Your Best Life Now: 7 Steps to Living at Your Full Potential*: "When God created us, he put His supernatural love in all of our hearts. He's placed in you the potential to have a kind, caring, gentle, loving spirit. You have the ability to empathize, to feel what other people are feeling. Because you were created in the image of God, you have the moral capacity to experience God's compassion in your heart. But too often, because of our own selfishness, we choose to close our hearts to compassion."[2]

We know that God put mirror neurons in our brains so we can overcome evil through compassion and experience God's goodness and mercy in our lives (Rom. 12:21). Also, God made mirror neurons in our brains so we can lay up treasures in heaven for eternity through compassion for others and good deeds. Eternity is our true life. After our flesh has died, we will be more alive in heaven, where God is glorified forever. Mirror neurons in our brains build potential for eternal reward. Jesus had perfect mirror neurons and great compassion for humanity. He paid the ultimate price, dying on the cross for our sins so we could have eternal life.

God loves a joyful giver. Overcome worry by finding someone else who needs your compassion. God created our brains with the ability to follow His commandments. He is asking us to clothe ourselves with compassion, because He had compassion (Col. 3:12). He is not asking us to do something too difficult. He knows we have mirror neurons that are activated through the power of God to follow His prescriptions. Pharmacists know how companies develop medications to bind with receptors or enzymes in the body to achieve the proposed therapeutic level for a certain condition. God, the supreme scientist and pharmacist, gave us the Holy Spirit to activate our mirror neurons to have compassion for needy people, as it is written: "Each one of you should use whatever gift you have received to serve others" (1 Pet. 4:10). Compassion was His ultimate goal.

We were created for His glory, and we will bring Him glory for eternity. There are benefits beyond this life. Do good deeds and have an honorable character, refreshing others in your community and internationally. Jesus was moved with compassion when He fed the hungry multitudes, healed the sick, delivered the captives from demonic oppression, and raised the dead. Jesus wept at the tomb where Lazarus lay dead, because He mirrored the family's brokenness. What can you give when everything comes from Him? Everything is from Him, including our mirror neurons. Consider His goodness and come to Him with a willing attitude.

Through our mirror neurons we are able to feel other people's emotions.[3] If someone laughs, we laugh; if people cry, we cry. The Holy Spirit touches our mirror neurons to show favor, mercy, kindness, and gentleness, and to help us feel the pain of vulnerable people. Jesus instructed us to pray for the sick and heal them in His name. He gave us authority to do that, because He knew we have mirror neurons built in us to feel their pain. Because of those mirror neurons, we are able to feel the pain of those who suffer, and rejoice with those who rejoice, according to God's prescriptions: "Rejoice with those who rejoice; mourn with those who mourn" (Rom. 12:15). Many times my eyes are filled with tears of sadness and my heart is moved when I see so many needs here in the United States (especially at the free clinic where I volunteer). Then I find myself with tears of joy, when I see people recovering from sickness, or when I feel God's presence in my life. I know that I do not do that by my own power; it is the Holy Spirit who activates my mirror neurons.

We also have the second commandment, to love our neighbors like ourselves.

You have the capacity to repair the world around you by helping others. (See Isaiah 58:6–14.) The entire Bible is about God's prescriptions for love. He wants us to love one another as He first loved us.

Jesus, our example, poured out His character to the people around Him. His passion for people drove Him to the cross. We must have the same passion for the human race. Passion in your heart leads you to help others, to pray, and to provide emotional and physical support. Beth Moore wrote in *Jesus, the One and Only*: "Your heart means far more to Christ than anything. That your heart is utterly taken with Christ is more important than any amount of service you could render or rules you could keep. If Christ has your heart, He will have your obedience (John 14:21). God wants to completely captivate your heart and cause it to burn with passion for Him. It is His absolute priority for you according to Mark 12:30; joy and satisfaction will elude you in its absence."[4] Your spiritual passion for Christ will be ignited through prayer and studying the Word of God, the only way for true joy and satisfaction.

When the fire is burning inside you, and when the mirror neurons are activated, all your heart, mind, and soul burn with the desire to help others. I grew up in a very poor family, although I did not realize we were poor. I saw my family as one of the richest in the village, even though our home had dirt floors, beds made of wood and straw, and no electricity or indoor plumbing. From a young age, I always had the desire to share what I had and to help those around me. It seems like my mirror neurons in my brain were activated very early in life!

Whenever I heard that a person was in need, I would share what I had. One time as a teenager, I felt compassion in my heart so strongly for others that I put what few clothes I had in a small box and sent it to a needy family who had nothing (keeping only two blouses, two skirts, one pair of shoes, two pair of socks, and one scarf). I did not buy new ones for a while, because I had enough compared with those who had nothing.

Another time in Bucharest, I visited a family with twelve children. As I scrutinized the house I saw on the kitchen table a fresh onion, with a few slices of very low quality salami (made of cartilage and fat) for dinner. I realized that was the single meal for that day for the whole family. Deep in my soul, I cried out in prayer to the Lord to help this family. At that time people could not prosper because of the tight controls of the communist dictators. God answered my prayers, and in a few years I received my visa to leave the country. God has blessed us richly, so we are able to help others now, including that family.

Don't ever give up when you pray. God hears your cries and gives you your heart's desires. He will either answer your prayers, or change the desire of your heart until you pray a different way. The passion of God overwhelms you and changes your thinking, language, attitude, work, and deeds. You cannot keep passion inside. It finds an outlet. As Psalm 42:1 says, "As the deer pants for steams of water, so my soul pants for you, my God." Passion is a continual desire to pray, to serve with all your heart, to love deeply, to drink from the Word of God's living water, to give with joy, and "not grow weary while doing good" (Gal. 6:9, NKJV).

Your stress level will decrease when you have the kind of servant's heart outlined in Mark 10:42–45, and as Jesus taught in John 13:34, to love as the Lord loved us. When you lay down your life for others, God's blessings will explode in your life (1 John 3:16). True servanthood is to serve not only when it is convenient. Jesus served His disciples and the people around Him to the end. He had a servant's heart to love, even to death on the cross. Do things you are not comfortable with, and you do not feel like doing. Many times I felt like I needed to stop spending my time volunteering in a small clinic for a disadvantaged and marginalized population, but the small voice inside me activated my mirror neurons and did not let me quit. Sometimes there were people who did not have even five dollars in their pocket to spend on food or medication.

Jesus loved the community where He lived, and He tells us to love our neighbors as ourselves. Our whole community is our neighbor. Jesus had a passion for His ministry and compassion for the people around Him. His heart was moved with compassion for people's physical and emotional needs, to the point of crying for them. When was the last time you cried for someone who had a great need? Love others as Jesus did.

God has a calling for each person on earth. He is patient for each of us to come to know Him, because He put the thought of eternity in mankind since creation (Eccles. 3:11). God also gives people gifts and talents. Time is the greatest treasure on this planet, but it passes by very fast. We must fulfill our calling for this short life by helping and serving others. We need to live with eternity in our thoughts and be heavenly minded.

It is not about us, but as Jesus said in Matthew 5:16, to shine our light to those around us. God put us in a community for a reason—to pray for that community, to serve with all our hearts, to spend our resources and energies on those in need and feel their pain. In our business we have opportunities to serve the underserved population, and we discover that many of these people were homeless at some point in their lives, or orphans given up for adoption, or abandoned in their childhood, living on the margins—a life full of discouragement. But God brings them into our care facility to spend their last years, months, and days with us, and we treat them like royalty. We do not differentiate between the homeless and the very rich, or a highly educated person with a PhD. We embrace them, give them hugs, and encourage them so they will feel accepted and loved. When I told one elderly patient he is special and I love him, he replied, "You make me smile. I did not smile for five years."

We understand that this is our calling in life. We can have compassion for people who live in very stressful situations—one person at a time. It pleases God when we are clothed with humility, serving others. Your stress level will diminish when you have the approach that "whoever wants to become great among you must be your servant" (Mark 10:43). Jesus instructed us to "Love one another. As I have loved you, so you must love one another" (John 13:34). When you lay down your life for others, blessings will chase you. "Jesus Christ laid down His life for us. And we ought to lay down our lives for our brothers and sisters" (1 John 3:16). When I'm volunteering, I get so busy I don't have time to focus on my problems. I am happy when I can make a difference in someone's life. I prefer to serve, rather than to be in their shoes. I count my blessings when I see so many needs and so much pain in others. God puts us in places to help others, and to tell our story.

God is there when you go through tough situations. Jesus is listening to what we have to say. He answers us in our pain. He weeps with those who are weeping. We are sometimes unemotional toward other people because of our own emotional pain. Sometimes I feel that—because of our busy lives—we are dehumanized and care too little for others. Jesus wept for Lazarus, and for his family's pain. Jesus wept for the entire city of Jerusalem, and for all the generations on earth until His coming again. What God put in us we must share with others.

As a primary care provider, I realized that I could help people who had fallen through the cracks (lost their jobs and/or their health insurance), and people who could not afford to buy insurance or could not qualify for social programs. Those people were desperate, suffering from many acute and chronic conditions, and without access to the health care system. I always wanted to be a missionary—to help people in need and to tell them about the love of Jesus. It never crossed my mind that I would come to the United States to serve needy minorities—immigrants from around the world who have no possible way to pay for their health services. Besides my business (providing care to elderly and frail people with multiple chronic conditions and neurocognitive disorders since 1990) I have accumulated more than five thousand hours taking care of patients in a free health clinic. In my private practice I serve the most vulnerable population: minorities who have no place to go for care. I choose to, because I was taught at church (the Romanian Church, and New Beginnings Christian Center in the Portland area) that if God blesses us, He does so with a purpose, so we can bless others.

TIME WELL SPENT

> Give, and it will be given to you. A good measure, pressed down, shaken together and running over, will be poured into your lap. For with the measure you use, it will be measured to you.
>
> —Luke 6:38

Time well spent is a huge factor in reducing stress. Have you spent time telling others about your hope in Christ? Those who are wise shall shine like the brightness of the firmament, and those who turn many to righteousness will be like the stars forever and ever (Dan. 12:3). That promise from God will bring you much peace and dissipate your frustration from the world's stressors. Statistics say that the average American spends a total of 14.6 years watching television during his or her lifetime.[5] Can you imagine 14.6 years of sitting in front of that box, clicking away time day and night, seven days a week? What a wasted life.

The Bible speaks of many rewards in heaven, even crowns, for those who have faithfully served the Lord. In fact, I think we will be shocked when the awards are presented in heaven. Each one of us will be judged based on our deeds on Earth. When you get to heaven, what will you have to show for your life? All of your accomplishments will be evaluated when you stand before Christ.

It is not so much a judgment for sin, because all sins if confessed are forgiven by Jesus, but a judgment of how we spent our time. Did you have more passion or excitement for your career, or for a sport, or your possessions, than you had for the things of God? Did you spend your time carelessly, doing nothing for the kingdom of God? Do not let anybody distract you or move you from your faithful walk with God. Be faithful in everything you do and your reward will be great. Your crown is waiting for you.

God wants to capture our attention and make a change in our schedule. He wants our heart to break for what breaks His. In Romania, when I was about seventeen, I traveled six hundred kilometers (about 370 miles) north from Bucharest to see my parents. I had very little money at that time—just enough for food and the trip. I heard about a family with many children (one of them was mentally ill) who lived six kilometers (3.7 miles) from my parents. I walked to their house to give them the little money I had saved from my meager income. When I arrived at their house the little girl (about six or seven) sat naked in the middle of the backyard, her little body so covered with dirt and mud that it was hard to distinguish even her beautiful, innocent eyes. The mother invited me into their house with a dirt floor, and we knelt and prayed with many tears. I left some money for clothes for her little girl. I felt so blessed. On the way back home I was "flying," praising God and leaping for joy because I had brought a ray of hope to that mother and her daughter.

I felt God's hand on me all the way home. Blessings started flowing in my life then, and have continued until today. It was because my heart was broken for that little girl. "Give, and it will be given to you. A good measure, pressed down, shaken together and running over, will be poured into your lap. For with the measure you use, it will be measured to you" (Luke 6:38).

That verse in Luke literally came true in my life. I see now that obeying the Word of God has become my biography. It is not about the "prosperity" mentality. It is God's economy, because God loves a cheerful giver. It is not only about money. If your heart is broken for the needy and suffering, God's heart is broken for you. God's Word doesn't fail. We still continue to give generously to those with a broken heart, or living in poverty, to honor God.

Evangelist, Bible teacher, and best-selling author John Bevere stated in his book *Honor's Reward: How to Attract God's Favor and Blessing*:

We are to value, esteem, respect, and reverence Him above anyone or anything. We dishonor Him if we value anyone or anything above Him. He is the Great King; He is worthy to receive all our respect, not just a portion. To God alone does our honor transcend to worship. Remember, the ultimate goal is to honor God.[6]

HE REJOICES OVER YOU

He will take great delight in you; in his love he will no longer rebuke you, but will rejoice over you with singing.

—ZEPHANIAH 3:17

To manage stress more effectively, sing and rejoice, because nothing can stop you when you have a happy attitude. Happiness and joy are contagious. People like being around joyful people who smile and laugh, and God instructs us to "shout and be glad" (Zech. 2:10). Sing and make a melody in your heart to the Lord, "and walk in the way of love, just as Christ loved us and gave himself up for us as a fragrant offering and sacrifice to God" (Eph. 5:2). Make a decision to glorify God. "May God who gives endurance and encouragement give you the same attitude of mind toward each other that Jesus Christ had" (Rom. 15:5). He is singing and rejoicing over you! Zephaniah 3:17 says He will take great delight us. He is looking for us to rejoice in Him as we follow His supernatural prescriptions.

God has encoded the ability to be joyful and to sing for joy into our DNA. We need revelation to stir the passion of Christ and the joy of the Lord. Everything we do with passion will be remembered in generations to come. Sometimes other people misunderstand our passion. Remember the story in Mark of the woman who broke the alabaster jar to anoint Jesus' head with oil? She sacrificed more than a year's wages because of her passion for the Lord. (See Mark 14:3–5.) When you sacrifice, your passion flows freely. We should live out our Christian life with joy—not out of obligation. During the communist era people would ask why I didn't serve the Lord secretly, so I could still get promotions. Although I had the degree needed for a managerial position, I couldn't get promoted because I believed in God. That went against the communist doctrine: "There is no God." But I had so much joy I wasn't able to hide it from people, and for me, God was first, promotion second.

In my heart I always desired to please God, even though I realized that the communists around me despised my Christian beliefs. At the same time, I observed that they liked the fruit of the Spirit in my life, flowing from the biblical standards I lived by. I was fascinated by that contradictory attitude of the communists toward me. I couldn't have had a Christian's walk without faith in the Lord Jesus Christ. God's Word changed my walk with God, through the power of the Holy Spirit. Since the age of thirteen, I've had that burning desire to tell others about Jesus and how His powerful Word changes people's lives.

During high school, I had communist friends living immoral, adulterous, miserable lifestyles, with no hope for the future. I remember one time during a break I was looking through an open window, feeling the breeze from outside on the third floor, when a fragile young girl who had watched me for a few years approached slowly and asked me with tearful eyes if she could be like me. In her brokenness, she started to pour out her heart. In her desperation, she wanted to find peace for her troubled heart and hope for her future.

The joy of salvation that Jesus has poured into us, we must pour into others' hearts. God loved us so we can love others; He forgave us so we can forgive others; had mercy on us so we can have mercy for others. When you receive Jesus Christ in your heart, He "will rejoice over you with singing" (Zeph. 3:17). There is a supernatural activation of your spiritual DNA. You receive a more tender heart, are able to forgive others, and you become a new creation with a new personality, a new character, a new joy.

Gain by Giving

> Then the King will say to those on His right, "Come, you who are blessed by my Father; take your inheritance, the kingdom prepared for you since the creation of the world. For I was hungry and you gave me something to eat, I was thirsty and you gave me something to drink, I was a stranger and you invited me in, I needed clothes and you clothed me, I was sick and you looked after me, I was in prison and you came to visit me."
>
> —Matthew 25:34–36

I want to be transparent about our walk with God, and how we dealt with high levels of stress in our own life, by giving. Since arriving in the United States, we have always given to ministries, to poor orphans and widows, and to churches and other charitable organizations. I have worked as a doctor and a nurse practitioner, volunteering for more than fifteen years, first as a registered nurse and later as a primary care provider after earning my doctorate in nursing from Oregon Health & Science University. I help organize annual health fairs for those with great needs, and provide free consultations. We help people who cannot afford health insurance and have no financial or material resources to pay for health care. We also have provided treatment to many needy people in the United States and abroad. We sent clothes and medications to Romania several times and conducted free consultations there when on mission trips. We have not stopped giving and serving since 1990. That was "bread cast on water," and now that bread is coming back to us in a rich harvest through so many blessings and unmerited favor from God, as His Word promises.

Pastor Joel Osteen refers many times to the story of his mother, Dodie. Diagnosed with cancer in 1981, she had just weeks to live. Naturally, she should have been on comfort measures and end-of-life care for her terminal condition, but she chose at that time to declare healing Scriptures. She enveloped herself in God's promises for healing. She also started to focus on other people's needs and prayed for their healing. She was healed by God's supernatural power and nearly four decades later was still alive and well.[7] When you serve others, your faith will increase. Your love will be contagious as you love unconditionally and serve those around you and become radically generous. You will generously care for others, have more influence in people's lives, and the world will see that you have a different spirit. You gain by giving.

COMPASSION CHANGES THE ATMOSPHERE

> Walk in the way of love, just as Christ loved us and gave himself up for us as a fragrant offering and sacrifice to God.
> —EPHESIANS 5:2

Caring for lost people is compassion in action. Jesus was moved with compassion each time He met people suffering from physical and spiritual diseases. Emotions are universal; in every culture people are crying and laughing. Everywhere in the world people need food, water, clothing, and shelter. Just as physical needs are universal, spiritual needs are universal too. We must share what we have with other people. People need Christ, wherever they live on the planet. To change the atmosphere, we must speak life and words of encouragement to everyone.

Be the voice for the most vulnerable and afflicted people, with compassionate love. The anterior cingulate is stimulated by compassion for others, keeping your brain healthy and active.[8] The parietal lobe keeps you separated from the world and helps you forget your problems when you are in fellowship with God the Father.[9] Prayer puts our focus on others rather than on ourselves and our own problems, thus reducing our stress.

Compassion changes the atmosphere in the brain—and in real life. Love requires compassion, and we can love lost people by praying and fasting for them. Seek the lost and watch for opportunities to help others. Your faith and your prayers will activate the compassion neurons (spindle neurons in the anterior cingulate) used for social skills, to help use your emotions in a positive way.[10]

Jesus came into our world to teach us how to live. When Jesus arrived in a place, the atmosphere there changed. In Nain, He encountered a widow at a funeral service. Moved with compassion by her pain, He raised her son from the dead (Luke 7:15). When Jesus enters your heart, soul, and mind, the spiritual atmosphere will change, and healthy amounts of neurotransmitters will be released in your brain. You will demonstrate more fruit of the Spirit and respond with more compassion. You will be different. Your thinking and the atmosphere in your brain will change in Jesus' presence. Compassion changes you, and your compassion changes the people in your sphere of influence. All we need is love. Because God is love, we need God. Never confuse love with the lusts of the world.

When you truly love, you are moved into action. When God pours love deep in your soul, it creates a new atmosphere in your brain and changes your heart toward each person you encounter. We know that sexual love is based on surging dopamine levels (the pleasure neurochemical) for a short moment in your brain, and later in your marriage as oxytocin (the love neurotransmitter). That is from God, and it is useful to sustain your marriage. Spiritual love is superior to fleshly love. A spiritually loving person says no to worldly things and temporary lusts and has a blessed life with a tender, caring, generous heart. Invest time in spiritual love that creates a place of recovery. As Galatians 6:9 teaches, we should never lose hope.

Start to care authentically for those in need. We are responsible on earth to help somebody in need (Phil. 2:19–21) because it matters to God. God cared for us. He came to earth and walked on the Via Dolorosa (way of sorrows) for all human beings. He shed His blood and gave His life for you and me. Where would all of us be if Jesus had not died on the cross for us? You know there is chaos in many parts of the world. Those are the regions where we must bring Jesus. Where Jesus is, the atmosphere is changed. Jesus was moved with compassion when He walked on this planet. We need to move into action. Compassion moves us to do something, even if it costs us in comfort, health, and resources.

When my doctor friend was on her deathbed, it stirred up so much compassion in my heart that I gave up my free time and embraced the inconvenience of helping her. I was available to her during the worst time of her life, when she was so vulnerable in her last days, dying of cancer. Compassion will move your heart. Driving home late at night, after long hours of work caring for sick people, then spending time at her house, rivers of tears would flow because of the compassion activated in me by Christ. I did not feel exhausted from those long hours of giving. I was just overwhelmed by emotion from seeing her suffering. The spindle neurons in my anterior cingulate were stretched to the maximum then, and the emotions in my amygdala were used in a positive way.

VALUE PEOPLE

> But when you give a banquet, invite the poor, the crippled, the lame, the blind, and you will be blessed.
> —Luke 14:13–14

Value everyone, even those who hurt you. People have values, even if they are different from yours. As a young girl in Bucharest, when everything was under the tight control of the communists, we were not allowed to communicate with people from other nations who came to study there. I remember the first time I met an African student. She visited our church and we became good friends. We visited each other, prayed together, and visited my parents in the northern part of the country, where people had never seen a black African. They were in awe and embraced her fellowship, giving her gifts. It was very risky, but it was amazing because we shared the same Jesus.

Here in the United States I have had close friends from Japan, the Philippines, Ethiopia, Vietnam, Russia, Ukraine, and Africa. Three years after I got to the United States, I met an international student from Japan named Hiro. She was completely different from me, but when we started to talk, we found we had many things in common. We spoke different languages, but only a little English. We had little money, but loved the same Savior. We were created by the same Father and both followed His culture. That brought us very close. She spent three months in our house for free to save some money for a mission trip. In similar ways, God activated my spindle neurons to develop social relationships and to have compassion for others in immediate need. The Bible instructs us to love the "strangers" beyond our own personal world. We have the potential, through the spindle neurons in our anterior cingulate, to "take" His prescription, develop social relationships, show compassion, and value people beyond science.

Look at life from Jesus' perspective and your attitude will change. Be open-minded. Open your heart for others of a different color, a different culture, a different nation, or a different profession. That's why we have those spindle neurons in the anterior cingulate of our brains. I worked with minorities, because they are the most vulnerable population. But we all are so much alike in our feelings. We all laugh, cry, have joy, and feel pain. We are created by the same Creator and have the same Father and same Savior. We all have feelings. He invites all of us to be like Jesus, who in Luke 14:12–14 taught us that when we give a banquet, we should invite the crippled, the lame, and the poor, and we will be blessed. When I started volunteering as a primary care provider, I did not know what kind of people I was going to serve. I just wanted to use my knowledge and my profession in the community, and I ended up serving the neediest from around the world. People have left me notes, thanking me for saving their lives when they had no access to medical care for their acute or chronic conditions. Reach out, be friendly, and God will honor your sincere efforts.

No Competition

Competition increases our stress. Without Jesus, we were enemies of God, but He showered us with His mercy and grace. Putting on the mind of Christ will reduce your stress level, and you can stop comparing yourself with others. The stress of competition dissolves when your mirror neurons (for compassion) are activated. Instead of struggling to please everyone, simply humble yourself, desire to please God, and have the attitude which was in Christ Jesus. Humble yourself and He will exalt you. Knowing Jesus and being more like Him will free you from desiring competition and all its stress. He is pleased when you say, "I want to be like Jesus." He likes that attitude. God is transforming people's lives and changing destinies. The potential is in you to change yourself, if you choose to do so.

Chapter 23

PRAYER REDUCES STRESS

Blessed is the one...whose delight is in the law of the Lord, and who meditates on his law day and night.
—Psalm 1:1–2

MEDITATION THROUGH PRAYER is the best way to cope with stress. Scientific literature has documented prayer's healthy impact on the brain. Prayer enhances your ability to perform and solve problems. It also reduces stress; decreases anxiety; prevents panic attacks, depression, and bad behavior; corrects unhealthy emotions; reduces pain; lowers blood pressure; promotes rapid healing; and prevents infection. Prayer promotes good behavior and wise choices. Prayer promotes a healthier lifestyle, triggering a positive attitude that leads to physical and emotional health.

Meditation through prayer will calm an overactive brain and positively stimulate its structure. Neuroscientists have discovered that the frontal lobe can shrink with aging, causing Alzheimer's disease, but prayer stimulates the frontal lobe and prevents shrinkage! Prayer is an antiaging exercise that causes new neurons to develop when you meditate in prayer. Through prayer you activate the mirror neurons and develop compassion for others, which positively affects the anterior cingulate, the brain area responsible for compassion and empathy.[1]

Prayer reduces activity in the parietal lobe, causing you to forget about your own problems and focus on other people's needs. The parietal lobe helps you separate from worldly things and forget your problems. Prayer activates the compassion center in your anterior cingulate area, suppressing worry about your own emotional and physical pain.[2]

SCIENTIFIC BENEFITS OF PRAYER AND MEDITATION

In one study, prayer significantly increased pain tolerance in 202 patients with chronic pain.[3] Scientists have proven that prayer and meditation help patients cope better with pain and stressful situations, and they can be included in pain management as coping mechanisms to manage stress from chronic diseases.[4] Scientists have proven that God's instructions and promises work in people's life. Prayer and meditation will create an atmosphere in your brain to create new neurons through neurogenesis, improve your cognition, positively affect your decision-making ability, slow the aging process, and increase your quality of life.

FREQUENT PRAYER AND YOUR HEALTH

"Pray without ceasing" is what God tells us we should do in 1 Thessalonians 5:17 (NKJV). The wisdom of this prescription is demonstrated by another study showing that patients who prayed more often, forgave more, and those who attended church services handled stress better by excreting less cortisol and lowering blood pressure.[5] Low cortisol will also preserve the function of the immune system, prevent diabetes, and prevent certain infections and cancer.

Prayer is important for children too. Children and teenagers need prayer to cope with stress and struggles with peer pressure. One study found that prayer influenced children positively in their health and social connections.[6] Children's behavior is affected by all the abnormal neurotransmitters and hormones released in the body during adolescence, causing more emotional and physical pain and more behavior problems. Prayer will calm the overactive brain, reduce anxiety, lower the cortisol level, and promote healthy growth in children.

PRAYER AND CHRONIC ILLNESS

Prayer works even for people who are dying from incurable diseases, shown by a study where long survival was related to both frequency of prayer (positively) and judgmental attitude (negatively), and that patients with AIDS who prayed experienced "less distress, more hope, social support, healthier behaviors, helping others, and lower cortisol levels."[7] It has been demonstrated through recent studies that people have better physical and psychological health when their mindfulness is at a higher level. These people experience fewer episodes of mood disorder and cope better with stress. But many people become vulnerable and experience the consequences of stress when their mindfulness decreases.[8] A high level of mindfulness is obtained through constantly studying the Word of God. Doing what it tells us to do promotes psychological and physical health. In addition, meditation has neurological benefits that are like a medical treatment, affecting the cingulate cortex, which regulates mood.[9]

Scientists agree that meditation is powerful in regulating the release of neurotransmitters and their receptors in the body. Beyond science, the Book of Joshua admonishes: "Keep this Book of the Law always on your lips; meditate on it day and night, so that you may be careful to do everything written in it. Then you will be prosperous and successful" (Josh. 1:8). Illness and disease cannot make you prosperous and successful. Physical and spiritual health will give satisfaction to your body and soul, and they are necessary for a prosperous and successful life.

Psalm 1:3 says the person who meditates on God's law is like "a tree planted by streams of water, which yields its fruits in season and whose leaf does not wither—whatever they do prospers." Meditate on the Word of God. When the Word is stored in your brain it "waters" your thoughts in the neurons, yielding the "fruit" of healthy actions. Healthy thinking will become a normal part of your being (your "spiritual" DNA), producing good fruit and helping you prosper in your body, mind, and spirit. Your dendrites in your neurons, the nerve cells you use for thinking and cognition, have the configuration of a tree where thoughts flow. If those neurons have the "living water" of the Word of God, your soul, body, and mind will prosper in health, your body will be healthy, your emotions and relationships with family, friends, and others in society will be healthy, and you will prosper. Our Lord delights when His servants prosper in health, family relationships, and friendships in the church and community: "May those who delight in my vindication shout for joy and gladness; may they always say, 'The LORD be exalted, who delights in the well-being of his servant'" (Ps. 35:27).

THE ATMOSPHERE FOR NEUROGENESIS

Scientific literature also verifies that meditation creates an atmosphere for neurogenesis in the brain. These new neurons improve memory and diminish the chances for neurocognitive disorders and Alzheimer's disease. It also slows the aging process. Meditation is a strong part of your lifelong antiaging formula. With such great benefits from meditation, people would be wise to follow God's prescription.

Thinking beyond your circumstances requires creativity and meditation that creates new neurons. The great psalmist, David, never knew about neurogenesis, but he was inspired by the Holy Spirit to write about a renewal of our minds when we hunger for the Word of God and meditate on His precepts.

All of God's prescriptions have positive outcomes, according to the promises written in the Word of God. All instructions found in God's Rx lead to positive results: "Whatever is true, whatever is noble, whatever is right, whatever is pure, whatever is lovely whatever is admirable—if anything is excellent or praiseworthy—think about such things" (Phil. 4:8). God put purpose in everything for your good, even though sometimes you may see only the opposite.

When memorized scriptures pop into your conscious mind, your life will be changed. There is a still, small voice—the Holy Spirit—who speaks to our conscience and transforms our lives if we obey. The Word of God is God's breath. He breathes life into every cell of your body, reprogramming your "spiritual" DNA. You receive Christ's "spiritual DNA" when you invite Him to come into your heart through His Holy Spirit. You need to "feed" your mind with the Bible. Read the Bible to nourish your spiritual soul. As you eat spiritual food you nourish your spiritual DNA, which makes you the person you are, spiritually, with the personality needed to fulfill your destiny.

Let the Word of God occupy your mind and heart and take control over your feelings, thoughts, and emotions. Life is in the Word of God. God wants the Word to live in us so we can live in truth, love, and peace and have a healthy body, soul, and mind.

Prayer... Beyond Science

> The LORD is my portion; therefore I will wait for Him. The LORD is good to those whose hope is in him, to the one who seeks him."
> —Lamentations 3:24–25

Professor and nurse practitioner Dr. Mary Helming explains, "Prayer serves as a connection to God but secondly, prayer bonds human beings to human beings. Surely a sense of oneness with humanity and oneness with the Divine were essential aspects of the lived experience of healing through prayer."[10] Medical and health care providers also recognize that there is good evidence supporting the physical and spiritual benefits from prayer.

Dr. David Levy, an award-winning neurosurgeon, said in his book, *Gray Matter: A Neurosurgeon Discovers the Power of Prayer... One Patient at a Time*:

> As I have addressed patients' spirituality and made prayer a regular part of my patient interactions, the response has been impressive. I have seen lives brought to a level of spiritual, emotional, and physical health that my patients had never enjoyed before. In the process, I have learned two important things: that there is a limit to what I can do as a highly trained and experienced surgeon and that there is no limit to what God can do to touch a person emotionally and spiritually, not just physically.[11]

When we pray without ceasing, we can expect supernatural results. Praying in the Holy Spirit brings supernatural results. The Holy Spirit intercedes for our needs and knows the answers to our prayers.

A new chapter in your life starts with prayer. Jesus prayed with a loud voice—He cried out and prayed earnestly. Jesus wrestled with God for His future, especially in the Garden of Gethsemane before giving His life for the sin of the world. Prayer becomes powerful when we wrestle with God, and then say, "Thy will be done" (Matt. 6:10, kjv). Many Bible characters wrestled with God and—like Jacob—refused to quit "unless You bless me" (Gen. 32:26). They knew God's will was to bless them. God had something good for them, and He has something good for you too. In fact, everything you have comes from God. Through prayer you can rekindle your passion for His presence and His blessings.

When you are passionate for God, all things become new, as 2 Corinthians 5:17 says. To follow God's will and stay on the right path to your goal, you must have a vision. A new passion will bring a new destiny and a life transformed. Transformation, new vision, and revelation for new things come through fervent prayer. When you pray, hearts are transformed, lives change, cities are blessed, and nations are revived. Do not give up in prayer. (See 2 Corinthians 4.)

Since arriving in the United States in 1990, I focused on the possibilities of open doors, yet realized that nothing happens without prayer. I faced all the challenges of a different culture, but because of Jesus I found out that in Christ there is the same culture—heaven's culture—and it is global. Having passion, praying and standing in the gap for the needs of others, and seeing opportunities to serve will transform you and those around you. For all your generous prayer, passion, love, caring, emotional support, experience, training, and devotion, the reward will be in heaven. The wise men sacrificed their time, energy, and material possessions, to come worship the King of kings and the Lord of lords when Jesus was born on earth. They came to worship. Worship is the most important part of your prayers.

I cannot wait to see what God will do in my future. For the past several years, I have been prompted by the Holy Spirit to pray for about an hour almost every morning. I know from my past that perseverance brings victory, and I am forceful in my prayers through the power of Holy Spirit. The assertive woman who had the issue of bleeding for twelve years reached out boldly, touched Jesus' garment as He walked by, and laid hands on her destiny. (See Luke 8:43–48.) Step into the future forcefully and boldly with a brand-new perspective for a safe and healthy future. God can do anything. Ask Him to do something supernatural, something beyond your own power.

To enter into the spiritual realm where the supernatural is normal, you need forceful prayer to break through the enemy's strongholds. Charles Stanley is a Bible teacher and senior pastor of a noted megachurch in Atlanta. In his book, *Handle With Prayer: Discovering God's Strength for Living*, he stated, "Our responsibility as Christians is to tear down these strongholds through Spirit-filled prayers. How? There is only one weapon—the sword of the Spirit. We must fight these lies with God's Word. We must fight specific lies with specific truths."[12]

You need God's power to know that God is with you when you pray. God gives you power to do things that you cannot do by yourself. He gives you everything you need when you access Him through the power of prayer. God will accomplish in us what He called us to do, more than we can ask or imagine. So everything you have—talents; profession; expertise; wisdom, your power to invent, create, and innovate; your network; and your relationships—are gifts from God. Step into His presence and access God's power for a new mind and a new thinking process. It is God's idea to bless you through prayer.

How was I able to overcome so many things in my life without compromising my faith? It was only through prayer. God has promises for you and your life. Finding God's way for your life takes discipline in prayer. It is like when physicians prescribe exercises for their patients that fit their condition. You start exercising to promote your health and prevent diseases in your body, including your mind. The doctor gives you directions about what kinds of food to eat, with the right nutrients for health. But the benefits from following the great physician's prescriptions, to pray without ceasing and walk in God's way, are eternal.

God wants to restore your physical and spiritual health through a life of prayer. His mercy is new every morning, restoring your future. "Because of the Lord's great love we are not consumed, for his compassions never fail. They are new every morning; great is your faithfulness. I say to myself, 'The Lord is my portion; therefore I will wait for him. The Lord is good to those whose hope is in him, to the one who seeks him" (Lam. 3:22–25). He wants to bless you when you hope in Him and wait for Him. Waiting for Him is an active process; do not let anything disrupt your connection with God. I have received showers of blessings through fasting and prayer. Try a new experience. Fasting and praying makes us strong spiritually. Faith and confidence in God's promises will bring joy and peace, and the love inside you will increase when you believe, trust, and continue to pray.

Prayer for His Glory

> Not to us, Lord, not to us, but to your name be the glory, because of your love and faithfulness.
>
> —Psalm 115:1

David's fame spread far and wide when God used him to destroy the enemy, because he did everything for the glory of the Lord. (Read the Book of Psalms.) David was constantly connected with Jehovah Elohim, the King of the universe, giving Him glory in his prayers. Nothing just happens or is an accident or a coincidence. We should never take the glory for what we have received from God because the glory belongs only to God. The highest calling in this world is to be like Jesus Christ, who prayed without ceasing and served others tirelessly. The Holy Spirit will give you the power to accomplish what you cannot do in your own abilities. To build and to heal your house, you must care for others, spend your life for your family, and pour out your life for others. Then it will be well with you for God's glory.

Chapter 24

GIVING THANKS

*Rejoice always; pray without ceasing; in everything give thanks;
for this is the will of God for you in Christ Jesus.*
—1 THESSALONIANS 5:16–18, NASB

Enter his gates with thanksgiving, and his courts with praise.
—PSALM 100:4

TRUSTING GOD AND His promises will create in us an attitude of thanksgiving. God promised in 2 Corinthians 9:8 that His children will be sufficient in all things. God will supply all your needs (Phil. 4:19) through prayer, if you believe (Mark 11:24). When discouraging thoughts flood your mind, claim the verse, "I can do all this through him who gives me strength" (Phil. 4:13).

In 2010, I was invited to speak at a women's conference for mothers of children with disabilities in Iași, Romania. Organizers asked me to encourage them and teach them ways to manage stress. You might have stress, but imagine having three disabled children who will never be able to walk, speak, or function normally in society for the rest of their lives. Those parents were devastated. They felt like they were always carrying a dying person on their shoulder. Fittingly, the conference motto was the words of Philippians 4:13.

Many tears flowed at that conference. I had to stay strong, even though inside I felt like crying the whole time. I had nothing to offer them but an abundance of tears of compassion, flowing down my face. They were crying more, mirroring my compassion for them! I felt like the least qualified person to speak at that conference, because I could give them nothing. Still, the Word of God and His promises were sufficient. Participants were encouraged because the Word of God has the power to comfort anyone through the power of the Holy Spirit. As Paul wrote to the Corinthians: "And He said to me, 'My grace is sufficient for you, for My strength is made perfect in weakness'", and, "Therefore I take pleasure in infirmities, in reproaches, in needs, in persecutions, in distresses, for Christ's sake" (2 Cor. 12:9–10, NKJV). Out of your painful situations and brokenness a great destiny is possible.

Like these children's parents, you may be asking why God allowed these children to be born with disabilities. I asked the same question myself. The answer: God wants to get our attention to remind us that life is short. We are not our own, and He wants to shine through our disabilities and brokenness. We need to stop, reflect, be thankful, and show love to those around us so God can receive the glory. All life is in God's hands. These children have their destiny too—to awaken the rest of us to live with eternity in mind and to be thankful for our lives. We are more than conquerors in Jesus. (See Romans 8:37.)

God answers your prayers so the Father will be glorified in the Son (John 14:13). He is ready to give us all things when we ask according to His will (Rom. 8:32). As Psalm 103:2–4 says, your iniquities are forgiven and all your diseases are healed. So nothing is held against you to hinder your prayer when you live in obedience. He who redeemed your life from destruction offers mercy and lovingkindness. A thankful heart will calm an overreacting mind.

GRATITUDE

> He who offers a sacrifice of thanksgiving honors Me; and to him who orders his way aright I shall show the salvation of God.
> —PSALM 50:23, NASB

Giving thanks to God with a grateful heart brings you peace, but many things can block our gratitude. The greatest quality of the human soul is thankfulness, which should be our basic Christian attitude. On one of my visits to Romania, the small voice inside me started insisting, "Bring thanksgiving as a sacrifice, because everything you asked God has done for you, and He will continue to give to you more than you ask." I did not need to hear that inner voice twice. Right away I began a "Daniel Fast." (This is a twenty-one or forty-day partial fast of fruits and vegetables only, to give the Lord thanks for everything He has done in our lives.) By offering praise and giving thanks in everything, we glorify God. As 1 Thessalonians 5:16–18 tells us, this is the will of God.

All our prayers should incorporate thanksgiving. In her book *The Armor of God*, author, Bible teacher, and actress Priscilla Shirer stated that "gratitude to God for who He is and what He's already done should thread throughout every prayer, because ultimately His name and His fame are the only reasons any of this matters."[1] Give thanks and praise to the Lord at all times. Shall we not accept adversity as we accept blessings? You must praise God no matter what you are going through, to release the blessings of God in your life.

What about when everything goes wrong? God ultimately programs everything in our lives according to His will. Paul's "thorn in the flesh," outlined in 2 Corinthians 12:7–9, strengthened his character. Jesus' crucifixion brought the joy of salvation and an eternal inheritance to the entire world. God develops endurance in us for the long run. He develops and strengthens our character. God plans events behind the scene to strengthen us. We put our hope in Him, not only here on earth but for eternity.

Keep looking ahead to what God has for you. Paul learned to be content with every circumstance in life. The key to a peaceful life without stress is thankfulness in every situation. This will keep all your brain neurochemicals in balance, as we know from Philippians. "Be anxious for nothing, but in everything by prayer and supplication with thanksgiving let your requests be made known to God. And the peace of God, which surpasses all comprehension, shall guard your hearts and your minds in Christ Jesus" (Phil. 4:6–7, NASB).

When you start to feel anxious, recognize the anxiety as a call to prayer to calm your overreacting brain. Beginning your prayer with thanksgiving will link your spirit to the peace of God, guarding and keeping you in Christ. Prayer is likened to incense in Scripture, and thanksgiving is the ingredient that makes your prayer a "sweet savor" to the Lord. You have so much to thank the Lord for that you could keep on thanking Him forever, and it wouldn't be long enough. The Bible's strongest prescription to prevent anxiety is the rejoicing theme of 1 Thessalonians 5:16–18. Giving thanks reminds us of good things and brings joy to our heart and soul. Neuroscientists have found that rejoicing causes the right atmosphere in the brain to release a healthy amount of natural antianxiety and antidepressant neurotransmitters (endorphins, serotonin, oxytocin and dopamine), which will heal the cells damaged by stress.[2]

GIVE THANKS

The Word of God says, "In everything give thanks." You must believe that "God causes all things to work together for good for those who love God, to those who are called according to His purpose" (Rom. 8:28, NASB). It's not easy to give thanks for all things, but if you do, you benefit from walking in faith, pleasing God, and showing Him that you trust Him.

Be thankful every day. Sing and rejoice! Nothing can stop you when you have a happy attitude. Happiness and joy are contagious. People enjoy being around joyful people who smile and laugh. The Book of Zechariah says, "Shout and be glad" (Zech. 2:10). Sing and make melody in your heart to the Lord "and walk in the way of love, just as Christ loved us and gave himself up for us as a fragrant offering and sacrifice to God" (Eph. 5:2).

Glorify God with your mind and your voice. "May God who gives endurance and encouragement give you the same attitude of mind toward each other that Jesus Christ had" (Rom. 15:5). Our joy encourages people around us.

Joyful thanksgiving can also save you from panic attacks, which come from our spiritual enemy. The first generation of Israel that left Egypt died in the wilderness without attaining the promised land. Their "grumbling and complaining" brought diseases among them. Grumblers and complainers will spend their lives in unhappiness and die anxious and depressed, because complaining brings bitterness, not joy. God wants us to walk in all the promises in His Word, but it takes faith, a contented spirit, and patience to inherit the promises (Heb. 6:12). So let us turn our complaining into thankfulness. It improves our physical and emotional health, and the people around us benefit from our gratitude through mirror neurons, mirroring our attitude.

One blind resident in our memory care unit often said, "I had such a good life and the Lord has been so good to me." He died peacefully at ninety-two years old, having never been bed-bound or suffering, not even one single day. His grateful heart ushered him into the presence of the Lord.

God's Presence in Thanksgiving

Let us come before His presence with thanksgiving.
—Psalm 95:2, kjv

Thanksgiving brings us into the presence of the Lord. In addition to Psalm 95:2, Psalm 100:4 tells us to "enter His gates with thanksgiving and His courts with praise." In these verses, we see that to enter His presence we must come with thanksgiving. Start your day by telling the Lord how thankful you are, and you can enter into His presence first thing. By keeping a thankful heart all day, you can abide in His presence. This is the happiest and most successful way to live. Neuroscientists talk about the importance of counting our blessings to maintain a peaceful mind, normal blood pressure, and normal blood sugar. It even improves the immune system, helping to prevent infections, even from the common cold.[3]

You have God's favor when you live in an atmosphere of thanksgiving. This is God's will for you. Thanksgiving has the power to transform your thinking and your mind. When you give thanks, it stops the plans of the enemy. You need insights from God. All my insights, inspiration, and discernment come when I spend time in prayer with thanksgiving.

I always start my prayers with thanksgiving, and I start to feel God's presence when I meditate on the amazing things God has done in my life. Confusion, anxiety, and worry disappear in His presence. I receive clarity and discernment in making decisions. In a world of uncertainty, insecurity, and confusion, we need clarity to hear from God. We need His presence in this postmodern era more than ever. He gives us wisdom, revelation, inspiration, and guidance through the power of the Holy Spirit when we spend time giving Him thanks.

Thanksgiving has the power to cast out fear, worry, anxiety, and depression, and to calm the brain. Thankfulness can change any situation. Your feelings, signs, and symptoms will change too. Your mind's eyes will open and start to understand the purpose of your life. You will become eternity-oriented and live with eternity in mind. Everything changes around you when you decide to have a life full of thanksgiving.

SACRIFICE OF PRAISE

> Through Jesus, therefore, let us continually offer to God a sacrifice of praise—the fruit of lips that openly profess his name.
> —HEBREWS 13:15

Have an attitude of gratitude, and offer the sacrifice of praise with your lips. The Lord's Prayer starts by praising the Father for who He is. We magnify His name because His is the kingdom, the power, and the glory forever and ever (Matt. 6:13). Praise Him for everything He has done for you, even when things do not go your way; it is a sacrifice of praise. I often like to fast, just to bring Him a sacrifice of praise and thanksgiving. God inhales our praises and then breathes His Holy Spirit over us in our worship time with His healing power. Extend your hands in thanksgiving. Raise up your hands with excitement, praise Him confidently with songs, and bless His mighty name, declaring the wonders of God. Sing in the spirit spontaneously. The Holy Spirit is prompting us to praise our Father in our heavenly language.

God gives us wisdom to discern His voice from the voice of the enemy. When you shout praises to God, the enemy gets confused. The walls of Jericho fell down when Israel's army shouted, as the Lord commanded (Josh. 6:20). The enemy got confused. Praise brings us victory in our lives at a specific time. When you praise Him continually and bring a sacrifice of praise, you build confidence in the power of the Lord. Then your fear will be gone and faith will increase, creating an optimistic atmosphere in the brain for a healthy amount of neurochemicals. The stress level will go down and healing and restoration will come. Cortisol levels decrease and serotonin levels increase to a healthy amount when you are joyful, and your depression and anxiety will be healed. Praising God occupies your mind with positive thoughts and connects your mind and spirit with heaven's power.

Follow God's prescription, giving thanks in all things, through all things. You are in control of your feelings. Be determined to have faith in the Word of God and you will be successful. Sing praises and give thanks to the Lord, for His love endures forever. Just a few months ago I took care of a dying resident who was blind her entire life, but still a strong believer. I spent time at her bedside during the dying process, and many times whispered into her ear the refrain of Psalm 136: "His love endures forever, His love endures forever." She knew exactly what I was talking about and what that meant. Her smiling face would glow as she looked up toward heaven. She won her spiritual battles through praising and singing worship songs throughout the day in her room, until her soul left her body and angels escorted her into the arms of Jesus.

In times of stress and worry, praise the Lord and affirm deep in your heart: "You are my hiding place" (Ps. 32:7). God wants people to praise Him all the time. He gave instructions throughout His Word not to forget the Lord's kindness and benefits. Everything you have is from Him, the Creator of the universe. Do not forget, He is the One who gives you breath in your lungs as well as everlasting life. We were created for His glory.

Praise Through the Trials

> But I will sing of your strength, in the morning; I will sing of your love; for you are my fortress, my refuge in times of trouble.
>
> —Psalm 59:16

Paul and Silas praised the King of the universe when they were chained in a prison. As they praised God in the midnight hour, He listened from heaven. Then the earth shook and the chains fell from Paul's and Silas' feet. (See Acts 16: 16–40.) God is shaking things on earth on your behalf when you praise His mighty name.

In the Book of Jonah we read that Jonah was in the fish's belly for three days. When he started to praise the Lord there in the deep sea, in the belly of that big fish, God heard him and delivered him. (See Jonah 2.) Praise Him through your trials. You cannot wait until the battle is over. God likes your new song, a new hymn of praise in trials. (See Psalm 40.) I have done this often when I am going through trials. I have praised God in my loneliness, even though many times my heart was filled with emotional pain and my soul was crying. I read all the Psalms in the Bible, and I praised Him, and He gave me victory so many times. With praises in our mouth, we overcome our struggles and spiritual battles victoriously. The "real estate" in our brains is filled with contentment, bringing peace, joy, and happiness because God's glory changes our thinking forever. Jesus praised God with His life on earth and in His humility received glory from the Father.

Through praise and thanksgiving God will open closed doors for you, because He holds the keys. It is reassuring to know that God opens doors for you that nobody can close. Likewise, it is He who closes doors. God has opened many giant doors for me and my family since I was a little girl in a poor village. I could write another book about that. Gloria Copeland, in her book *Blessed Beyond Measure: Experience the Extraordinary Goodness of God*, emphasized the importance of thanksgiving during prayer:

Fill your mouth with thanksgiving. Jesus said in Mark 11:24 to believe you receive when you pray. What do you do when you receive something? You say, "Thank you!" The appropriate and powerful thing you do after you pray is to be thankful. Maintain a thankful attitude all the time, and it will go a long way in undergirding faith and patience.[4]

Chapter 25

LIFESTYLE CHANGE

This day I call the heavens and the earth as witnesses against you that I have set before you life and death, blessings and curses. Now choose life, so that you and your children may live.
—DEUTERONOMY 30:19

WHETHER OR NOT we follow God's high potency prescriptions really becomes a life-and-death situation. To obey God—or not—becomes a critical lifestyle choice with eternal consequences, as outlined in Deuteronomy 30:19. A. V. Rzheshevsky of the Restorative Medicine Center in Dnepropetrovsk, Ukraine, asserted in an article for the publication, *Biochemistry*:

> Negative factors, such as the "magnificent" five that includes alcoholism, smoking, unhealthy food, lack of movement, and negative emotions, accompany a person almost from birth and trigger powerful internal biochemical reactions leading to disastrous consequences. Those new deleterious reactions force the organism to mobilize all of its internal reserves to neutralize, at least temporarily, the destructive effects of these negative factors. As a result of this continuous struggle for survival, body parts degenerate, starting from connective tissue protein molecules to entire newly formed organs (such as adipose tissue). Today we can state with certainty that the reason for the majority of widespread pathologies causing premature aging and death, such as atherosclerosis and arterial hypertension, is exactly those external negative factors that a person voluntary introduces into their life. However, the margin of safety that Nature enclosed in the human body is really amazing, allowing light-minded and self-destructive people to live up to 60 years and longer. It is quite possible that the lifespan will increase up to 100 years and more if a person stops destroying

themself with negative emotions and bad habits, including unhealthy food and overeating. This article examines possible interconnection between unhealthy overeating and the theory of programmed aging and phenoptosis.[1]

God will enable us to live a longer, better quality life with our family and children under His blessings—if we follow His prescriptions that reach far beyond science.

People dislike change because they are comfortable with their old ways. They do not want to get out of their comfort zones or alter their lifestyle. Perhaps for many years your lifestyle has led you into a rut, and you cannot seem to make changes. The failures in your life have given you an identity that threatens your future, and you are losing control of your life and feeling hopeless. Hopelessness keeps you from reaching your maximum potential and fulfilling your purpose and destiny.

By understanding the disease process in the human body, you can reverse many diseases with lifestyle changes. Most diseases are due to bad habits and an unhealthy lifestyle. For example, atherosclerosis (coronary artery disease), myocardial infarction (heart attack), cerebrovascular accidents, congestive heart failure, diabetes, cancer, obesity, and high cholesterol—all are caused by high levels of stress. Thus, complications of stress are responsible for all physical and spiritual pain and premature deaths in the world.

While studying for my doctorate at Oregon Health & Science University, I found that "the most widely recognized of the metabolic risk factors are atherogenic dyslipidemia, elevated blood pressure, and elevated plasma glucose."[2] In addition, metabolic syndrome (MSDR) is a major risk factor for stroke, chronic kidney disease, and the complications from these conditions.[3] Patients with MSDR also are susceptible to other conditions such as polycystic ovary syndrome, fatty liver, gallstones, asthma, and sleep disturbances. "Atherogenic dyslipidemia consists of an aggregation of lipoprotein abnormalities including elevated serum triglyceride and apolipoprotein B (apoB), increased LDL particles, and a reduced level of HDL cholesterol."[4] An elevated glucose can be in the range of impaired fasting glucose (IFG), which is called pre-diabetes, or at the level of diabetes. Other risk factors are advancing age, physical inactivity, hormonal imbalance, endocrine dysfunction, smoking, high levels of stress, alcohol intake, and genetic or ethnic predisposition.[5] Operationally, the risk factors that exacerbate MSDR are elevated blood pressure $\geq$ 130/85, elevated glucose $\geq$ 100 mg/dl, increased serum triglyceride $\geq$ 150 mg/dl, reduced HDL cholesterol (HDL-C) < 40 mg/dl, elevations of plasminogen activator inhibitor-1 and fibrinogen, and a pro-inflammatory state.[6]

Patients with MSDR need treatments to control blood sugar, blood pressure, and cholesterol. They also need coaching in lifestyle changes to stop smoking, follow a healthy diet, get regular exercise, and take antiplatelet medicines (such as low-dose aspirin).[7] They need an eye exam, dental care, foot care, and stress management. Patients with MSDR need regular follow-up visits for their conditions:

regular physical exams, counseling on medication use, educational classes, and referrals to a nutritionist, ophthalmologist, podiatrist, and dentist.

Identification and modification of lifestyle risk factors associated with the syndrome is important for its effective prevention and for reducing the risks of cardiovascular disease (CVD) in this population. The beneficial effect of lifestyle intervention on the metabolic syndrome components "provides important evidence of the value of this approach to those with blood pressure, weight, and lipid disturbances in general."[8] Although most lifestyle change interventions have proven effective in achieving short-term adherence, "the evidence is limited regarding specific strategies that are most helpful…for the long-term maintenance of lifestyle changes."[9] "The evidence…lacks the respective attention to specific behavioral or motivational factors in helping patients to adhere to the multifaceted lifestyle changes."[10]

Motivation to change one's lifestyle is the key to improving physical and spiritual health. Take to heart God's divine prescription, given to motivate us to choose life and blessings, as the words of Deuteronomy 30:19 urge: "This day I call the heavens and the earth as witnesses against you that I have set before you life and death, blessings and curses. Now choose life, so that you and your children may live."

Bad behavior, stress from fear and worries, and unhealthy diet negatively alter the gene expression through epigenetic mechanism. All these increase the risk for physical diseases, such as heart disease, diabetes, obesity, and stroke, and emotional diseases, including anxiety, depression, and dementia later in life. Science has discovered that second and third generations can be affected by those diseases.[11] The Bible calls them "generational curses" that can be broken through new good habits. Our DNA contains the genetic code, the blueprint in our cells for protein synthesis necessary for life, which is influenced by our lifestyle. For example, healthy foods—fish, whole grains, green vegetables, and citrus fruits—are rich in methyl and will suppress (through methylation) those bad genes that are pre-programmed to trigger chronic diseases.[12] Hydration is extremely important for mood regulation and cognition.[13] It is recommended for adults to drink 1,500–2,000 mL during the day. (Avoid drinking after 5:00 p.m. so you do not need to wake up at night to void, and interrupt your sleep).

SLEEP WITH THE LORD AT YOUR SIDE

> When you lie down, you will not be afraid; when you lie down, your sleep will be sweet. Have no fear of sudden disaster or of the ruin that overtakes the wicked, for the LORD will be at your side and will keep your foot from being snared.
>
> —PROVERBS 3:24–26

> In peace I will lie down and sleep, for you alone, Lord, make me dwell in safety.
>
> —Psalm 4:8

Sleep is one of the most important factors for healthy brain regulation. Excessive amounts of adrenaline, norepinephrine, and anxiety keep the brain very busy and awake, causing sleep disturbances and leading to insomnia. The deep sleep phase is affected by excess cortisol due to a high level of stress, which makes people very tired. Their energy is low, they cannot concentrate, and their emotions are fragile, leading to depression. Major depression and extremely severe and prolonged stress will further increase cortisol. Excess cortisol is toxic for the brain and further impairs emotional regulation, damaging the brain and shrinking the hippocampus area.

To sleep well, you must avoid caffeine (drink less than 500 mg in the morning), alcohol, tranquilizers, narcotics, and prescription drugs for sleep; even an over-the-counter melatonin sleep aid can cause depression in some people.[14] Exercise regularly (at least two hours before bedtime) and keep calm, with no TV or computer use before bedtime (follow instructions for sleep hygiene).

To sleep in peace is a divine order. Do not go to bed angry. Anger causes stress, disrupting the neurotransmitter balance in the brain. This will create sleep disturbances. A German research group led by Thomas Unbehaun, using an electroencephalogram in their study, concluded:

> Specific sleep stages are defined which occur in a distinctive order during the night. Sleep regulation means mechanisms to induce wakefulness and sleep as well as the alternative occurrence of REM and nonREM sleep. In this regulation a specialized neuronal brain network is involved, including the ascending reticular activating system (ARAS), the Raphe nuclei, Locus coeruleus, ventrolateral praeoptic nucleus, tuberomammilare nucleus, the laterodorsal and pedunculopontine tegmental nuclei. Several neurotransmitters like acetylcholine, norepinephrine, serotonine, dopamine, GABA, histamine, orexin and adenosine are mediating the interaction between these brain centers. Reciprocal inhibition and circadian rhythms are two regulating principles within this network. Conclusion: Any external influence upon this interaction of neurotransmitters could induce sleep changes and may be the mechanism by which several substances induce or disturb sleep.[15]

God's prescription—beyond science—is: "In your anger, do not sin. Do not let the sun go down while you are still angry, and do not give the devil a foothold" (Eph. 4:26). We are programmed to sleep seven to nine hours a night. We read in Isaiah, "He wakens me morning by morning" (Isa. 50:4). The neurotransmitter adenosine builds up daily to just the right level to allow us to fall asleep after a day of work or a day of rest. Then we can sleep through the night, be rested, and wake up in the morning. Adenosine is a neuromodulator with an inhibitory mechanism in the central nervous system that suppresses arousal, promoting sleeping at night.[16] When the adenosine level is raised, dopamine is low and blood pressure is naturally lowered.[17] People who sleep too little or too much can develop depression due to the unhealthy amounts of several neurotransmitters,[18] including serotonin, acetylcholine, norepinephrine, dopamine, orexin, histamine, GABA, and adenosine.[19] We can correct or prevent insomnia through good sleep hygiene, including physical activity during the day, limiting liquids before bedtime, avoiding naps, and meditation and prayer to reduce fear and anxiety, thus calming the overactive brain.

The Word of God tells us we must sleep in peace, because He promised to watch over us. Worry, anxiety, and stress will keep us awake and activate genes that lead to depression. Sleep is an amazing phenomenon. The cells enter into a sleeping phase, and the whole body is refreshed and restored upon waking up. The brain performs right where it left off just before falling asleep. The brain at night regulates our sleep time through different phases, including (as I call it) a "natural anesthesia" phase that reduces blood pressure, constricts our bronchioles, and then wakes us up without a post anesthesia rehabilitation phase, and without side effects.[20] Then the brain commands the liver to produce new glucose, increasing the blood sugar level automatically through glycogenesis for the right amount of energy to get out of bed in the morning.[21]

We wake up refreshed and renewed with energy, ready to start the tasks where we left them. Everything is programmed to accomplish our normal daily routine of rest at night and work during the day. At the unconscious level, through apoptosis during the night, our bodies are cleansed from damaged cells and eliminate the cells that are programmed to die, not causing inflammation or cell proliferation and keeping our bodies in homeostasis. The brain is sculpted by this process of neural apoptosis during embryonic development.[22] This astonishing process renews our strength every morning.

RENEWING OUR SPIRIT AND BODY

> Because of the LORD's great love we are not consumed, for his compassions never fail. They are new every morning; great is your faithfulness.
> —LAMENTATIONS 3:22–23

The process of apoptosis as a built-in feature programmed in our DNA is an astonishing example of how God cares for us and what our bodies do at the unconscious level to keep us alive, even after all our destructive behaviors and bad choices. God renews our strength every single day by His Spirit, and through apoptosis. Apoptosis is "a genetically directed process of cell self-destruction that is marked by the fragmentation of nuclear DNA, is activated either by the presence of a stimulus or removal of a suppressing agent or stimulus, is a normal physiological process eliminating DNA-damaged, superfluous, or unwanted cells, and when halted (as by genetic mutation) may result in uncontrolled cell growth and tumor formation—called also...*programmed cell death*."[23]

DEFEATING THE DISUSE SYNDROME

> The LORD God took the man and put him in the Garden of Eden to work it and keep it.
> —GENESIS 2:15

> All hard work brings profit, but mere talk leads only to poverty.
> —PROVERBS 14:23

Advanced technology has opened the door for the "disuse syndrome." This inactive, sedentary lifestyle kills millions. Advanced technology in developed countries has displaced much of the traditional workforce—and work—yet physical labor is a healthy activity that we need. As Genesis 2:15 tells us, when God placed Adam in the Garden of Eden, it was to "work it." Scientists continue to discover physiological benefits of an active lifestyle, proving the benefits of following God's plan. There are many physiological rewards for our obedience to the Word of God, even for the active lifestyle. I tell all my patients that it is extremely important to be active, even if they live in luxury and do not need to work.

For example, during physical activity the chemical neurotrophin is released, helping to repair the brain. Physical activity increases blood and lymph flow to all organs, including the lungs and heart, to clean them from the buildup of toxins. Benefits from physical activity are multifaceted and are mentioned in the Word of God. God tells us to be active always; as Proverbs 14:23 says: "All hard work brings profit, but mere talk leads only to poverty." The Word also says, "The one who is unwilling to work shall not eat" (2 Thess. 3:10). It is ethical to work to obtain our food and not be a burden on others, or on the government. In the health field, scientists have found that a lack of physical activity results in calories deposited as fats. Moreover, toxins from inside the body and the environment will be deposited in the fatty tissue.

I started to work at about six years of age, helping my parents with farming. I would wake up early and do whatever needed to be done: take care of the animals, work in the garden or the field, or inside the house cooking, cleaning inside and outside, and even painting the walls of the house. I knitted my own clothes and did many other things. At the same time I attended school full time through the eighth grade in my home village, then moved to Bucharest to attend a vocational school and high school, to be able to support myself. After two years of school, before I was seventeen, I got a full-time job and continued school as a full-time

Lifestyle Change

student to finish high school. Then I attended the Academy of Economic Studies in Bucharest. I have never stopped working.

When I arrived in the United States, even though I was a professional economist, I began by cleaning toilets and making beds in a nursing home because I did not speak English. I washed and painted the walls of my friends' houses, and helped the elderly as a nursing aid. How many healthy young people, full of energy, are now on welfare, without working? This is so detrimental for their health and for society as a whole. We must take on responsibilities in life to live more abundantly. Jesus died on the cross to give us life more abundantly. He did everything for us. We must just enter in to fulfill what was done for us at Calvary. You can rise up from your situation, pray, and change your thoughts, attitudes, and habits. God can bless you with many blessings you never dreamed of, if you change your attitude and follow God's Word.

One Bible story tells about a weak, disabled man lying on a mat. Jesus told that person to take up his mat and walk. And the sick person obeyed, and got up and was healed. (See Matthew 9.) God is asking us to take action, move, get up and have an active life that will benefit our health, as well as others in our community and society as a whole. Jesus will help us, but we need to obey, change our attitude, and keep moving.

One day my daughter heard me praying on my knees, asking God to protect me from the spirit of laziness. She started to laugh, asking me, "Protect you from what?" Then I explained to her that many people struggle all their lives with the spirit of laziness. She then understood and followed my example, studying hard at school, working hard at home, and volunteering at a very young age. She still continues to work hard for her family and at her job, where she has huge responsibilities as a Doctor of Pharmacy and clinic manager at The AntiCoagulation Clinic—and volunteering at church.

In *A Woman After God's Own Heart*, prolific author and speaker Elizabeth George advises the reader:

> *Keep moving*—Remember the principle of momentum: "A body at rest [human or otherwise] tends to remain at rest, and a body in motion tends to remain in motion." Use this law of physics to your advantage. Tell yourself, "Just one more thing…just five more minutes." Keep moving and you can cross one more thing off your to do list![24]

Taking Action

Many people, by their own choices, fall prey to diseases that will kill them, either suddenly or slowly. The way you choose to live, what you eat, how much you exercise, how you manage your level of stress, and other habits—such as drinking, sleeping, using drugs, having premarital sex, adultery, smoking, and your choice of friends—will determine who you become in the future. Take responsibility for your health to prevent disability and premature disease, suffering, physical and emotional pain, stress, and premature death of the body, soul, and spirit. For example, it is a fact that by lowering your low density lipoprotein (LDL) to less than 100 mg/dl, and your blood pressure to less than 120/80 mmHg, and quitting smoking, you will reduce your risk of heart attack before age sixty-five by more than 80 percent.[25] You must take action today to reduce the risk for heart attack or stroke. You can see the difference even after four to eight weeks of dietary changes.

The "Daniel Fast" works extremely well, since you eat only fresh fruits, vegetables, and legumes. In one year I was able to follow this fast six times, which helped me and my husband to lower our total cholesterol, LDL (bad cholesterol), and triglycerides by half, and also to raise the high density lipoprotein (good cholesterol). We lost eight to twelve pounds each time we fasted. Besides lowering all the numbers, we also received answers to our prayers, reduced our worry and stress, and improved our immune system. We were able to exercise more and became more efficient in our jobs, providing care for the elderly and others, became more relaxed and calmer, and our quality of life increased.

In the clinic I see many patients suffering from metabolic syndrome, and I teach them (besides prescribing medication as needed) to also try the "Daniel Fast" for better results. Those who follow my instructions usually see benefits. After adjusting their lifestyle, many of my patients using several medications for their medical conditions were able to decrease their number of meds.

Diabetes, hypertension, and high cholesterol, and their complications, can be prevented with lifestyle changes (as discussed earlier). Statistics shows that one out of seven Americans are dying from heart disease, due to an unhealthy lifestyle. In 2019, about eighty-four million adults were prediabetic, and if not addressed, will become diabetics, with all the complications of diabetes.[26] Studies show that coronary artery diseases result from a diet high in sugar, fat and cholesterol, high levels of stress, and lack of exercise.[27]

These diseases are on our plates every single day when we eat sugary, fatty foods, high in cholesterol, with extra calories. Studies show that patients on a very strict vegetarian diet actually widened their arteries, and the heart muscle received increased oxygenation. Heart disease even reversed itself with a healthy diet and lifestyle changes. We must go beyond the American Heart Association's recommended diet.[28] A healthy diet rich in fibers (fresh fruits and vegetables, legumes, and whole grains) prevents many diseases and their complications. Beyond science the Bible has been teaching that for thousands of years. For example, Daniel's fast (Dan. 1:8–14) was written in the Bible thousands of years ago—namely, a diet low in cholesterol and high in fiber and antioxidants, needed to detoxify the cells to prevent cancer.

To reverse heart disease, it is recommended to reduce the LDL levels in your blood to 100 mg/dl, lose weight, drop your blood pressure to 120/80 mmHg, stop smoking, reduce stress, stop drinking alcohol, and avoid other destructive habits.[29]

Lifestyle Change

You can achieve that goal by reducing fats in your diet, reducing simple carbohydrates, substituting with healthy foods (fresh vegetables, legumes, fresh fruits, whole grains, and complex carbohydrates), and exercising regularly. Even walking thirty to sixty minutes a day has great benefit. Eliminate sweets, reduce salt, resist temptations, and cook at home. Your food can be your medicine. How much extra it costs us to buy unhealthy food from the store, and then go see the doctor and buy the prescribed treatment for the diseases caused by our unhealthy food choices!

Check your blood pressure. Hypertension is the silent killer, because the body compensates slowly and you don't experience symptoms until a stroke or sudden heart attack. More than seventy-five million (nearly one in three) American adults have hypertension, but about one in five do not know they have it.[30] The body compensates until the heart becomes very weak, developing congestive heart failure and cardiac insufficiency. The higher the blood pressure, the greater the risk for heart disease. Salty food consumed daily is a major cause of high blood pressure. When we eat too much salt, our electrolyte balance is affected, also leading to heart disease.[31]

Excess weight causes the heart to work harder to administer nutrients to the body, and blood pressure goes up. It's like attaching a big truck to a small engine, and then expecting it to work normally. Too much fat and cholesterol in our diet causes stenosis in the arteries, blocking them and causing a heart attack or stroke. Lack of exercise, high stress, smoking, alcohol, and estrogen[32] affects your heart condition. Obesity will impair blood circulation, affecting your thinking process and leading to dementia.[33]

Drugs will not cure hypertension; they can only control it. They cannot prevent arteriosclerosis or heart attack. Only lifestyle changes can quickly reverse hypertension without drugs. When you reduce salt in your diet and lose weight, your blood pressure will drop without medication. Reducing weight sometimes is the only needed treatment. If you take medication and make a major change in your lifestyle, your blood pressure will improve. But *do not stop* taking medication or heart pills without consulting your doctor, even if your blood pressure is lowered by the changes you make. The damage to your heart was done a long time ago. You may need both medication and lifestyle change, but remember that medication alone will not cure your diseases. Talk to your doctor about any changes.

To avoid diseases, you must read the labels of the food you buy. Cerebrovascular accidents (strokes) occur due to atherosclerosis. Plaque in the blood vessels cause the occlusions or thrombosis. During the occlusion process the plaque that is formed can be dislodged, or a clot can form, blocking the small arteries that supply blood to the brain. Then the artery can break and cause a hemorrhage in the brain—a stroke. High blood pressure may cause the arteries to break when forcing blood through the small, stiffened arteries, causing them to rupture. Hemorrhage cuts off oxygen to that portion of the brain, and it dies, causing paralysis. Stroke can be severe, or fatal. High blood pressure, high cholesterol, high triglycerides, elevated sugar, uncontrolled diabetes, sedentary lifestyle, obesity, high levels of stress, and smoking are all serious risk factors for cerebrovascular accidents or stroke.[34]

Stroke, like heart attacks, can be prevented through lifestyle changes to decrease blood pressure and promote healthy arteries. Check your blood pressure regularly, do not smoke, lose weight, reduce your salt intake, exercise regularly, eat a very low fat diet, increase fruits and vegetables to four or five servings a day, increase fiber, and manage stress; then you will enjoy a good, healthy life. It is God's will for you to have a healthy body, soul, and spirit. Read your Bible every day to find God's prescriptions for a healthy spiritual heart that will support your emotional and physical health.

Americans consume tons of aspirin. Aspirin can help with atrial fibrillation, *but ask your primary care provider if aspirin is OK for you.* I recommend a baby aspirin (81 mg) daily for patients with a history of diabetes, myocardial infarction, or stroke, for secondary prevention. Thickened arteries can open again when you start a diet very low in fat and higher in fiber. You also can develop collateral circulation when you exercise regularly. Even walking for thirty to sixty minutes a day will make a huge difference in the circulation of blood to your heart, and your whole body will improve.

A Mediterranean diet contains anti-inflammatory nutrients because of its emphasis on healthy foods, such as fruits, vegetables, whole grains, legumes, flaxseeds, omega-3 fatty acids, and nuts, as well as spices like chili, black pepper, cumin, ginger, and sage. They may reduce the risk for heart diseases, depression, and dementia. Stress management will also keep your neurotransmitters at a healthy level to protect your heart. You need to be serious about adopting a healthy lifestyle before the damage is done.

During exercise, the brain produces the natural antidepressant—the "feel good" hormone—endorphin, making you feel well and think clearly. Work on reaching a healthy body weight. Monitor your risks for diabetes, check your blood sugar regularly if you suffer from diabetes already, and consume less than 300 mg/dl cholesterol per day. Eating more fruits and vegetables and food rich in omega-3 (salmon, nuts, mackerel) increases circulation of blood in the brain and prevents not only heart disease but Alzheimer's. If you change the conditions of your blood vessels, you can prevent dementia. Avoid fatty meats, butter and creams, high synthetic sugar, or simple carbohydrate products, such as starches. All of them are artery-clogging foods. Keep your blood pressure under control, as it is the number one risk factor for stroke.

If you experience tightness in your chest, chest pain, shortness of breath upon exertion with activities, fast heartbeat, indigestion, nausea and unusual stomach pain, drooping face, weakness in one arm or leg, or difficultly in speaking, call 911 and go to the emergency room immediately.

Change your bad habits today. Throw away saltshakers, salty snacks, and fast foods. You need to do a U-turn in your life to prevent disaster. No matter how old you are, or your health history, you can add quality years to your life by starting today to make changes in your lifestyle. You will be healthier, have more energy, and be more efficient in everything you do. Your thinking process will improve with all the healthy neurotransmitters in your body, making you look younger. Lifestyle change is the least expensive antiaging treatment.

You are in control of your life through the power of your thinking process. You can make changes using your willpower and your gift of free choice. If you have a chronic disease, such as diabetes, high blood pressure, asthma, arthritis, depression, bladder incontinence, immunodeficiency disease, or another condition, keep your follow-up visits with your health care provider. Act on your lifestyle changes (even losing two pounds can make a difference in improving your health condition) as described above. You can improve your health and decrease the stress level in your life. Attend a nutrition class and talk to your health care provider about all the changes you need to make in your lifestyle, and adjust your treatment accordingly.

Many cancers develop as a consequence of unhealthy habits and the environment. Up to 80 percent of cancers can be prevented through improved lifestyle. For example, cancer of the lungs, lips, mouth, tongue, throat, esophagus, and bladder can be prevented.[35] Colon cancer in men and women, prostate cancer in men, and breast cancer in women are related to overeating, being overweight, having too many fats, and having a low level of melatonin, causing a lack of sleep.[36] The following are risk factors for cancer: tobacco, red meat, junk food, inactivity, overeating, alcohol, and high levels of stress. Changing those risk factors and not smoking, not drinking alcohol, and following a Mediterranean diet, one low in fats and high in fibers, can reduce your cancer risk. A diet low in fat and cholesterol reduces the risk of heart disease, stroke, diabetes, and cancer. Fasting was prescribed by God in ancient times, and it is still His prescription for us today—beyond science—to maintain our well-being, stay in balance, and get closer to God for better physical and spiritual health.

Chapter 26

PRAYER AND FASTING

If you remain in me and my words remain in you, ask whatever you wish, and it will be done for you. This is to my Father's glory, that you bear much fruit, showing yourselves to be my disciples.
—John 15:7–8

PRAYER TRANSITIONS YOUR spirit, passing beyond the threshold of the natural world into God's supernatural sphere. Bondage can be broken and attitudes can be changed through prayer when you surrender and let Christ live in you. Prayer changes the atmosphere, even when you are tempted to have a bad attitude, and keeps you away from temptation. When you pray, you turn 180 degrees from your filthy thoughts and destructive habits. You cannot pray sincerely and then resume a bad habit.

I remember my first prayer in public. I was in fifth grade, and my uncle asked me to pray aloud at a prayer meeting. That launched me into a life of prayer. I also remember that as a child I longed to get closer to God, to know Jesus more, and to receive the power of the Holy Spirit. I sought out prayer meetings and spent time in prayer, but I knew I needed to do something more. Then I heard some teaching about fasting, and I knew in my heart that I needed to fast in order to get closer to God. That began a life of prayer and fasting, which God honored. I have seen His protection and favor over my life.

I could have been arrested many times in communist Romania for speaking publicly about my faith in God. The police threatened and investigated me a few times, making me give an account for my Christian walk and my values and beliefs. I was scared because the communist police in Romania at that time were very mean, rude, and rough. One time as a teenager, when I went to a prayer meeting at my grandmother's house with some relatives and friends, a policeman took us from my grandmother's house and forced us to walk five kilometers through the snow to the police station for a day-long investigation. It was winter and bitter cold, and we had nothing to eat or drink that day. They threatened us, then let us go back home—under police supervision. Through all of those trials God's eyes were upon me, and I felt His divine protection everywhere I went. Prayer and fasting bring spiritual breakthrough and divine intervention.

PRAYER—THE ANTIAGING EXERCISE

Exercise prayer and faith for a victorious life, for "without faith it is impossible to please God" (Heb. 11:6). If you do not have faith, Jesus says He cannot hear your voice. Faith in Christ is a spiritual gift. You can know God more through prayer. On Mount Sinai, Moses asked God who He was, and Jehovah showed a glimpse of His glory to Moses (Exod. 33:21–23). He will do just the same for you when you ask with a sincere heart and are desperate for His presence. He is the great "I AM" (Exod. 3:14), today and forever, as He was for Moses more than thirty-four hundred years ago.

You must be willing to know Him to receive a greater revelation, because whoever has more knowledge will be given more knowledge about Him (Matt. 13:12). We are blessed to have eyes to see and ears to hear. In our facility, many of our residents are blind or hard of hearing, and it is heartbreaking to see them live with such devastating disabilities. We must accommodate the surroundings for them to meet their needs. In order to rearrange our vision, Christ is willing to rearrange our surroundings. He took Peter, John, and James to the mountain to see His glorious transfiguration. (See Matthew 17:1–2; Mark 9:2–4; and Luke 9:28–30.) Ask God to let you see who He truly is, and to recognize Christ.

We know very little about prayer. When I was a teenager in Bucharest, a Christian woman whom I considered a prayer mentor would pray for one hour every day. She prayed for many people by name, then for churches, for communities, for cities, for nations, for presidents, leaders in government, judges, teachers, doctors, nurses, lawyers, businesspersons, and more. She had a notebook, just like a student, listing all the countries around the world, and interceded for each one of them by name every morning. I am sure that her prayers, and those of many others, contributed to the entire communist system collapsing in the surrounding countries only a few years after her prolonged times of intercession.

One day one of Jesus' disciples made a request: "Lord, teach us how to pray just as John taught his disciples" (Luke 11:1). Prayer will change your relationship with God. God never will change, but we will. God's ways are still higher than ours (Isa. 55:8–9). God wants to train us to pray, even though we do not see results. We must practice continual prayer.

When I examined my first patient, I was a bit unsure how to start the exam. Even though I felt confident in my knowledge (after more than ten years of medical education), I was trembling at first, because any beginning is stressful. But after a while I became an expert. With prayer, it is similar. You become more confident spiritually by spending more time with God. You will know Him better, and learn to discern His distinct voice. I wanted to hear God, to know Him and learn how to hear Him speaking to me. I needed to know Jesus. Missionary Heidi Baker, PhD, stated in her book *Birthing the Miraculous: The Power of Personal Encounters With God to Change Your Life and the World*: "Without Him our efforts produce nothing spectacular, no matter how much we strive. The one thing we can do is respond to the Father's words over our lives. We can position our hearts in humility and hunger. Hunger always delights the heart of God."[1]

You must spend time with Him to know Him. Engage in a personal relationship with your heavenly Father. Choose to meet with God in prayer and expect Him to meet you in that place of humility, dedication, and surrender. Our Father God is a consuming fire. He is holy. Establish a priority in your prayers that His will should be done on Earth, as it is in heaven. When you delight in the Lord, He will give you your heart's desire. (See Psalm 37.) If you abide in Jesus, you may ask whatever you wish and He will give it to you. It is for God's glory that your prayers will be fruitful (John 15:7–8). Surrender to *His agenda*, pray for His will to be done in your life, and develop a day-by-day mentality in prayer. Prayer calms your brain, reduces worry and fear, increases peace, and keeps you healthy on a daily basis.

On the other hand, fear causes death. Fearful thoughts, worries, and anxieties damage your body. Psychologist David Stoop, PhD, in his book *You Are What You Think*, says, "The key to breaking the paralyzing cycle of worry and anxiety is to find something solid in which to trust. For me, the only thing worth trusting for the future is God himself. Jesus points out the obvious choice we have to make when it comes to solving the patterns of worry and anxiety."[2] When you trust God and pray, your faith will increase and fear, anxiety, and depression will resolve. Jesus prayed in the Garden of Gethsemane one night before His death on the cross, and the fear of death vanished. Death was defeated forever, bringing eternal life for all those who believe in Him. When fear is defeated, anxiety and depression will have no place.

Scientific literature has documented that resolving depression or feelings of depression will lead to lower blood pressure, decreased pain, and a more positive outlook on life. Lack of fear, anxiety, and depression will give you a longer, healthier, and happier life. Prayer impacts your brain, enhances your ability to solve problems, and prevents mental decline or Alzheimer's.[3] Neuroscientists have proven that prayer also decreases stress and negative emotions, stroke risk, heart attack events, neurocognitive disorders, and panic attacks. It enhances your ability to think clearly and function well, increases lifespan, and increases physical and emotional health overall.[4]

The promises of God are positive affirmations that lead to a positive attitude. Strengthen your brain through the power of prayer and claim God's promises. What is going on in your brain affects your physical body. Thoughts of faith affect your mental and physical being in a positive way. When you do not pray, fear settles in and degrades your mental condition. The frontal lobe can shrink with aging, causing mental decline and Alzheimer's disease, but prayer stimulates the frontal lobe, preventing shrinking. Prayer is an antiaging exercise.[5]

PRAY WITHOUT CEASING

> Rejoice always, pray without ceasing, in everything give thanks; for this is the will of God in Christ Jesus for you.
> —1 THESSALONIANS 5:16–18, NKJV

Prayer connects us with God at a deeper level, and fasting requires even more self-discipline. We need to disconnect from the world in order to get closer to God. Jesus prayed often, and He asked the disciples to pray. God created in us the ability to pray continually, and He is asking us for unceasing prayer. So how is that possible? Texas physician Dr. Larry Dossey remarked in his book *Healing Words: The Power of Prayer and the Practice of Medicine*, "A state of prayerfulness has infiltrated not just the conscious mind but the unconscious as well, including sleep and dreams."[6] We learned the activities in the unconscious mind are taking place 24/7, without ceasing. If you have a prayer life and meditate day and night on the Word of God, your unconscious mind is in the mode to pray without ceasing. The disciples, who traveled and lived alongside Jesus—who prayed throughout the night—tasted the power of prayer. They gave us instructions through the power of the Holy Spirit to pray without ceasing.

When the Holy Spirit is in us we cannot stop praying, because He is praying in us without ceasing, whether when we are awake or asleep. The devil will try to interrupt your prayers, because he knows the power of prayer. The devil wants to steal your peace, bringing unexpected disturbances. Everything around you becomes dark when you lose your peace. You see things from the world's perspective and negative thoughts flood your mind. Anger can build up and sour your spirit, releasing unhealthy amounts of neurochemicals, with unpleasant symptoms, killing neurons and modifying the brain's structure.

How much better it is for us to seek God's face and His presence. When you pray and enter into the presence of God, great joy will flood your soul. You have had an audience with the CEO of the universe! When you pray, the presence of God brings you peace, even in the middle of a "storm." God uses storms to wake us up, to seek His presence. No one can sleep through a disastrous storm, and serious action is immediately required. Prayer is hard work. Sometimes you must pray for the strength to pray. When you go through difficult times, whether in physical or emotional pain, or discouragement, you can receive peace deep in your heart when you pray. God's ways are beyond our understanding, but if you pray and choose not to worry, you will receive the peace that only God can give through Jesus Christ, the peace that passes all understanding.

When I was in seventh and eighth grade, if I did not like a person's character, my mind would be full of anxiety, anger, selfishness, and unhappiness. Even though I lived in a Christian family, I still struggled with wrong thoughts. I kept trying to get closer to God, memorizing His Word and meditating day and night. Then, when I had my amazing encounter with God, it transformed my thought life.

Only the power of the Holy Spirit can change our insight. This happens by the washing of the Word of God and unceasing prayer. Invite the presence of God into your life and pray for God's mercy and power. Believe that He hears your prayer for your specific needs. Change and shape the world around you through the power of prayer and fasting. We can overcome all circumstances through prayer, the power that changes things. Through prayer and fasting we can expect something out of the ordinary. God will give you power, but you need to know what to do with that power from heaven (Acts 1:8). God instructs us in the Bible how to receive the Holy Spirit through prayer and fasting. Step out in faith, and God can do miracles.

The Lord Fights for You

> The Lord shall fight for you, and ye shall hold your peace.
> —Exodus 14:14, kjv

As a young child I believed that God could do anything, so I prayed. I remember that during the communist regime a few friends and I frequently attended all-night prayer meetings, crying out to God for a clean heart so we could fight the enemy of our souls. Now I wonder what would have happened to us if we had not prayed. Where would we be today? God listens to your prayers—just ask. He answered Joshua's prayer, when he was distressed at the enemies' attack (Josh. 10), and the sun and the moon stopped miraculously for about one day until they had won the battle.

It is easy to get discouraged during the battle, but God is fighting your battle for you when you pray. People in the Bible (Nehemiah, King Asa, King David, the apostle Paul, and others) prayed often, even all night long, when they were surrounded by enemies. The most powerful people on earth were people who prayed. They overcame fear. Whom should we fear? Fear paralyzes us—but it is not from God. The devil wants to reduce us to silence, but the power that created the world is in us. In the beginning, the Spirit of God moved over the chaotic universe and organized our world. He can create order in your life too, as He has done many times in mine.

Through prayer we activate the promises of God. To illustrate, I prayed the prayer of Jabez (1 Chron. 4:9–10) every single day for a few months, asking God to enlarge my territory. He did, and He continues to work in our lives. Heaven is open for business, and the angels are waiting to be released on your behalf—sent through by prayers—to fight the battle for you. They are waiting to receive the assignment from the Father, at your request.

Pray a Big Prayer

> "'If you can'? said Jesus. "Everything is possible for one who believes."
> —Mark 9:23

When you are stressed, pray a big, bold prayer. Cry out to God from the depths of your heart, and He will have compassion on you. When I arrived in the United States without my daughter or husband, the only thing I knew to do amid all my troubles was pray big prayers. Leaving Romania in 1990, I woke up early in the morning to catch the train to Bucharest. My two-year-old, Andreea, was still sleeping in my mother-in-law's house and I knew I would not see her again soon. Needless to say, like any mother I wanted to be there for her every moment—to watch her waking up every morning, playing, learning new things, and then tucking her into bed at the end of the day. I even had her sleep with me until she was one year old. I wanted to hear her breath, to feel every move she made. But that morning I left, I knew it would be a long time until we were reunited and I could once again enjoy her childhood. I did not have a clue then about God's plans for our future life. But He gave me strength that morning to kiss her goodbye, not knowing I wouldn't see her again for a few years. I needed to pray a big prayer.

During those years I had so many struggles. Negative thoughts would bring me to the point of panic. My body suffered all kinds of signs and symptoms from anxiety and depression. These biological responses to my thoughts of fear and worry caused neurotransmitters to be released in unhealthy amounts. The devil whispered so many lies in my ears, bringing all kinds of accusations and threats on my life. But I kept praying the promises of God over myself and my family, every single day. I kept on believing and declaring, "If God is for us, who can be against us?" (Rom. 8:31). I believed His promise: "Never will I leave you. Never will I forsake you" (Heb. 13:5). I believed that the God who took care of my needs and my future during the communist era would continue caring for my family.

I remember when I left my parents' house and went to Bucharest for vocational school. I was a stranger in the city at just fourteen years of age, with no family around me. I felt lonely and threatened by the corrupt communist society, but I prayed, "Lord, help me have a clean heart; help me know You more." I was living in a dormitory, and we were not allowed to have any religious material. But I had the New Testament with me, hidden under some books and clothes in my closet, or sometimes under the mattress when I read late at night.

I had the Word of God in my heart, but I needed to learn more. I also found time during breaks at school to pray in the bathroom. Everywhere I went I first located the bathroom, because I needed a place to hide and pray. My number one priority as a teenager was to learn the Word of God and to pray. God helped me so much in school that I became one of the best students. The adults around me noticed that my behavior and character were different from the other boys and girls. They could trust me with anything.

The Lord answers prayers; as Psalm 138:3 says, "When I called, you answered me." He has answered so many of my prayers and He will answer yours too. Through prayer and the power of the Word of God you can push the limits of your life. Believe God for big things. I have pushed the limits in my life since I was young, through prayer and fasting. Nowadays I am still harvesting the fruit of all the prayer and fasting in my early years. God has worked miracles in my life. He knows everything about your life, so do not give up on prayer. Pray until something happens. There is no expiration date on God's promises or on His prescriptions for your health and prosperity.

Glorify His Name

> Answer me, Lord, answer me, so these people will know that you, Lord, are God, and that you are turning their hearts back again.
> —1 Kings 18:37

God allows things to happen in your life to get your attention. You can pray, and He will answer your prayer, so you will know that He is God, and He will receive the glory. The world can be changed through your prayer. Remember the prayer of Elijah in 1 Kings 18:37. God answered Elijah's prayer so all the Israelites would know that He was and is God, and always will be. Prayer changes things in your life and people around you will know that God is in control of all things. Through prayer you can accomplish things of eternal significance for God's glory.

God Hears Impossible Prayers

> So do not fear, for I am with you; do not be dismayed, for I am your God. I will strengthen you and help you; I will uphold you with my righteous right hand.
> —Isaiah 41:10

God will take the broken pieces of your heart and make everything new. So make a break with the past, because He makes all things new in your life. I have heard testimonies and seen people facing all kinds of catastrophes:

- lost jobs
- broken relationships

- business failures
- natural disasters
- health problems
- addictions
- criminal behavior

But when they started to obey the Word of God, their lives began to change. Through divine restoration things started to turn around in their favor, to a life of victory in Jesus Christ, the Savior of the world.

I was one of those people. I am a living testimony of God's work. When we see lives being transformed, we do not need more scientific evidence or proofs. Just get on your knees, lift your hands, and cry out to God. Repent first, and ask for forgiveness to be reconciled with God. Best-selling author Lee Strobel, in his book *The Case for Christ: A Journalist's Personal Investigation of the Evidence for Jesus*, explains, "Jesus has done for us on the cross what we cannot do for ourselves: he has paid the death penalty that we deserve for our rebellion and wrongdoing, so we can become reconciled with God."[7] Your prayer can be, "Lord, I cannot sustain myself. I need strength from You." Wicked ways only bring destruction, and people perish. Do not forsake your family or church, but serve them with a pure heart because Jesus paid the death penalty for you.

God gives us reassurance when we pray big prayers, like the one above from Isaiah 41:10. He has continued to uphold our family with His right hand and fulfilled our dreams. Do not be afraid and do not fear, but be bold and bring your big prayers to God. He honors bold prayers. "Let us then approach God's throne of grace with confidence so that we may receive mercy and find grace to help us in our time of need" (Heb. 4:16). Let the Word of God occupy your mind, and ask the Holy Spirit to fill you so your impossible prayers are heard. "'If you can'? said Jesus. 'Everything is possible for one who believes'" (Mark 9:23).

DO NOT GIVE UP

As I've said before, there is no expiration date on God's promises, so do not listen to people who speak discouraging, negative things into your life. Keep your prayer line open at all times. If other people share their doubts, and negativity and unbelief enter your heart, your brain will perceive that as a threat, raising your stress level and producing physiological symptoms (a biological response to those stressors) and causing more distress.

Pray out loud, because life and death is in the power of your tongue. Our faith will be built on our words. Faith comes by hearing. If you hear negative words, your faith becomes negative, producing fear. When you speak positive words and pray God's promises out loud, you will build your inner faith and develop a constructive attitude. God loves people with great faith and is pleased with their faithfulness. From Hebrews 11:6, we know that without faith it is impossible to please God.

We live in a world with so much chaos, violence, war, catastrophic weather events, earthquakes, famines, nuclear breakdown, political crises, terrorists, occupiers, and accelerating sexual perversion. Whole nations are scared and overstressed. In the middle of all these situations there is hope in Jesus Christ. He is the answer to every stress in life. Jesus, ruler of the kings of the earth, is the King of kings, Judge, Redeemer, Savior, Healer, Intercessor, and Counselor. He is the head of the church. He functions as the greatest prophet and priest. He has power and authority over the world, dispatching angels to earth to help those who please Him. Your attitude toward God must be right at all times.

Jesus governs the affairs of the earth and is in control over the entire world. Satan has no autonomy or authority on this planet. God shakes the earth to destroy the work of the devil when you pray. Have discernment and take refuge in Him through constant prayer. He is incredibly powerful; in his last letter, John included a greeting "from Jesus Christ, who is the faithful witness, the firstborn from the dead, and the ruler of the kings of the earth" (Rev. 1:5). The earth is in His care. Worship the Lord.

MANAGE STRESS THROUGH FASTING

Fasting is also recommended for recovering your health and preventing diseases, physically and spiritually. *New York Times* best-selling author Dr. Don Colbert, in his book *Toxic Relief: Restore Health and Energy Through Fasting and Detoxification*, stated: "I believe that many diseases are the direct result of an excessive buildup of these toxins." He gives a list of "diseases that are often directly linked to a buildup of toxins: food and environmental allergies; asthma; headaches; fatigue; fibromyalgia; chronic back pain; eczema, chronic acne, and other skin conditions; insomnia; depression; irritable bowel syndrome; decreased sex drive; menstrual problems; abdominal bloating; belching; gas; memory loss; chronic diarrhea; Crohn's disease; ulcerative colitis; atherosclerosis; hypertension; obesity; constipation; angina; multiple sclerosis; coronary artery disease; cancer; mental illness; diabetes."[8]

Fasting is recommended for a healthy lifestyle. However, any time you plan to fast without food or water for more than twenty-four hours and you are on medications for any of those diseases, you must consult your primary care provider first. A partial fast is the most beneficial for your body, especially if you are taking medication for different conditions. But fasting should be for a spiritual benefit, even though the side effect of a partial fast will benefit your health by eating only fresh fruits, vegetables, and legumes in moderation for twenty-one days at a time. The aforementioned "Daniel Fast" gets its name from its mention in Daniel, chapters 1 and 10. I also recommend reading *Toxic Relief* for more details about detoxification through fasting, as well as restoring your physical and spiritual health, your energy, and preventing physical and spiritual diseases.

God, wanting us to be healthy, gave us prescriptions to stay healthy and prevent diseases. (See 3 John 2.) While earning my master's and doctoral degrees, I was fascinated with classes about health promotion and disease prevention. They were the catalyst for writing this book. God gave us instructions long ago on how to stay healthy and how to regain our health again if we become ill. The Bible gives directions from God about what to eat, what to wear, how to behave, how to stay calm in the storm, trust Him and obey His instructions, in order to improve our health and prevent diseases. Those instructions are in our DNA. But disobedience will lead to unhealthy behaviors, destroying our God-given DNA. Many times we try to do things by ourselves and fail, because we do not rely on God's instructions. Deceptions in the world blind people's eyes so they cannot see God's intentions for our health.

Your lifestyle can have a deeper meaning when you fast. (See Isaiah 58:3.) Do not focus on food but on your dependence on God. In order to get results, do not do as you please. (See Isaiah 58:8–9.) Let a new chapter in your life begin. Fasting brings deliverance from selfishness. According to the Word of God, in order to break the spirit of heaviness related to depression, oppression, condemnation, worry, and fear, one must fast and pray, and help others. Pastor Jentezen Franklin stated in his book *Fasting: Opening the Door to a Deeper, More Intimate, More Powerful Relationship With God*: "Americans use drinking, smoking, drugs, medications, overeating, and other harmful behaviors to try to lift the spirit of heaviness.... Instead of looking for more stuff to put *into* our bodies to ease the pain, we should fast and seek the God who gives us a garment of praise for the spirit of heaviness that afflicts so many"[9]

A Newswise article reported on research by Dr. Benjamin Horne under the headline, "Fasting Reduces Cholesterol Levels in Prediabetic People Over Extended Period of Time, New Research Finds." According to Dr. Horne, studies showed that "decades of routine fasting was associated with a lower risk of diabetes and coronary artery disease, [leading] us to think that fasting is most impactful for reducing the risk of diabetes and related metabolic problems.... The fat cells themselves are a major contributor to insulin resistance, which can lead to diabetes.... Because fasting may help to eliminate and break down fat cells, insulin resistance may be frustrated by fasting."[10]

The first time I fasted at age sixteen, I went for two days (forty-eight hours) without food and water. I did not understand much about fasting, but felt the physical and the spiritual benefits right away, even though I was hungry and thirsty and felt discomfort from the detoxifying process. After fasting physically I felt lighter, able to run better, move faster, and think clearer. Meditation on the Word of God amplified all those benefits.

By following God's prescriptions for a healthy life I was able to concentrate more on spiritual things and focus more on my attitude and behavior. I started to have more compassion for people around me and was able to focus more on good things and to discern right from wrong. Then I realized that fasting could bring more positive results, so I read the Bible more about fasting and developed a lifestyle of prayer and fasting.

One time in Bucharest I was in a Max, a common transportation vehicle, with a group of believers from our church. I heard some older women whispering to each other about a missionary in Africa who visited Romania and told about a revival going on there. They said people in Africa were fasting three days and nights without food or water for a spiritual breakthrough, to break the bondage and yoke of witchcraft in that region. I was stunned to hear people could fast that long. I read the Book of Esther and found out that Esther, and all the Jews at that time, also fasted three days and nights with no food or water, and God took note of their sacrifices and gave them a miraculous victory over their enemy. After reading Esther many times, I began to understand the power of fasting for three days and three nights.

I started to consider this possibility to see God's hand work in my life, to obtain victory in my own spiritual battles. I thought it would be impossible for me to fast that long. But I prayed and asked God to help me, and He did. After that I fasted many times like Esther, and God intervened to show Himself strong on my behalf. He opened many closed doors that needed to be opened for me, and closed many doors that the devil would open to try to deceive me and lead me into temptations and destruction.

Fasting for Spiritual Health

Fasting will help you solve problems and remove limits that hinder God's plan and blessings in your life. We have been blessed in our lives because of a lifestyle of fasting and praying. We still continue to fast and pray, both in the good times, and any time we have a problem, and the burden is removed. Ezra 8:23 tells us that when the Jews wanted to rebuild the walls for their old city, the enemy of Israel opposed the progress for restoration and renewal. But "we fasted and petitioned our God about this and he answered our prayer." God brings revival and harvest during stressful times through fasting and prayer.

Fasting and prayer will bring us from darkness to light and restore our emotions. Following God's prescriptions develops a heart that is clean, humble, joyful, thankful, kind, trusting, open, forgiving, confident, pure, wise, sincere, sensitive, happy, undivided, tender, whole, fervent, and secure. You can have that kind of heart through consistent prayer and fasting. Proverbs 4:23 advises: "Above all else, guard your heart, for everything you do flows from it." There must be a hunger for change. During the time of the prophet Samuel, people fasted one whole day (1 Sam. 7:6) and confessed their sins. They confessed to sinning against the Lord and found forgiveness. God spared their lives.

Your fasting can also influence others positively and change their future, bringing them blessings. "Thy righteousness shall go before thee" (Isa. 58:8, KJV). As a young girl I had the opportunity to lead to Christ a few atheist girls who were able to understand my righteousness in Christ. Their lives were completely changed, and the lives of their extended families and close friends. Through fasting "the glory of the LORD shall be thy reward" (v. 8, KJV).

In March of 1993, during my studies at Multnomah Bible College (now Multnomah University) in Portland, I heard a radio announcement about a catastrophic earthquake projected to hit Portland. At that time my family was still in Romania. Fear overcame me, my heart started racing, and I became very anxious—almost panicking. Because of my experience in the 1977 Bucharest disaster, I knew what an earthquake of such a high magnitude could do. My knees started shaking, epinephrine rushed through my body, anxiety grabbed me, and I could not eat or sleep. As my stress increased so did my depression. So I decided to fast the "Esther's Fast" described in Esther 4:16: "Go...and fast ye for me and neither eat nor drink three days, night or day: I also and my maidens will fast likewise; and so I will go in unto the king, which is not according to the law: and if I perish, I perish" (KJV). Ultimately Esther obtained favor in the king's eyes and he held out his golden scepter to her.

It was really hard to fast at that time, because I was providing round-the-clock care by myself in my home to four elderly residents with multiple chronic conditions. I had to cook for them three daily meals and snacks for good nutrition; I had to give them showers and provide personal hygiene; transfer them in and out of their bed, chair, and toilet; and do all the laundry and housekeeping. I was tempted to give up fasting, but when I thought about a possible catastrophic earthquake, and that I might not see my family again, I humbled myself to seek God's face with all my heart. I cried out to God and called upon His name to intervene and prevent a catastrophic event. Rereading the Book of Esther strengthened my spirit, and I believed God for a divine intervention for our city. An earthquake did strike, but it measured just 5.6 on the Richter scale. Who knows if those three days and nights of fasting did not prevent a worse disaster? I'm sure many other Christians also fasted and prayed about that.

Another example is the biblical city of Nineveh. As I mentioned in a previous chapter, when the whole city repented, fasted, and prayed for three days and three nights, God spared their city. Do not underestimate the power of fasting when everything is going well—and even more in terrible circumstances.

When Daniel fasted he did not want to defile himself with the king's meat or with his wine (Dan. 1:8). Daniel and his friends, who ate only fruits and vegetables, appeared healthier than those who ate meat and drank wine at the king's table. Isaiah 58:8 says when you fast, "thine health shall spring forth speedily" (KJV).

If you have a medical or mental condition, you must consult your doctor before you fast. I guarantee you will have only benefits from a healthy fasting diet of fresh fruits, legumes, and vegetables. I have always been very healthy all my life and worked very hard. I've never been to the emergency room. I am still very healthy and strong to this day. Through fasting, God has helped me make many crucial decisions in stressful times.

After Paul met the Lord on the road to Damascus, he did not eat or drink for three days and three nights. His entire life changed in a moment. He made the decision to follow Christ, even though previously he had been extremely zealous in persecuting Christians. The will of God had grabbed hold of his life, and he became the greatest evangelist of all the ages. (See Acts 9:1–9.) If you are worried about your future and do not know which direction to go, start fasting; "then thy light shall break forth as the morning" (Isa. 58:8, KJV). For me the light came when my husband won an unexpected visa lottery—a miracle from God—and we all received green cards and became American citizens. After a six-year struggle, our deliverance came from above.

Through fasting you can help others who are going through stressful situations. During your fast you can put aside food for hungry people and "deal thy bread to the hungry" (Isa. 58:7, KJV). When you share your food with the hungry during your fast, God will make you prosperous and bless you miraculously. In 1 Kings 17:16, "the barrel of meal wasted not, neither did the cruse of the oil fail" (KJV), as the Lord promised to the widow and her son who were preparing to die from famine. She prepared the food for the hungry man of God from the last resources they had. They gave away their last meal and received, in turn, bountiful provision for their lives and prosperity.

You can start with fasting two or three days a week, or with no food or water for twenty-four to seventy-two hours, or try three–four days with liquids only, or twenty-one to forty days of the "Daniel Fast" with fruits, vegetables, and legumes. Overall, begin to use more whole grains and cereals, many fresh fruits, and fresh vegetables and legumes. While they don't have as much as dairy products, green vegetables do contain calcium; yellow vegetables contain vitamin A; use nuts sparingly; and use beans, soy products, quinoa, and peas for protein. You can have a protein drink during this time of fasting; your muscles need protein to function. Eat foods rich in Vitamin D (about 600–800 IU a day) to modulate your cell growth, reduce inflammation, and improve your immune system and neuromuscular function. Antioxidants found in fresh fruits and fresh vegetables neutralize free radicals, which cause cancer.

You do need to consult with your doctor before you start any diet, or fast, or other changes in your life. You must do your blood tests as appropriate; even test your vitamin D_3 level. I must emphasize that vitamin deficiencies are unhealthy, but excessive amounts of vitamins cause toxicity that can be harmful too. And, before you start any extended period of fasting (more than three days fasting), talk with your doctor or nurse practitioner to make sure all your labs are within normal limits.

Your medications may need adjustment during this time. Many patients have the perception that if they have a condition such as diabetes, high blood pressure, or high cholesterol and are treated with medication they are not supposed to fast. I tell my patients that it was the overeating and unhealthy diet that caused almost all heart disease and diabetes in the first place. The body uses the necessary amount of energy from the calories we ingest, and the rest of the extra calories will be deposited in the fatty tissues, increasing the circulation demands for maintenance and the deposit of toxins in the fatty tissues.

For example, when we eat too much sugar, the pancreas must produce more insulin. Sometimes we "shock" the pancreas with all the desserts rich in sugar, and then the cells from the pancreas will be damaged by those extra demands and soon will die. Then there will be no insulin available to carry the sugar particles, causing damage at the macro and microscopic levels in all the organs, including nerves, cells, eyes, kidneys, and blood vessels. Fasting actually will improve your condition at the micro and macroscopic level, and your lifestyle change can help you reduce the number of meds you take. But you need close monitoring by your provider to change your medication, whether you fast or not.

Because of multiple chronic conditions, or increased responsibilities in life that are above one's ability to perform, many people feel stressed, and as a result get depressed. You can treat your situational or major depression with medication and counseling. But a spiritual lifestyle change, and reducing your stress, is needed to help combat your depression. You are the person who needs to initiate looking for help.

Increased health care costs increase the financial burden on everyone. Researchers say that reducing the rates of diabetes and high blood pressure by 5 percent would save about $9 billion a year in health care costs. The study estimated $24.7 billion would be saved over time by a corresponding reduction in health problems related to those diseases.[11] How about a 50 percent or 100 percent improvement? We must revolutionize the health of people around us by teaching them to change their lifestyle, not only eating right and exercising regularly, but educating them about healthy habits and behavior. For example, we can teach teenagers about abstinence from drugs, alcohol, gambling, smoking, and sex until they get married.

We must focus on healthy behaviors and then lead by example, teaching, and influencing the younger generation so the devil will not steal and destroy our children. If we are ignorant, it will cost us our future: our children, their children, and the generations after them through the epigenetic mechanism discussed earlier. It is our responsibility to educate the future generation. By having compassion for people who live in stressful situations, we can help one person at a time. God's way is the best way for a healthy lifestyle. To be successful and able to overcome the challenges in the world, change your spiritual nutrients. Feed on the Word of God by radical obedience and discipline, and God will give you wisdom and strength to change your habits and your lifestyle.

Chapter 27

RELATIONSHIPS

*And let us consider how we may spur one another on toward
love and good deeds, not giving up meeting together, as some
are in the habit of doing, but encouraging one another.*
—HEBREWS 10:24–25

NEUROSCIENTISTS HAVE STUDIED in depth how mirror neurons in people's social life can affect a healthy lifestyle. The mirror neurons in our brains enable our social relationships and allow for healing to take place. Our brains, in fact, are reshaped through the mirror neurons according to the power of our relationships. Psychology professor Louis Cozolino concluded:

> Our understanding of mirror neurons and their significance to human relationships has continued to expand and deepen....A great deal of neural overlap has been discovered in brain activation when we are thinking about others and ourselves. This raises many questions, including how we come to know others and whether the notion of an "individual self" is anything more than an evolutionary strategy to support our interconnection.[1]

We are just beginning to see the larger implications of all neurological processes—how the architecture of the brain can help us to better understand individuals and our relationships.[2]

MANAGE STRESS THROUGH HEALTHY CONNECTIONS

God honors connections, and high on His list is friendship. God's plan includes relationships between people, for we are not meant to do life alone (Acts 5:2). Jesus' disciples were involved in preaching publicly, as well as going from house to house.

When our plans go wrong and we need advice, we must seek the right connections and study God's Word for direction. When I was going through my "valley," I read the Psalms every day and prayed and fasted, seeking God's direction for my future and for the right connections and friendships.

Our spiritual vision and social connections need constant adjustments and corrections. When we lose our way in life, we need a higher wisdom than our own; Proverbs 15:22 says, "Plans fail for lack of counsel, but with many advisers they succeed." We must encourage one another to find the right direction and the solution for our disorientation. (See Hebrews 10:23–25.) In my work with people disoriented by neurocognitive disorders, I find myself reorienting and redirecting all the time—not only my patients and residents, but even their families, who are directly affected by the struggles of their loved ones. I must remind them all the time to seek connections and stay connected with support groups. Church networks and loyal friends provide strong connections and healthy relationships to prevent depression, fear, and anxiety. We need each other.

Scientists have recently discovered that support groups are effective in rehabilitation from drugs, tobacco, and alcohol abuse.[3] But we know the Word of God—beyond science—instructs us not to neglect the saints' gatherings. We are to encourage each other with the promises of God, singing psalms and songs, and lifting each other up. (See Colossians 3:8–17.) Christians grow stronger when supporting each other and caring for each other's needs. It is the empathy in the mirror neurons, enabling us to feel other people's pain and taking action to help. We are created to have healthy connections and to help each other.

God's Word is the ultimate prescription for healing relationships. Nothing is more effective. Jesus was the Word in the beginning, and the Word became flesh (John 1:1). This reality amplifies Psalm 107:20: "He sent out his word and healed them; he rescued them from the grave." Jesus came to revive us and restore our relationship with the Father in heaven, as well as our relationships with one another. Even when people hate each other and their relationship is broken, Jesus has the power to redeem and restore. The cross is the place where we learn what love and surrender mean. God promises in His Word that He will never forsake us in our emotional and physical distress. His Word promises that He is with us, and will bless us with complete physical and spiritual restoration in our time of trouble. The Word of God, the same power that raised Jesus from the dead, lives in us. Through the power of prayer, He can heal and transform our relationships. My whole life has been changed by the power of the Word, transforming my perspective on life and for eternity. We must embrace and appropriate God's unmerited grace and favor, activate our mirror neurons, and consolidate healthy, positive emotions in our limbic system. When all our brain structures align with the miraculous Word of God, we receive physical and spiritual healing in our connections and relationships.

Everyone has a God-given capacity to see the unseen world through faith, and to understand and access God's kingdom principles. Memory has a huge impact on our daily life. What we remember from the Word (deposited in our brain structures) determines and directs how we live. Caring for people with dementia and Alzheimer's disease, we observe this every day. Neuroscientists know that to maintain a healthy brain we must socialize and stay connected with friends. Stress is lower when we have support from family and friends through healthy relationships. Communication with healthy people exercises the brain and helps keeps our memory healthy.[4]

Say No to Destructive Behaviors

It is a mystery how God uses natural inhibitory neurochemicals and neurotransmitters in our physical bodies to protect us from destructive behaviors, such as GABA that works automatically in our subconscious when we approach a potentially harmful situation (touching a hot stove or electric socket).[5] When we activate our spirituality through fasting and prayer, we create the atmosphere in our brains for more discipline to prevent us from wrong behavior. Fasting, according to Isaiah 58:6, can "loose the bands of wickedness" (KJV) that stress our lives. That means we can be delivered from the power of sin and the strongholds on our lives through *the power of saying no* to lying, lust, doubt, laziness, discouragement, covetousness, addictions, envy, inconsistency, anger, discontentment, resentment, impulsiveness, judgment, harshness, self-indulgence, hypocrisy, pride, apathy, and more. You can have the power to overcome any addiction through prayer and fasting. You will live victoriously when you say no to destructive behaviors.

When discussing His disciples' inability to cast out a demon, Jesus said, "This kind can only come out by prayer and fasting" (Mark 9:29). Prayer and fasting have strengthened my ability to resist sin. I have been invited to many parties where my colleagues were indulging in harmful behaviors, but I had the strength to say no because I had spent time in prayer and fasting. Who knows where I would be today if I had not said no to those harmful invitations? The seed of sin and misbehavior is planted in everyone because of Adam and Eve's fall. Will you produce bad fruit, destroying your entire future and your eternity? Or will you overcome your sin nature? Read the Word of God, plant a new seed, and powerful spiritual thoughts that bring good fruit will remain forever. With fasting and prayer you reprogram what I call your "spiritual GABA" in your brain to say no to destructive behaviors.

Manage Stress With Passionate Worship

> Praise ye the Lord. I will praise the Lord with my whole heart, in the assembly of the upright, and in the congregation.
>
> —Psalm 111:1, kjv

Jesus tells us in Matthew 6:33 to seek first the kingdom of God. He must be our ultimate passion. The best example is the woman in the New Testament who broke an alabaster jar to anoint Jesus' feet with oil. She sacrificed something precious to worship Christ with passion. Jesus in His passion for us left His glory in heaven and chose to come to earth to humble Himself and die on the cross. God loved us so we can love others; He forgave us so we can forgive others; He had mercy on us so we can show mercy to others. His love was perfect.

When you meet Jesus face to face in worship your life will be changed. You will become a new person and leave behind all the old things that kept you from experiencing a glimpse of heaven. You enter God's kingdom through passionate worship. That gives you authority over your stressors in life. Leif Hetland, president and founder of Global Mission Awareness, stated in his book *Seeing Through Heaven's Eyes: A Worldview That Will Transform Your Life*:

> Those who have the keys to the castle of a king, for example, can access any part of it, from the front door to the back door, from the pantry to the treasury. Those who have been given *"the keys of the kingdom of heaven"* have access to the castle of the King of Kings, which is another way of saying that they have the power and authority of heaven over things in the spiritual realm.[6]

In passionate worship the kingdom of God fills your heart and helps you overcome fear, loneliness, rejection, intimidation, shame, loneliness, addiction, perversion, dysfunction, and emptiness—everything that brings high levels of stress and a chemical imbalance in your brain. When all the prodigal son's resources were gone and the fear of destruction crippled his soul, he had to radically change his thinking and return to his father's house. Thoughts that ruined his life changed to thoughts of a bright future when he returned to his father's house. (See Luke 15:11–32.) Worldly thoughts can ruin your life, but passionate worship will restore hope for your life and for eternity. Connect with God's treasure in worship and "set your minds on things above, not on earthly things" (Col. 3:2).

Chapter 28

OUR HOPE IS IN HEAVEN

Then I saw "a new heaven and a new earth," for the first heaven and the first earth had passed away, and there was no longer any sea.
—Revelation 21:1

He will wipe every tear from their eyes, there will be no more death or mourning or crying or pain, for the old order of things has passed away.
—Revelation 21:4

Death is the most undemocratic thing on earth, and it raises the stress level in our lives without preference. We all leave this planet sooner or later. We can't choose when we come into the world, and we can't decide when we leave it. The Word of God informs us about heaven; we had better believe what the Word of God says about life after death. God's Word has the power to transform us into a new creation, and to give us a relationship with God, our superintelligent designer, while we are here on earth. He designed our physical bodies to function as a whole, and to progress from birth to death, living with purpose and a hope for heaven in our hearts and minds.

From the day we are born, billions of our cells die daily through the process of apoptosis, ridding the body of unnecessary toxic materials and debris. When the body dies, the soul is freed from its earthly shell to live forever in eternity. Over and over again I have seen the pain and suffering of people with multi-organ failure at the end of life. All their systems shut down, and their souls leave their bodies in their last breaths.

INTERNAL THOUGHTS ARE ETERNAL

> My son, pay attention to what I say; turn your ear to my words. Do not let them out of your sight, keep them within your heart; for they are life to those who find them and health to one's whole body.
> —Proverbs 4:20–22

Live with eternity in mind, because your life is in God's hands. Listen to His Word, the wellspring of life, as outlined in Proverbs 4:20–22. Words can bring healing to your heart, body, soul, and mind. You are not what people around you say you are. You are a child of God, with a purpose on earth and a destiny in heaven. Even facing death, you can have peace and hope with God. (See Psalm 23.) When we walk with God, we won't fear death.

A close friend had Parkinson's disease and knew that he was slowly dying, day by day. He said, "I know I am dying, but whom shall I fear when I have served a mighty God my entire life? Now I will go and meet Him." He spoke with so much confidence and with a smile on his face. He had lived his entire life with purpose and hope for eternity, despite living under communist persecution in Romania. The Word says that whether we live or die, we are the Lord's. He loves us in all circumstances.

Fear has no room when His love fills your heart and mind. Feel the love of our Father. Jesus said, "The one who loves me will be loved by my Father, and I too will love them and show myself to them" (John 14:21). Even though the devil puts his seed of fear in people's minds to frighten them, the love of God casts out fear. "Do not be afraid" is the most quoted instruction in the Bible.[1]

HE FIGHTS FOR YOU EVEN IN DEATH

> When you pass through the waters, I will be with you; and when you pass through the rivers, they will not sweep over you. When you walk through the fire, you will not be burned; the flame will not set you ablaze.
> —Isaiah 43:2

> The Lord your God, who is going before you, will fight for you.
> —Deuteronomy 1:30

God promised in Isaiah 43:2 that you would not be harmed, whether going through water or fire. In Deuteronomy 1:30, He promises to fight for you and show Himself strong on your behalf. Second Chronicles 16:9 says, "For the eyes of the Lord range throughout the earth to strengthen those whose hearts are fully committed to Him." Turn away from foolish things and do not believe the deceiving lies of Satan. This entire world loses the battle at the end. Nobody leaves earth alive. Only in Jesus will we find eternal victory.

Jesus said that He has gone to prepare a place for us in heaven. Our true citizenship is not of this earth. In His time, Jesus will come again to take all of us to heaven. Have hope in God, and He will bless you. You have the anchor of your soul in the hope of Jesus, the High Priest, "so that what you hope for may be fully realized" (Heb. 6:11). First Thessalonians 4:16–17 states: "For the Lord Himself will come down from heaven, with a loud command, with the voice of the archangel and with the trumpet call of God, and the dead in Christ will rise first. After that, we who are still alive and are left will be caught up together with them in the clouds to meet the Lord in the air. And so we will be with the Lord forever." This is our hope and purpose, and we must encourage each other with this truth.

The Lord is sovereign, and the universe proclaims and declares His majesty and glory. He created you, and He will call you to heaven when He decides. Our hope is anchored in His promises. The righteous, even in death, have hope (Prov. 14:32). For Christians, dying is gain. Those who die in Christ have hope in death, because they will rest from their work after this life on earth is done. Life and death are real, as we see with our own eyes, but heaven is real too. You do not know what day your life will end and the Lord will call you to heaven. You must be ready at any time. We read in the Book of Luke chapter 12 about the wealthy man who neglected the real purpose of life and lost his soul at the end. The purpose for our lives here on earth is to prepare us for eternity.

Where Your Heart Is, There Is Your Treasure

> Do not store up for yourselves treasures on earth, where moths and vermin destroy, and where thieves break in and steal, but store up for yourselves treasures in heaven, where moths and vermin do not destroy, and where thieves do not break in and steal. For where your treasure is, there your heart will be also.
>
> —Matthew 6:19–21

Jesus' purpose on this earth was to provide salvation and eternal life in heaven, through His death on the cross and His triumphal resurrection. Jesus, the author of social transformation, carried all of humankind's sorrow, grief, and mourning. Jesus Christ indeed fulfilled His purpose. We are His treasure. After His departure from earth, His followers began serving others, developing Christian communities and charitable services, such as hospitals and organizations with biblical names that are relevant to this day: Good Samaritan, Emanuel, Providence, Adventist, St. Mary, and Mt. Sinai are good examples. Christians through the ages have followed God's Rx to care for others with compassion, dignity, love, and respect. Even today this is what medical and nursing schools teach practitioners and health care providers. Jesus Christ changed the world entirely. He started a new culture on earth, showing us how to live life with purpose.

These days we live in the Christian era that began when Christ was born more than two thousand years ago. Time on most countries' calendars is divided into "before Christ" (BC) and *"anno domini* (in the year of our Lord)," or AD. We have traveled in Europe, visiting all the ancient ruins and cathedrals, and the guides always refer to the "Before Christ" and "After Christ" eras when talking about what was built there. But Jesus' kingdom is forever and has no end (Luke 1:32–33). Jesus' philosophy even inspired kings to apply kingdom principles. He was without sin, but He still befriended tax collectors and sinners to bring them into His kingdom. Wisdom and knowledge are gained only when you love God with your entire heart, mind, and soul. Jesus valued training and education, and we need to prepare our minds to focus on the eternal treasure in heaven.

We were created with built-in desires to be like Jesus. People pray in Jesus' name in their desperation. Jesus was and is the most recognized person on Earth. He is the center of the universe. He is the light of the world and the hope for mankind, giving us a life with purpose. The Bible tells us that we are citizens of heaven, and we must treasure that which cannot be destroyed, as Jesus tells us in Matthew 6:19–21.

Not Afraid to Die

> Put to death...sexual immorality, impurity, lust, evil desires and greed, which is idolatry....Rid yourselves of all such things as these: anger, rage, malice, slander, and filthy language from your lips.
> —Colossians 3:5, 8

It is time to seek knowledge and wisdom from God and follow Jesus' principles for kingdom living. Love God and seek wisdom and understanding through the Word of God. We have no excuse for not seeking wisdom from Him, for we must eventually give account for ignoring God's prescriptions in His Word. As Romans 1:20 says, "For since the creation of the world God's invisible qualities— His eternal power and divine nature—have been clearly seen, being understood from what has been made, so that people are without excuse."

We have no excuse for not knowing God, because we can see His creation. The universe declares His majesty. All mankind is created in the image of God and reflects His image. Those who knew Jesus and His power were not afraid of dying. Only our guilt of not living according to the Word of God causes us to fear death. We must follow His instructions in Colossians 3 to rid ourselves of sinful, unhealthy habits. All of these cause us to fear death, and they will bring down the wrath of God.

Everything on earth must be done from heaven's perspective. Live your life to affect eternity, and invest in the invisible spiritual world by ministering with a heart that is focused on your treasure. Living according to God's instructions and prescriptions for life will reduce your stress from fears, including guilt and fear of death. Power is released in your life when you respond to the Word of God that is working in you, transforming your thinking and life. God wants to deliver you from the fear of death "so that by his death he might break the power of him who holds the power of death—that is, the devil—and free those who, all their lives, were held in slavery by their fear of death" (Heb. 2:14–15).

Joy in Death

> But…we are looking forward to a new heaven and a new earth.
> —2 Peter 3:13

As a teenager I always looked for wholesome, trustworthy relationships, longing to belong to a group I could trust. While searching for that perfect group I felt lonely and insecure—even hurt by colleagues and friends who did not understand my longing for an unpolluted spiritual environment. One night as I went to bed feeling sad and disappointed, the Holy Spirit touched me. I felt my soul and spirit lifting from my body and into the spiritual realm. I was immersed in "a sea of multitudes of souls" (Rev. 19:6) in perfect unity, peace, and unspeakable joy. I saw my earthly body lying down as if numb. I did not want to leave that indescribable moment of great joy and perfect peace in my soul and spirit. I even recognized some of the spiritual heroes of earlier eras, who served God reverently on earth. It was only a glimpse, but that was enough for me to have an impression of the atmosphere in heaven.

We should not fear death, "because through Christ Jesus, the law of the Spirit, who gives life, has set you free from the law of sin and death" (Rom. 8:2). Set your mind on the Spirit's desires, because the mind set on the flesh is death. The Spirit of God can deliver you from the fear of death. Even thinking about the dying process can be joyful. Your life is like a moment to God; each of us is but a breath (Ps. 39:5). We have an obligation to prepare for our lives after death. People get very busy and do not spend enough time to know God more. God shakes us to wake us up and get our attention. We are not on this planet forever. God loves this generation and wants us to put our trust in Him.

We must be filled with overflowing joy. Jesus said, "I have told you this so that my joy may be in you and that your joy may be complete" (John 15:11). The devil can make you bitter when you think about how someone you loved has died. Some people turn to drugs to numb their emotional pain after a close friend dies, but we must be realistic about how quickly life passes. As 2 Peter 3:13 says, we are looking forward to a new heaven and a new earth. Jesus has promised us a new world filled with God's righteousness. When you close your eyes in this life, you open them in another life. Entrust your life into God's hands. Be reassured in every moment that "if God is for us, who can be against us?" (Rom. 8:31).

Jesus went to the cross to give us eternal life. Even when you are threatened by disease, violence, or painful emotions, you must be determined to finish the race well. There will always be pressure to give up and not finish the race. Press on, despite all circumstances. God will respond to you when you seek Him. Your Creator will provide the strength and resources you need to physically and spiritually fulfill your destiny and prepare for heaven.

He who created you will give you joy. God knows the effect of joy in our spirit, soul, and body. "Rejoice in the Lord always. I will say it again: Rejoice!" (Phil. 4:4). Our great commission on this earthly journey is to be filled with the knowledge of the Word of God and lead other people to Jesus, which produces great joy in heaven. You will feel His joy and goodness. God's glory is God's goodness; you are made to be profoundly affected by God's presence. During our journey to heaven, He is pruning us to be more effective. God called us to continue to pour out what we have received so that at the end of our lives our joy will be complete.

The apostle Paul considered death as something to be gained. He said, "I am torn between the two: I desire to depart and be with Christ, which is better by far" (Phil. 1:23). When your days are finished, your physical body will die, because your days are numbered. If you have lived according to the Word of God, then when your days are finished, you will move into your eternal home in heaven with the Lord.

Heaven as described in the Book of Revelation is real. One day you will step right onto the streets of gold. There is a glorious, shining city with mansions, streets of gold, rivers of living water, trees with healing leaves, and animals that harm no one. Many books have been written about heaven based on people's near-death experiences—even by medical providers, such as cardiologists and neurosurgeons.

You and I are all going to die. Even kings die sooner or later. One hundred years from now none of us will be here. It is important that we finish well. John stated in Revelation 14:13, "I heard a voice from heaven saying unto me, Write, Blessed are the dead which die in the Lord from henceforth: Yea saith the Spirit, that they may rest from their labors; and their works do follow them" (KJV). All your deeds will follow you.

The rewards in heaven are great. Rejoice, for we are going to heaven when our temporary "visa" on this planet expires. There will be eternal peace. There will be a glorious day when we will meet all our loved ones. When our lives on earth finish, we will be raised from death on the resurrection day. "Brothers and sisters, we do not want you to be uninformed about those who sleep in death, so that you do not grieve like the rest of mankind, who have no hope" (1 Thess. 4:13). In heaven you will meet all those who died in the Lord—your close relatives and friends. Live with hope in eternal life, in resurrection. Jesus was the first resurrected One who ascended to heaven.

There will be a day when all of us will see God and give an account for our lives. Check yourself. Are you ready for the day when you're called to heaven, your eternal home? In his book *Heaven*, Dr. Randy Alcorn, founder and director of Eternal Perspective Ministries, emphasized:

> *Home* as a term for Heaven isn't simply a metaphor. It describes an actual, physical place—a place promised and built by our bridegroom; a place we'll share with loved ones; a place of fond familiarity and comfort and refuge; a place of marvelous smells and tastes, fine food, and great conversation; a place of contemplation and interaction and expressing the gifts and passions that God has given us. It'll be a place of unprecedented freedom and adventure.[2]

Persevere according to the Word of God that releases you from stress and from worrying about death. He is calling you to live at peace with Him. Your stress will be lowered, your entire physical body will relax, and the signs and symptoms of fear will diminish or disappear completely. If your life ended today, where would you go? God longs for you to go to heaven and live with Him. Paul lived a life filled with the Holy Spirit. He knew that for him it was better to go to heaven to be with the Lord, but for others on earth, it was better for him to remain here, to keep preaching about eternal life through Jesus Christ. You have not yet finished your assignment that you were called to do on earth.

Live for Christ while you can, and when you leave, heaven will gain. Over the last three decades of providing end-of-life care in our facility, I have often seen people dying. I could fill a whole amphitheater with the people who have passed on in our foster homes and our memory care facility. I sense their fear of death and their struggle in the last days or hours of their lives. I whisper in their ears when they are on their deathbed: "Do not be afraid to go. The Lord is sending His angel to usher you home to heaven in His presence." Then I pray for them so the angel will come to take their souls to heaven when they are ready. I continue to pray for forgiveness for each dying person. The atmosphere changes each time I pray where a person is dying.

Once at a funeral service where I was invited to speak, I told the congregation how I talk to these special people when they are dying, and how I pray for them at their bedside, in addition to the medical and health care we provide. We play music and worship songs throughout the day for their physical and spiritual comfort. You can feel the presence of God in the room. At the end of that service, one lady said to me, "I know where I will go to die when my life is almost finished—Tabor Crest" (the name of our business). Natural death demands courage, but death is part of your destiny and your life story.

The Bible is about dying to self and becoming alive in Christ Jesus. When you live with eternity in mind, you will live forever. It is written:

> Brothers and sisters, we do not want you to be uninformed about those who sleep in death, so that you do not grieve like the rest of the mankind, who have no hope. For we believe that Jesus died and rose again, and so we believe that God will bring with Jesus those who have fallen asleep in him. According to the Lord's word, we tell you that we who are still alive, who are left until the coming of the Lord, will certainly not precede those who have fallen asleep. For the Lord Himself will come down from heaven, with a loud command, with the voice of the archangel and with the trumpet call of God, and the dead in Christ will rise first. After that, we who are still alive and are left will be caught up together with them in the clouds to meet the Lord in the air. So we will be with the Lord forever. Therefore encourage one another with these words.
>
> —1 Thessalonians 4:13–18

What a fascinating, joyful promise! God, knowing we would be afraid of death, wrote this to encourage us. We will be with the Lord forever, even though we must face the pain of separation from death. We are also instructed to encourage those around us. I hope you are encouraged by this clear message about life after death.

If the Spirit who raised Christ from the dead lives in you, then you are not afraid to die, for in Genesis 26:24 God promised that He is with you: "That night the Lord appeared to him and said, 'I am the God of your father Abraham. Do not be afraid, for I am with you; I will bless you.'"

God is with you in all seasons of your life. Trust His promises and do not despair in your tribulations. We learn in the Word of God that all the Bible characters faced death with courage—Esther, Daniel, Shadrach, Meshach, Abednego, Joseph, and many prophets—as well as many Christians through the centuries. All the apostles took courage when threatened with death. Their Lord, whom they loved and served with a pure heart, was with them. Take courage. God promised all of us, "I am with you." His presence is with you. Appreciate the presence of God and enjoy His presence in your life.

Manage Stress With Courage

Can you imagine living without fear, weakness, or vulnerability? Strive for a noble character. Esther had noble character in the face of an enemy and made a stand for what was right, for herself and her nation. She did everything in her power to save their lives and stated, "If I perish, I perish" (Est. 4:16). The enemy is threatening you over and over again with the thing you fear the most. You may have many "ifs" in your mind right now, like all of us: "What if" my child, my husband, my business, my job, my church, my parents, my friends, my nation, my world (fill in the blank)? What if? In all situations, God wants us to trust Him. Courage comes when our heart is convinced we are loved. Love casts out fear when you take courage. God loved us so much that He gave His only Son to come to earth and die for us in humiliation, hanging on the cross. There is no greater love on the face of the earth than the Father's and the Son's. God's pleasure is to give you the kingdom, to invite you to live with Him in eternity after your physical body dies. Live with no fear of death.

The prophet Isaiah foretold of God creating a new heaven and a new earth: "See, I will create new heavens and a new earth. The former things will not be remembered, nor will they come to mind. But be glad and rejoice forever in what I will create, for I will create Jerusalem to be a delight and its people a joy. I will rejoice over Jerusalem and take delight in my people; the sound of weeping and of crying will be heard in it no more" (Isa. 65:17–19). God's prescription for us is to rejoice in Him when our lives are finished.

God did not give us a spirit of fear. Before he died, my father gave instructions for my oldest brother to read Psalm 91 at his funeral service so everyone attending would know not to fear death. We just need to position ourselves under the shadow of the wings of El Elyon, the Most High God, where there is no fear.

Going to Heaven

Insecurity and uncertainty about your last days on earth, and where you will spend eternity, will cause more fear. If you prepare now, the fear of death will disappear. You do not need to go through stress and emotional pain because of such fear. Recently at the gym I met a young Christian mother with three children. During our conversation she said, "I cannot wait to get to heaven." I considered this with a professional ear and mind, and clearly that was not a suicidal thought—it was genuine happiness, knowing where her journey on earth will end and where she is heading. She was so excited about God. As my silent evaluation continued, I realized that she loves her children and is reading books on how to raise children and how to be the wife God wants her to be. She wants to help her husband reach his full potential and fulfill his destiny here on this planet.

When you know where you will spend eternity, you will be at peace. You will desire to see your future real estate in heaven, even though you are committed to earthly assignments and obligations. You can persevere and live according to the Word of God, while waiting to meet your Creator. God promised eternal life to all who obey Him and follow His prescriptions beyond science—His commandments, instructions, and directions. God is calling you to live at peace with Him during your short time on earth. He wants you to serve Him. Nobody will avoid seeing death. King David asked the Lord to tell him when the end of his life would be so he could count his days on earth. David lived with eternity in mind. God's answer was that life is extremely short, like a vapor, and one day we will go to heaven.

Trust the Lord and have confidence that He cares for you. Even with my strong faith, I have had to remind myself over and over again of the words of Hebrews

13:6: "The Lord is my helper; I will not be afraid. What can mere mortals do to me?" and verse 8: "Jesus Christ is the same yesterday and today and forever." We look forward to heaven because our current location is not an enduring city (vv. 12–14).

Preparing for the Last Move

Although most people look at death as a tragedy, it is meant to be a move to your eternal home in heaven, to live forever with your Lord. We have had to move many times, both in Romania and here in the United States. Maybe you have moved a lot too. Each time we had to make huge preparations for moving day, it was stressful getting everything ready.

Our last move will be when we leave this earth, but for that day we must make a major spiritual preparation. We all have real estate waiting for us in heaven, promised by Jesus Christ and prepared by Him for those who follow His teaching. It is important that you and I finish as more than conquerors. All the saints in the Bible kept eternity in mind and followed God's plans for preparation. That will indeed be a glorious, peaceful day. No spirit of fear, and no more stress. heaven is a "Stress Free Zone."

Hope in Eternity

> For the Spirit God gave us does not make us timid, but gives us power, love and self-discipline.
> —2 Timothy 1:7

Many are anxious and frustrated at the thought of facing death. Proverbs 12:25 states: "Anxiety weighs down the heart but a kind word cheers it up." Emotionally you are affected by fearful thoughts. Proverbs 14:10 explains, "Each heart knows its bitterness, and no one else can share its joy." But God has not given you a spirit of fear, according to 2 Timothy 1:7. We will feel the pain of a temporary separation—no one can avoid that. But in God we have hope that in eternity we will be together again with our loved ones. Paul Manwaring, registered general and psychiatric nurse, former prisoner manager in England, and former Global Legacy overseer, said in his book *What on Earth Is Glory? A Practical Approach to a Glory-Filled Life*:

> We are all called to an eternal journey that will take us from glory to glory and ultimately to the great cloud of witnesses, where we will watch as those who follow us continue and complete the work of revealing the fullness of God's glory in the earth, culminating in the most glorious wedding and family reunion, which will last for eternity.[3]

Your Days Are Numbered

> Your eyes saw my unformed body; all the days ordained for me were written in your book before one of them came to be.
> —Psalm 139:16

As the psalmist said, your days are numbered. Before you were born, God wrote your life on earth and your destiny. Before you were born, you were in God's thoughts. That eternal thought of God materialized when it crossed the threshold of your parents' emotions, and oxytocin rushed through their brains. Their physical bodies united, releasing a half-cell from your mother and another half from your father to form an amazing, new little baby human in just over nine months—you! Learn more about that by reading about embryology. It is fascinating. Your life starts and ends with God. He knows your destiny. Check yourself. Are you ready for that day when you are called back home to heaven?

The Reality of Heaven

You were born because you are important. You must stay here until the Lord decides for you to go. As Paul contemplated the decision between life and death, he said if he lived he wanted to lift up the name of Jesus. (See Philippians 1.) We must stay here to lift up the name of Jesus Christ so more souls will be saved for eternity. Your death is controlled by the power of the Holy Spirit. He decides your time to go. You do not need to worry about the timing. Your days are numbered and must be fulfilled, until the angel is sent to escort you to the throne room of God. Live for Jesus Christ now, here on earth. Rely on God's promises and He will wipe every tear from your eyes. There will be no more death or sorrow or crying or pain (Rev. 21:4). All these things will be gone forever. Our citizenship is not here. Heaven is real, as described in Revelation. Have faith, and hope in God. He will bless you and give you victory, even in death.

Thinking About Heaven

Fear of death, and the unknowns of life after death, can trigger anxiety. This fear prompted the statement: "Death anxiety is the mother of all religions."[4] People do become more spiritual when they approach the end of life. Medication will not take away the fear of death. In uncertain situations and unpleasant circumstances you must have faith in God and experience His transforming power. Faith comes from hearing, and hearing by the Word of God (Rom. 10:17). The Word becomes alive in your heart, and when you live accordingly, it becomes your biography. You are not the same anymore when you have faith. The righteous live by faith.

I have had to live by faith all my life. I couldn't live without faith. When doubt and unbelief tried to come in, I cried out to God to increase my faith, and He did. From Hebrews 11:6, we know that without faith it is impossible to please God. Unbelief puts fear in your heart, with all its unhealthy symptoms. Have faith, resist the devil, and he will flee from you. Through faith you defeat the devil, which is why Paul said he preached the gospel, so that "your faith might not rest on human wisdom, but on God's power" (1 Cor. 2:5).

HEAVEN'S CULTURE

> He has made everything beautiful in its time. He has also set eternity in the human heart; yet no one can fathom what God has done from beginning to end.
> —ECCLESIASTES 3:11

You and I were born with eternity (heavenly citizenship and heaven's culture) in our DNA. I had to change my citizenship after I moved to the United States. In order to get my US citizenship, I had to learn everything about America's history and its laws. I also had to adopt American culture to be able to function here. I did that with much joy and gladness, knowing all the benefits and advantages I would have to live as an American citizen on American soil. Spiritually, our citizenship is in another, supernatural realm, with a heavenly culture based on God's character. We need to follow heaven's laws to get our heavenly citizenship. We also must adopt heaven's culture to live in God's kingdom. God puts desires in our heart that cannot be satisfied here on earth. This is because we must desire things from above and seek the supernatural, eternal kingdom of God.

Thousands of years ago Solomon wrote the eloquent words that led off this section. We know that earth is not our home. You and I are here with a temporary visa. When our earthly visa expires, we must move to our eternal home, where our permanent citizenship resides. It is very easy for me to go on a mission trip to Romania or Europe, where I have been before. I have a picture already in my mind about those places. But it is very hard to go places where I have never been. It is difficult to yield to something unseen. I have a picture in my mind of those places based on others' descriptions, but I am sure the idea I have in my mind is far from reality. We are afraid of the unknown, so we need God's supernatural power to overcome that fear.

ON THE WAY TO HEAVEN

When the first Europeans landed in North America hundreds of years ago, they did not know what the continent would be like in a few hundred years. America exists because long ago people from Europe desired to come here at any cost. They were motivated to start over in a different land. When I left Romania in 1990, I came with hopes and expectations, yet not knowing exactly what my future would hold. You must live with hope, desire, expectation, and motivation to move on to your heavenly home when your life here is over. Whatever happens in the natural happens in the spiritual. Thinking about heaven, we do not know how we will get there, but God has promised us a new heaven and a new earth, with streets of gold. We must live with expectations. What we believe, we receive.

We are on the way to heaven during our entire life. We are on the way to the promises of God. Walk like a person who belongs in heaven, a member of a royal priesthood, part of God's family, created in His image. In our heavenly kingdom there are no graves. The devil will never enter there. Heaven is prepared for those who have accepted heaven's identity through the blood of the Lamb. We travel around the world and we see people who desire to go abroad; they desire a new land. There is power in desire. Our desire must be driven by our thought of eternity in our DNA, to go to the land prepared for us by Jesus. Do not lose your focus. Those who believe in Jesus will overcome the world. Delight yourself in the Lord and He will give you the desires of your heart. It all begins with a desire in your heart. You can overcome huge mountains if you have the desire.

Character for Heaven

> For physical training is of some value, but godliness has value for all things, holding promise for both the present life and the life to come.
> —1 Timothy 4:8

The only thing you take to heaven is your character. Do not waste your time on earth with unnecessary things. Train yourself to develop a godly character. You must work hard and do what is right according to the highest standards, and God will build your character. Eternal issues are the most important things in life. First Timothy 4:8 tells us training for godliness is important. All training is good, but training for eternity is the most beneficial.

Many people get distracted and waste their eternal, God-given gifts. A hurting generation needs godly training and character to heal the broken souls. People deceive themselves with temporary pleasures. One day they will be on their deathbed, asking the tough question: "Where will I spend eternity?" He promised we would walk on streets of gold, but first we must live intentionally to obtain godly character. You are in the right place to obtain God's promises right now, if you are willing to invest in and develop your heavenly character.

DEATH IS THE BEGINNING OF YOUR TRUE LIFE

> Jesus said to her, "I am the resurrection and the life. The one who believes in me will live, even though they die; and whoever lives by believing in me will never die. Do you believe this?"
> —John 11:25–26

Dying looks like the end, but it is just the beginning of an eternal new life. Sooner or later, all of us will die. Kings, presidents, politicians, businesspeople, intellectuals, actors, rich, and poor—all will die at the end of their lives. The time will come for all of us to go to our eternal home. There will be a weeping for those who are not ready. You must surrender to God's plan. When you surrender, your stress will decrease because you have put your trust in God's promises. Jesus answers our questions about life after death, like He did for the woman at the well in John 11:25–26.

God gave us His prescription to treat fear: "So do not fear, for I am with you; do not be dismayed, for I am your God. I will strengthen you and help you; I will uphold you with my righteous right hand" (Isa. 41:10). That prescription can be used in any situation, even on our deathbed. When Jesus' love opens our spiritual eyes, we realize earth is not our home; we are just passing through to a new heaven and a new earth. The aging process is a downsizing process, preparing for our exit from this world to our eternal home.

People stress themselves when they hear that a family member or close friend is dying. I see people dying all the time, and I see the stress that family members and friends experience. One day each of us will leave this earth. People need to be ready. We cannot move on to a new earth and new heaven with an old body. We will enter the throne room of God with a new body. If we come boldly to Him in faith, Christ will make us perfect and He will do it according to His pleasure. Death is necessary; it is not a punishment. Our souls will join our spirit, and we will leave the body behind. We need to make sure our souls and spirits are ready.

NO SHORT CUTS

> Jesus said, "Look I am coming soon! My reward is with me, and I will give to each person according to what they have done."
> —Revelation 22:12

People want to know their calling and purpose on earth. God doesn't want anyone to die eternally. God wants us to see His kingdom come, His will to be done on earth as in heaven, as described in the Lord's Prayer. We need the gift of the Holy Spirit to see the manifestation of the kingdom of God on earth. The Holy Spirit works to positively encourage people. People need to seek wisdom from God. "For those who find me find life and receive favor from the Lord" (Prov. 8:35). Wait on God and see what He wants to say. Take time with the Holy Spirit. There is no substitute for time with God. In medicine, if a practitioner uses short cuts, the outcome can be severe, even resulting in unexpected death. We must spend real, sincere time with God. The heart and nature of God is of a Father with a true love. We cannot be what He is, but we can have what He has—His love, wisdom, inspiration, and anointing.

We need to honor those people who can teach us how to get into God's presence. Observe where the presence of God is resting and go there. When I hear about God showing His power at a saints gathering, my husband and I go there, even though we have to drive one or more days or fly on an airplane. When we travel, I like to read the Word of God, memorize verses, and read inspirational books. God's motivation for each human being is love. His love motivated Him to send Jesus to die on the cross for the world's sins.

As you get ready for heaven, allow God to change your "spiritual DNA" and character through His love. Jesus is building His church for Himself from heavenly minded people. He is ready to come and get us soon. Jesus said, "Look I am coming soon! My reward is with Me, and I will give to each person according to what they have done" (Rev. 22:12). We must accept our heavenly citizenship, walk in the right path, and live in a heavenly culture.

Dangerous Zone

Refuse to stay frustrated because of failures in your life. Do not allow frustration and anxiety to consume you. While a sense of insecurity and uncertainty from careless living will devastate you, God will always use somebody to help you up. Train your senses to notice when God sends somebody into your life to help you. Your senses are trained to discern right from wrong. Get up and move away from dangerous situations. I was afraid of the unknown in Bucharest, and later in the United States, but God brought many people into my life who shared good advice. I had to choose those people with godly advice and avoid dangerous ideas.

You must be willing to pay the price to fulfill your destiny. Your efforts, hardships, and personal sacrifice will give you a story that motivates others. The story of your life and your testimony, with all the difficulties you are going through, must be written so others will be encouraged. Jesus wrote His story with His own blood, with the power to transform the world. Have faith like a little child, receive Jesus, and worship Him in prayer and in truth. Trust and obey God. Guard your heart with all diligence and your stress levels will decrease.

ETERNAL REWARD

> If we live, we live for the Lord; if we die, we die for the Lord. So, whether we live or die, we belong to the Lord.
> —ROMANS 14:8

We were born needing to belong to our superintelligent designer. To belong to the Lord is an eternal prescription. Many of us at some point in life pass through a valley of discouragement, or get depressed about bad news, or bad things happen to us, or disabilities and infirmities happen with no apparent reason. Your struggle is God's instrument to convince you, to discipline you, and to catch your attention to prepare you for heaven.

God uses human instruments to prepare us for eternal life. My friend Dr. Lea stated that nothing could catch her attention for heaven "except getting cancer." Only a diagnosis of cancer motivated her to come to Christ and get saved. God knows exactly what will move you to seek salvation. In the middle of suffering, it is hard to see eternal victory. You may see your life as ruined, but God gives you a crown that will last forever. He has more in heaven for each of us. You just need your spiritual eyes to be opened and to trust in His powerful hands, because He holds your soul in His everlasting love. Only in heaven will we find out why God allowed so much suffering in our lives. Each one of us has questions for God in heaven. Save your questions for that time.

If you are not sure if you are saved, and not sure where you will spend your eternity, do not wait for that incurable diagnosis to force you to come to the Lord. You can lift your hands toward heaven right now and say from the bottom of your heart:

> *Father God in heaven, I sinned against You. I recognize and confess all my sins, since I was born until today. Please forgive all my sins and wash them away with the precious blood of the Lamb. I bring all my sins to the cross. Cleanse me with the precious holy blood that was shed by the Lamb of God, Your Son, Jesus Christ. Come into my heart through the power of the Holy Spirit and be my personal Lord and Savior. Transform my life. Today I want to start a new life with You, Jesus Christ, who died on the cross for my sins, was resurrected on the third day and ascended to heaven, and who is sitting at the right hand of God, the Father, the Creator of the universe, to intercede for me, my family, and the entire world. Thank You. In Jesus' name I pray.*

That powerful prayer will change your spiritual DNA and make you a new creation in Christ Jesus. You will receive unspeakable joy and peace—and no stress!

I pray that our heavenly Father will seal your decision to live for eternity from this moment on. I pray that God will give you a pure faith, courage, boldness, and authority over worldly temptations. Your pain and suffering are not without purpose. Your faith is more "precious than gold" (Ps. 19:10) and will bring you honor and glory when Jesus Christ comes. Keep your faith and look at all your circumstances with heavenly eyes. All the stories in the Bible are examples of great people who trusted God, believed in eternal life, and overcame worldly temptation.

God Is Not Finished With You

> It was good for me to be afflicted so that I might learn your decrees. The law of your mouth is more precious to me than thousands of pieces of silver and gold.
>
> —Psalm 119:71–72

God wants you to be victorious, even when you feel that your heart is broken into pieces. God puts all the small pieces from your broken heart together to fulfill His plan in you for eternity. He has not finished with you yet. "If we live, we live for the Lord; if we die, we die for the Lord. So, whether we live or die, we belong to the Lord" (Rom. 14:8). Many times discouragement, pain, suffering, and brokenness overwhelm our heart and we don't see anything good from our disaster. But in eternity you will see that this suffering was a precious opportunity to turn your attention to the Word of God, for the salvation of your soul.

The psalmist said, "It was good for me to be afflicted so that I might learn your decrees. The law of your mouth is more precious to me than thousands of pieces of silver and gold" (Ps. 119:71–72). God knows what is best for you, more than you know. Sometimes He allows even catastrophic events to wake us up.

Death Is Part of Your Destiny

> But if Christ is in you, then even though your body is subject to death because of sin, the Spirit gives life because of righteousness. And if the Spirit of him who raised Jesus from the dead is living in you, he who raised Christ from the dead will also give life to your mortal bodies because of his Spirit who lives in you.
>
> —Romans 8:10–11

If you believe the Word of God, you are already dead to sin, and you need not fear death anymore because Christ lives in you by faith. As Paul writes, "I have been crucified with Christ and I no longer live, but Christ lives in me. The life I now live in the body, I live by faith in the Son of God, who loved me and gave himself for me" (Gal. 2:20). We are redeemed and have a house in heaven. Ephesians 2:6 says, "And God raised us up with Christ and seated us with him in the heavenly realms in Christ Jesus." In His legendary prayer right before His crucifixion, Jesus said, "Now this is eternal life: that they know you, the only true God, and Jesus

Christ, whom you have sent" (John 17:3). Thinking of eternity gives you courage, and death demands courage. Death is part of life.

Take courage, because the Lord will not abandon you. You are the work of His hands. He is with you every moment. We can find encouragement in these words from the psalmist: "The LORD will vindicate me; your love, LORD, endures forever—do not abandon the works of your hands" (Ps. 138:8). And also from Paul, who declares: "In all these things we are more than conquerors through Him who loved us. For I am convinced that neither death nor life, neither angels nor demons, neither the present nor the future, nor any powers, neither height nor depth, nor anything else in all creation, will be able to separate us from the love of God that is in Christ Jesus our Lord (Rom. 8:37–39).

That reassurance allows us to live life without fear, weakness or vulnerability.

Full of Courage

There are many examples of courageous people in the Bible. One that amazes me is the story of Esther. Esther was full of courage and determined that nothing could be against her when she decided to go into the "king's presence to beg for mercy" (Est. 4:8), despite all the rules and regulations of that time. The king's rules were unbearable for his close family, and the queen herself said. We read in the Book of Esther: "All the king's officials and the people of the royal provinces know that for any man or woman who approaches the king in the inner court without being summoned the king has but one law: that they be put to death unless the king extends the gold scepter to them and spares their lives. But thirty days have passed since I was called to go to the king" (Est. 4:11).

Even though she knew that the probability she would die was very high, she was willing to take the chance after three days and three nights of fasting for the Jewish nation, with no food or drink. Verse 16 adds: "Go, gather together all the Jews that are present in Shushan, and fast ye for me, and neither eat nor drink three days, night or day: I also and my maidens will fast likewise; and so will I go in unto the king, which is not according to the law: and if I perish, I perish" (KJV).

She was determined to stand in the gap for her people selflessly, and thus fulfilled her destiny to save a nation from annihilation. Her courage preserved the lineage of the coming Messiah to bring salvation and eternal life to the entire world. We are called away from self-preservation to be courageous, determined to fulfill our calling. You can make choices; you can decide not to look back. The power of choice has an impact on your destiny and where you will spend your eternity. You are fully responsible to God for your life.

You are called to be courageous. "Be strong and courageous. Do not be afraid or terrified because of them, for the LORD your God goes with you; He will never leave you nor forsake you" (Deut. 31:6). You are one decision away from starting a new chapter in your life. You can be brave. Your narrative and your spiritual résumé can be changed. Become a courageous person, overcoming your old thoughts through a divine exchange, choosing thoughts that can change your life now and for eternity. Nobody is an obstacle to your destiny but yourself. God has no intention of leaving you this way. One brave decision can turn your path toward a healthy body, soul, and spirit. Bravely follow God's supernatural prescriptions to manage stress from the worry, fear, anxiety, and depression that can kill you. *Do not be afraid. Fear not.*

CONCLUSION

WE ARE NOW convinced by science that our emotions influence our thinking process, which dictates our lifestyle as well as the amount and quality of the neurotransmitters and neurochemicals released in our bodies. Thus, our emotions, thoughts, and lifestyle keep changing the structures of our brains. Science has demonstrated that we can rewire our brains through a process called neuroplasticity by renewing our minds and our thoughts and emotions. Dr. Jeffrey Barsch stated in his book *Praying for the Brain: Rewiring the Brain Through Prayer*:

> We now know that the brain has the ability to reorganize itself by forming new neural connections throughout life. The brain is not limited by age or by past learning, rather it adjusts to new situations and new environments in life. The more stimulation the brain receives the more likely it is to be vibrant and ready for life. Our life experiences rewire us. It will be very exciting to have our brains rewired by the Lord through brain exercises and prayer.[1]

He emphasized throughout this book that "brain rewiring" can be achieved by renewing our minds, as written in Romans 12:2.

With a mind renewed (one of the powerful supernatural prescriptions in the Word of God) through meditation on God's promises—prayer, fasting, compassion, gratitude, worshipping, and rejoicing in the Lord—we receive the supernatural solution—beyond science—to manage stress from fear, worry, anxiety, and depression. In her book *From Panic to Power*, Lucinda Bassett, the founder of the Midwest Center for Stress and Anxiety, said:

> Prayer can give you the opportunity to clarify what is bothering you, to put it into perspective, and to know that somebody else is sharing the burden. Prayer is God's gift to us and when we know how to use it most effectively, it can offer us great rewards. A wise person once said…when you pray, look for specific answers.[2]

However, scientists have also discovered that our brains' structures are hardwired to be resistant to changes, thus preserving a consistent personality.[3] But worries of all kinds, as well as our belief system, dictate our emotions and contribute to the development of our character and personality. Brian King, PhD, neuroscientist and comedian, in his seminar, "The Habits of Happy People," cited Corrie ten Boom's statement: "Worry does not empty tomorrow of its sorrow. It empties today of its strength."[4]

Worry creates fear, distress, anxiety, panic attacks, and depression. It greatly reduces our potential years of healthy life. We have read that "the joy of the Lord is your strength" (Neh. 8:10). Through joy and happiness we can reduce the damage that high levels of stress have caused to our brains and our physical bodies. Joy, happiness, and gratitude will reduce fear, anxiety, and depression by calming an overactive brain through healthy amounts of neurochemicals released as a result. Happiness has recently become the focus of new scientific research. We know that—beyond science—"merry heart" is the best medicine.

Body, soul, and spirit form our personality on earth. A spiritually transformed mind plays a huge role in promoting health in our physical bodies and souls. Body, soul, and spirit cannot be separated and must be preserved entirely until the coming of Jesus Christ. Bethel Church Pastor Bill Johnson stated in his book *The Power That Changes the World: Creating Eternal Impact in the Here and Now*:

> There is also a great hunger among us to see the medical community thrive with excellence, while its workers maintain the heart of a servant. It would be a dream come true if we found that this great part of every community had discovered the connection between spirit, soul and body. Part of that dream would be seeing them provide healthcare to the whole person through divine wisdom.[5]

By following God's supernatural prescription, depositing God's promises into your conscious and unconscious mind, and meditating on His Word day and night, you can reprogram your brain. Through protein synthesis and neurogenesis its capacity will increase, creating new, stronger neurons for a healthier life, physically and spiritually, both here on earth and in heaven forever.

NOTES

Preface

1. Kirsty L. Spalding et al., "Dynamics of Hippocampal Neurogenesis in Adult Humans," *Cell* 153, no. 6 (2013): 1219–1227, https://www.ncbi.nlm.nih.gov/pmc/articles/PMC4394608/; Britta K. Hölzel et al., "Mindfulness Practice Leads to Increases in Regional Brain Gray Matter Density," *Psychiatry Research* 191, no. 1 (2011): 36–43, https://www.ncbi.nlm.nih.gov/pmc/articles/PMC3004979/; Kendra Cherry, "5 Surprising Ways That Stress Affects Your Brain," Verywell Mind, March 27, 2019, https://www.verywellmind.com/surprising-ways-that-stress-affects-your-brain-2795040.

2. Debbie Hampton, "How Your Thoughts Change Your Brain, Cells and Genes," *HuffPost Life* (blog), March 24, 2017, https://www.huffpost.com/entry/how-your-thoughts-change-your-brain-cells-and-genes_n_9516176; Melanie Greenberg, "How to Prevent Stress From Shrinking Your Brain," *Psychology Today*, August 12, 2012, https://www.psychologytoday.com/us/blog/the-mindful-self-express/201208/how-prevent-stress-shrinking-your-brain.

3. Dina Aronson, "Cortisol—Its Role in Stress, Inflammation, and Indications for Diet Therapy," *Today's Dietitian* 11, no. 11 (November 2009): 38, https://www.todaysdietitian.com/newarchives/111609p38.shtml; M. Reuter, "Impact of Cortisol Under Stress and Nonstress Conditions: A Pharmacopsychological Approach," *Neuropsychobiology* 46, no. 1 (August 2002), abstract, https://www.karger.com/Article/Abstract/63575.

4. Cherry, "5 Surprising Ways That Stress Affects Your Brain."

5. Aronson, "Cortisol," 38; Sok Kuan Wong et al., "The Relationship Between Metabolic Syndrome and Osteoporosis: A Review," *Nutrients* 8, no. 6 (June 7, 2016): 347, https://www.ncbi.nlm.nih.gov/pmc/articles/PMC4924188/.

6. Ryan Hurd, "How Does Serotonin Affect Sleep?," LiveStrong, accessed July 16, 2019, https://www.livestrong.com/article/136959-how-does-serotonin-affect-sleep/; University of Pittsburgh Medical Center, "Serotonin May Play Role in Hardening of the Arteries," *Science Daily*, March 4, 2006, https://www.sciencedaily.com/releases/2006/03/060303205220.htm.

7. David Hellerstein, "Depression and Anxiety Disorders Damage Your Brain, Especially When Untreated," *Psychology Today*, July 14, 2011, https://www.psychologytoday.com/us/blog/heal-your-brain/201107/depression-and-anxiety-disorders-damage-your-brain-especially-when.

8. Hampton, "How Your Thoughts Change Your Brain, Cells and Genes"; "Harnessing Neurogenesis: How to Change the Adult Brain Through Meditation," EOC Institute, accessed June 5, 2019, https://eocinstitute.org/meditation/the-neurogenesis-guide-how-meditation-changes-the-adult-brain/; Rebecca Gladding, "This Is Your Brain on Meditation," *Psychology Today*, May 22, 2013, https://www

.psychologytoday.com/us/blog/use-your-mind-change-your-brain/201305/is-your-brain-meditation.

9. Connor Wood, "A New Theory for Why Buddhist Meditation Makes Us Feel Good," Science on Religion, Patheos, December 4, 2014, https://www.patheos.com/blogs/scienceonreligion/2014/12/a-new-theory-for-why-buddhist-meditation-makes-us-feel-good/.

10. TED, "You Can Grow New Brain Cells. Here's How," *HuffPost*, October 20, 2015, https://www.huffpost.com/entry/neurogenesis-how-to-grow-new-brain-cells_n_56253c16e4b0bce347019a2c.

11. Siresha Bathina and Undurti N. Das, "Brain-Derived Neurotrophic Factor and Its Clinical Implications," *Archives of Medical Science* 11, no. 6 (2015): 1164–1178, https://www.ncbi.nlm.nih.gov/pmc/articles/PMC4697050/.

12. "How to Manage Stress: Reducing Daily Stressors to Increase Longevity and Well-Being," SciLife Biosciences, accessed June 5, 2019, https://scilifebiosciences.com/blog/how-to-manage-stress-reducing-daily-stressors-to-increase-longevity-and-well-being.

13. Cherry, "5 Surprising Ways That Stress Affects Your Brain."

Introduction

1. "The Effects of Stress on Your Body," WebMD, reviewed December 10, 2017, https://www.webmd.com/balance/stress-management/effects-of-stress-on-your-body; Mohd Razali Salleh, "Life Event, Stress and Illness," *Malaysian Journal of Medical Sciences* 15, no. 4 (2008): 9–18, https://www.ncbi.nlm.nih.gov/pmc/articles/PMC3341916/#b7-mjms-15-4-009.

2. "Hazards," Occupational Safety and Health Administration, US Department of Labor, accessed May 20, 2019, https://www.osha.gov/youngworkers/hazards.html; "The Effects of Stress on Your Body," WebMD.

3. "Workplace Stress," American Institute of Stress, accessed May 20, 2019, https://www.stress.org/workplace-stress; "The Effects of Stress on Your Body," WebMD.

4. Carl Sagan, "Why We Need to Understand Science," *Mercury* 22, no. 2 (March/April 1993): 52–56, http://plaza.ufl.edu/trishak/Carl%20Sagan%20-%20Why%20We%20Need%20To%20Understand%20Science.pdf.

5. Mary Blaszko Helming, "Healing Through Prayer: A Qualitative Study," *Holistic Nursing Practice* 25, no. 1 (2011): 33–44.

6. James E. Stahl et al., "Relaxation Response and Resiliency Training and Its Effect on Healthcare Resource Utilization," *PLOS ONE* 10, no. 10 (October 13, 2015), https://journals.plos.org/plosone/article?id=10.1371/journal.pone.0140212.

7. Christopher Bergland, "Chronic Stress Can Damage Brain Structure and Connectivity," *Psychology Today*, February 12, 2014, https://www.psychologytoday.com/us/blog/the-athletes-way/201402/chronic-stress-can-damage-brain-structure-and-connectivity.

Chapter 1

1. Billy Graham, *The Journey: How to Live by Faith in an Uncertain World* (Nashville: W Publishing Group, 2006), 63.
2. Shaneen Clarke, *Dare to Be Great: Forget Your Past! Live Your Dream!* (Charlotte, NC: LifeBridge Books, 2009).
3. Anil Kumar et al., "Stress: Neurobiology, Consequences and Management," *Journal of Pharmacy and Bioallied Sciences* 5, no. 2 (2013): 91–97, https://www.ncbi.nlm.nih.gov/pmc/articles/PMC3697199/.
4. "Stress Effects," American Institute of Stress, accessed May 29, 2019, https://www.stress.org/stress-effects#effects; Jim Folk, "Pupils Anxiety Symptoms: Dilated or Contracted," Anxietycentre.com, April 3, 2019, https://www.anxietycentre.com/anxiety-symptoms/pupils-anxiety-symptoms.shtml.
5. American Institute of Stress, "Stress Symptoms," WebMD, July 11, 2017, https://www.webmd.com/balance/stress-management/stress-symptoms-effects_of-stress-on-the-body#1.
6. "Stress Effects on the Body: Cardiovascular System," American Psychological Association, accessed May 29, 2019, https://www.apa.org/helpcenter/stress/effects-cardiovascular.
7. "Tachycardia: Fast Heart Rate," American Heart Association, September 30, 2016, https://www.heart.org/en/health-topics/arrhythmia/about-arrhythmia/tachycardia--fast-heart-rate.
8. Jim Folk and Grace Lian, "Anxiety Attack Symptoms and Panic Attacks, How to Stop," Anxietycentre.com, June 19, 2019, https://www.anxietycentre.com/anxiety-attack-symptoms.shtml.
9. Holly Blake, "How Your Body Reacts to Stress," Smithsonian, August 9, 2017, https://www.smithsonianmag.com/science-nature/what-happens-your-body-when-youre-stressed-180964357/; Julie Ryan Evans, "Everything You Should Know About Stress-Induced Asthma," Healthline, September 18, 2017, https://www.healthline.com/health/asthma/stress-induced-asthma#diagnosis.
10. Jim Folk, "Anxiety Symptoms, Signs, Disorders, Types, Causes, Treatment," Anxietycentre.com, July 3, 2019, https://www.anxietycentre.com/anxiety-symptoms.shtml#9.
11. Hurd, "How Does Serotonin Affect Sleep?"
12. Richard J. Wurtman and Judith J. Wurtman, "Brain Serotonin, Carbohydrate-Craving, Obesity and Depression," *Obesity Research* 3, no. S4 (November 1995): 477S–480S, https://onlinelibrary.wiley.com/doi/abs/10.1002/j.1550-8528.1995.tb00215.x?sid=nlm%3Apubmed.
13. Ari Shechter et al., "Alterations in Sleep Architecture in Response to Experimental Sleep Curtailment Are Associated With Signs of Positive Energy Balance," *American Journal of Physiology: Regulatory, Integrative, and Comparative Physiology* 303, no. 9 (2012): R883–889, https://www.ncbi.nlm.nih.gov/pmc/articles/PMC3517705/.
14. "Lack of Sleep Increases Your Risk of Some Cancers," National Sleep Foundation, accessed July 16, 2019, https://www.sleepfoundation.org/articles/lack-sleep-increases-your-risk-some-cancers; Lara G. Sigurdardottir et al., "Circadian Disruption, Sleep Loss, and Prostate Cancer Risk: A Systematic Review of

Epidemiologic Studies," *Cancer Epidemiology, Biomarkers and Prevention* 21, no. 7 (July 2012), http://cebp.aacrjournals.org/content/21/7/1002.

15. Bruce S. McEwen, Carla Nasca, and Jason D. Gray, "Stress Effects on Neuronal Structure: Hippocampus, Amygdala, and Prefrontal Cortex," *Neuropsychopharmacology* 41, no. 1 (2016): 3–23, https://www.ncbi.nlm.nih.gov/pmc/articles/PMC4677120/.

16. Betty Zimmerberg, "IA1. Acetylcholine: A Representative Small Molecule Neurotransmitter," Williams College Neuroscience, 1998, https://web.williams.edu/imput/synapse/pages/IA1.htm; Rachael D. Rubin et al., "The Role of the Hippocampus in Flexible Cognition and Social Behavior," *Frontiers in Human Neuroscience* 8 (2014): 742, https://www.ncbi.nlm.nih.gov/pmc/articles/PMC4179699/.

17. Kristin Della Volpe, "High Evening Cortisol Levels Linked to Increased Risk for Type 2 Diabetes," Endocrine Web, March 14, 2016, https://www.endocrineweb.com/professional/type-2-diabetes/high-evening-cortisol-levels-linked-increased-risk-type-2-diabetes.

18. "Cortisol and Bone Loss," Osteoporosis and Bone Health, July 12, 2018, https://mavendoctors.io/osteoporosis/bone-health/cortisol-and-bone-loss-nNDSjj89cUyitv21oY4X8g/.

19. Amy Myers, "The Adrenal-Thyroid Connection," Amy Myers MD, May 21, 2019, https://www.amymyersmd.com/2017/03/adrenal-thyroid-connection/.

20. "Homeostasis," Human Physiology/Print Version, Wikibooks, August 17, 2017, https://en.wikibooks.org/wiki/Human_Physiology/Print_Version; "The Thyroid Gland," Boundless Anatomy and Physiology, Lumen, accessed June 11, 2019, https://courses.lumenlearning.com/boundless-ap/chapter/the-thyroid-gland/.

21. Jill Eisnaugle, "Stress and Your Thyroid: What's the Connection?," Healthline, January 2, 2019, https://www.healthline.com/health/hypothyroidism/stress-and-your-thyroid#1.

22. William Blahd, "Effects of Stress on Your Skin," WebMD, June 15, 2017, https://www.webmd.com/beauty/the-effects-of-stress-on-your-skin.

23. William C. Shiel Jr., "Does Stress Affect Lupus?," eMedicineHealth, accessed July 5, 2019, https://www.emedicinehealth.com/does_stress_affect_lupus/article_em.htm#in_what_ways_may_stress_affect_the_patient_with_lupus.

24. Ljudmila Stojanovich and Dragomir Marisavljevich, "Stress as a Trigger of Autoimmune Disease," *Autoimmunity Reviews* 7, no. 3 (January 2008): 209–213, https://www.sciencedirect.com/science/article/abs/pii/S156899720700170X?via%3Dihub.

25. Robert Kress, "Stress, Inflammation, Immunity," AMN Healthcare Education Services, 2018, https://www.rn.com/featured-stories/stress-inflammation-immunity/.

26. Marijke Vroomen-Durning, "The Link Between Stress and Rheumatoid Arthritis," Everyday Health, October 16, 2015, https://www.everydayhealth.com/rheumatoid-arthritis/living-with/rheumatoid-arthritis-stress/.

27. Boudewijn Van Houdenhove and Ulrich T. Egle, "Fibromyalgia: A Stress Disorder?: Piecing the Biopsychosocial Puzzle Together," *Psychotherapy and*

Psychosomatics 73 (2004): 267–275, http://kendal-tackett.www.uppitysciencechick.com/van_houdenhove_fm-psyther.pdf.

28. Folk, "Anxiety Symptoms, Signs, Disorders, Types, Causes, Treatment"; Vikram Bhatia and Rakesh K. Tandon, "Stress and the Gastrointestinal Tract," *Journal of Gastroenterology and Hepatology* 20, no. 3 (March 2005): 332–339, https://onlinelibrary.wiley.com/doi/full/10.1111/j.1440-1746.2004.03508.x.

29. Rice University, "21.1 Anatomy of the Lymphatic and Immune Systems," Anatomy and Physiology, accessed July 20, 2019, https://opentextbc.ca/anatomyandphysiology/chapter/21-1-anatomy-of-the-lymphatic-and-immune-systems/.

30. "What Happens When Your Immune System Gets Stressed Out?," Cleveland Clinic, March 1, 2017, https://health.clevelandclinic.org/what-happens-when-your-immune-system-gets-stressed-out/.

31. Katie Gallant, "The Lymphatic and Immune Systems," Quizlet, accessed June 11, 2019, https://quizlet.com/73298649/the-lymphatic-and-immune-systems-flash-cards/.

32. "Phagocytes," Boundless Microbiology, Lumen, accessed July 20, 2019, https://courses.lumenlearning.com/boundless-microbiology/chapter/phagocytes/.

33. Stephen Stahl and Mike Briley, "Understanding Pain in Depression," *Human Psychopharmacology: Clinical and Experimental* 19, no. S1 (September 20, 2004): abstract, https://onlinelibrary.wiley.com/doi/abs/10.1002/hup.619.

34. Caroline Leaf, "The Science of Thought," *Joy!*, February 2012, https://www.joymag.co.za/article.php?id=352; "Understanding the Stress Response," Harvard Health Publishing, May 1, 2018, https://www.health.harvard.edu/staying-healthy/understanding-the-stress-response.

35. Jeanie Lerche Davis, "Patient, Heal Thyself?," WebMD, September 7, 2000, http://www.webmd.com/balance/news/20000907/patient-heal-thyself.

Chapter 2

1. "The Nervous System: Teacher Pages," e-Mission: Cyber Surgeons, Wheeling Jesuit University/Center for Educational Technologies, accessed June 13, 2019, http://www.e-missions.net/cybersurgeons/?/nerv_teacher/.

2. Eric H. Chudler, "The Hows, Whats, and Whos of Neuroscience," Neuroscience for Kids, accessed June 24, 2019, https://faculty.washington.edu/chudler/what.html.

3. Kenneth Maiese, "Neurotransmission," *Merck Manual: Professional Version*, March 2019, https://www.merckmanuals.com/professional/neurologic-disorders/neurotransmission/neurotransmission.

4. Luke Mastin, "Neurons & Synapses," The Human Memory, accessed June 17, 2019, http://www.human-memory.net/brain_neurons.html.

5. "Biology of Emotion," Boundless Psychology, Lumen, accessed June 17, 2019, https://courses.lumenlearning.com/boundless-psychology/chapter/biology-of-emotion/.

6. "The Hypothalamus," Indiana University, accessed June 17, 2019, http://www.indiana.edu/~p1013447/dictionary/hypothal.htm.

7. Jillian Levy, "What Is the Limbic System?," Dr. Axe, September 27, 2016, https://draxe.com/limbic-system/.

8. Asociación RUVID, "Dopamine Regulates the Motivation to Act, Study Shows," *Science Daily*, January 10, 2013, https://www.sciencedaily.com/releases/2013/01/130110094415.htm.

9. Nora D. Volkow et al., "Decreased Dopamine Brain Reactivity in Marijuana Abusers Is Associated With Negative Emotionality and Addiction Severity," *Proceedings of the National Academy of Sciences of the United States of America* 111, no. 30 (2014): E3149–56, https://www.ncbi.nlm.nih.gov/pmc/articles/PMC4121778/.

10. "How Stress and Anxiety Affect the Brain," Neurocore, July 26, 2018, https://www.neurocorecenters.com/blog/depression-anxiety-stresseffects-of-stress-anxiety-on-brain.

11. Laurie Vazquez, "What Fear Does to Your Brain—and How to Stop It," Big Think, July 31, 2016, https://bigthink.com/laurie-vazquez/what-fear-does-to-your-brain-and-how-to-stop-it.

12. Brian Luke Seaward, *Managing Stress: Principles and Strategies for Health and Well-Being*, 5th ed. (Sudbury, MA: Jones and Bartlett, 2006), 35–36, https://books.google.com/books?id=I9B4dG4XJ8AC.

13. Charles Stangor, "4.4 Putting It All Together: The Nervous System and the Endocrine System," Introduction to Psychology—1st Canadian Edition, accessed June 17, 2019, https://opentextbc.ca/introductiontopsychology/chapter/3-4-putting-it-all-together-the-nervous-system-and-the-endocrine-system/.

14. Caroline Leaf, *Switch On Your Brain: The Key to Peak Happiness, Thinking, and Health* (Grand Rapids, MI: Baker Books, 2013), 125.

15. Eric H. Chudler, "How the Nervous System Interacts With Other Body Systems," Neuroscience for Kids, accessed June 18, 2019, https://faculty.washington.edu/chudler/organ.html.

16. Betsy Chesnutt, "Apoptosis in the Cell Cycle and Cancer," Cell Biology Study Guide, Study.com, accessed July 17, 2019, https://study.com/academy/lesson/apoptosis-in-the-cell-cycle-cancer.html.

17. "Homeostasis and Regulation in the Human Body," High School Biology Textbook, CK12 Foundation, accessed June 18, 2019, https://opencurriculum.org/5385/homeostasis-and-regulation-in-the-human-body/.

18. *Merriam-Webster*, s.v. "laminin," accessed June 18, 2019, https://www.merriam-webster.com/dictionary/laminin; Ranjay Jayadev and David R. Sherwood, "Primer: Basement Membranes," *Current Biology* 27 (March 20, 2017): R207, https://www.cell.com/current-biology/pdf/S0960-9822(17)30141-0.pdf.

19. "17.62 The Excretory System—Advanced," CK-12 Biology Advanced Concepts, CK-12 Foundation, accessed July 20, 2019, https://www.ck12.org/book/CK-12-Biology-Advanced-Concepts/section/17.62/.

20. Colleen Moriarty, "Vitamin D Myths 'D'-Bunked," Yale Medicine, March 15, 2018, https://www.yalemedicine.org/stories/vitamin-d-myths-debunked/.

21. E. Wehr et al., "Association of Vitamin D Status with Serum Androgen Levels in Men," *Clinical Endocrinology* 73, no. 2 (August 2010): 243–248, https://onlinelibrary.wiley.com/doi/full/10.1111/j.1365-2265.2009.03777.x; Jed Diamond, "Male Anger, Testosterone, and Depression: What Women and Men Need to Know

Before It's Too Late," *Men Alive* (blog), June 29, 2018, http://menalive.com/male-anger-testosterone-and-depression/.

22. Lana Barhum, "How Do You Boost Testosterone Naturally?," *Medical News Today*, July 18, 2018, https://www.medicalnewstoday.com/articles/322508.php.

23. Seaward, *Managing Stress*, 35–37.

24. Richard Gordan, Judith K. Gwathmey, and Lai-Hua Xie, "Autonomic and Endocrine Control of Cardiovascular Function," *World Journal of Cardiology* 7, no. 4 (2015): 204–214, https://www.ncbi.nlm.nih.gov/pmc/articles/PMC4404375/.

25. Seaward, *Managing Stress*, 37; Gordan, Gwathmey, and Xie, "Autonomic and Endocrine Control of Cardiovascular Function."

26. Seaward, *Managing Stress*, 39.

27. Seaward, *Managing Stress*, 46.

28. Leaf, "The Science of Thought."

29. Caroline Leaf, *Who Switched Off My Brain?: Controlling Toxic Thoughts and Emotions* (Southlake, TX: Improv Ltd., 2009), 52.

30. Leaf, "The Science of Thought."

31. "The Neuron," Micropsychology, accessed June 24, 2019, http://www.micropsychology.org/the-neuron/.

32. Leaf, "The Science of Thought."

33. Saul McLeod, "What Is the Stress Response?," Simply Psychology, 2010, https://www.simplypsychology.org/stress-biology.html; Karen Bruno, "Stress and Depression," WebMD, April 12, 2011, https://www.webmd.com/depression/features/stress-depression#1.

34. Seaward, *Managing Stress*, 43, Figure 2.6.

35. Charlotte Lillis, "What Can Cause Stomach Churning?," *Medical News Today*, March 13, 2019, https://www.medicalnewstoday.com/articles/324695.php.

36. Seaward, *Managing Stress*, 45.

37. Seaward, *Managing Stress*, 45; Deepak Chopra, "Stress and the Brain," *HuffPost*, updated December 6, 2017, https://www.huffpost.com/entry/effect-of-stress-on-health_b_907029.

38. Frank J. Jenkins, Bennett Van Houten, and Dana H. Bovbjerg, "Effects on DNA Damage and/or Repair Processes as Biological Mechanisms Linking Psychological Stress to Cancer Risk," *Journal of Applied Biobehavioral Research* 19, no. 1 (2014): 3–23, https://www.ncbi.nlm.nih.gov/pmc/articles/PMC4039216/.

39. Frederico A. C. Azevedo et al., "Equal Numbers of Neuronal and Nonneuronal Cells Make the Human Brain an Isometrically Scaled-Up Primate Brain," *Journal of Comparative Neurology* 513, no. 5 (April 10, 2009): 532–541, https://www.ncbi.nlm.nih.gov/pubmed/19226510.

40. "How Does the Nervous System Help Us Respond?—OCR21C," Bitesize, BBC, accessed June 25, 2019, https://www.bbc.com/bitesize/guides/zq8bqhv/revision/1.

41. "How Does the Nervous System Help Us Respond?—OCR21C," BBC.

42. Linda J. Vorvick, "Nerve Conduction," Medline Plus, US National Library of Medicine, May 10, 2019, https://medlineplus.gov/ency/anatomyvideos/000089.htm.

43. "Blood Vessels," The Franklin Institute, accessed June 25, 2019, https://www.fi.edu/heart/blood-vessels.
44. Maiese, "Neurotransmission."
45. Mastin, "Neurons & Synapses."
46. Society for Neuroscience, "Brain Changes Associated with Casual Marijuana Use in Young Adults, Study Finds," Science Daily, April 15, 2014, https://www.sciencedaily.com/releases/2014/04/140415181156.htm; .
47. Volkow et al., "Decreased Dopamine Brain Reactivity in Marijuana Abusers Is Associated With Negative Emotionality and Addiction Severity."
48. "The Dangers and Consequences of Marijuana Abuse," Drug Enforcement Agency, US Department of Justice, May 2014, https://www.getsmartaboutdrugs.gov/sites/getsmartaboutdrugs.com/files/publications/The_Dangers_and_Consequences_of_Marijuana_Abuse%20May2014_Accessible%20version.pdf.
49. Scott Gottlieb, "Statement From FDA Warning About Significant Health Risks of Contaminated Illegal Synthetic Cannabinoid Products That Are Being Encountered by FDA," Commissioner of Food and Drugs, US Food and Drug Administration, July 19, 2018, https://www.fda.gov/news-events/press-announcements/statement-fda-warning-about-significant-health-risks-contaminated-illegal-synthetic-cannabinoid.
50. "The Dangers and Consequences of Marijuana Abuse," US Department of Justice.
51. "How to Manage Stress: Reducing Daily Stressors to Increase Longevity and Well-Being," SciLife Biosciences.
52. Zimmerberg, "IA1. Acetylcholine: A Representative Small Molecule Neurotransmitter."
53. Betty Zimmerberg, "IA5. Clinical Application: Acetylcholine and Alzheimer's Disease," Synaptic Transmission: A Four-Step Process, 2000, https://web.williams.edu/imput/synapse/pages/IA5.html; W. A. Pedersen, M. A. Kloczewiak, and J. K. Blusztajn, "Amyloid Beta-Protein Reduces Acetylcholine Synthesis in a Cell Line Derived From Cholinergic Neurons of the Basal Forebrain," *Proceedings of the National Academy of Sciences of the United States of America* 93, no. 15 (1996): 8068–8071, https://www.ncbi.nlm.nih.gov/pmc/articles/PMC38876/.
54. "Stress: Fight or Flight Response," *Psychologist World*, accessed July 26, 2019, https://www.psychologistworld.com/stress/fight-or-flight-response.
55. "What Are MDMA's Effects on the Brain?," National Institute on Drug Abuse, National Institutes of Health, September 2017, https://www.drugabuse.gov/publications/research-reports/mdma-ecstasy-abuse/what-are-mdmas-effects-on-brain.
56. "Know Your Brain: Reward System," Neuroscientifically Challenged, January 16, 2015, https://neuroscientificallychallenged.com/blog/know-your-brain-reward-system.
57. Rajita Sinha, "Chronic Stress, Drug Use, and Vulnerability to Addiction," *Annals of the New York Academy of Sciences* 1141 (2008): 105–130, https://www.ncbi.nlm.nih.gov/pmc/articles/PMC2732004/.
58. "Why Stress Causes People to Overeat," *Harvard Mental Health Letter*, Harvard Health Publishing, July 18, 2018, https://www.health.harvard.edu/staying-healthy/why-stress-causes-people-to-overeat.

59. "Understanding Addiction: How Addiction Hijacks the Brain," Harvard Health, HelpGuide.org, accessed July 2, 2019, https://www.helpguide.org/harvard/how-addiction-hijacks-the-brain.htm.

60. "The Science of Drug Use and Addiction: The Basics," National Institute on Drug Abuse, National Institutes of Health, July 2018, https://www.drugabuse.gov/publications/media-guide/science-drug-use-addiction-basics.

61. "Schizophrenia," Mayo Clinic, April 10, 2018, https://www.mayoclinic.org/diseases-conditions/schizophrenia/symptoms-causes/syc-20354443; J. P. Kesby et al., "Dopamine, Psychosis, and Schizophrenia: The Widening Gap Between Basic and Clinical Neuroscience," *Translational Psychiatry* 8, no. 30 (January 31, 2018), https://www.nature.com/articles/s41398-017-0071-9.

62. Dena Westphalen, "What Does Gamma Aminobutyric Acid (GABA) Do?," Healthline, October 26, 2018, https://www.healthline.com/health/gamma-aminobutyric-acid.

63. "Natural GABA," Integrative Psychiatry, accessed July 2, 2019, https://www.integrativepsychiatry.net/natural_gaba.html; "GABA Receptors in Status Epilepticus," Epilepsy Foundation, February 13, 2018, https://www.epilepsy.com/article/2018/2/gaba-receptors-status-epilepticus.

64. Stephanie Liou, "About Glutamate Toxicity," Huntington's Outreach Project for Education, at Stanford (HOPES), June 26, 2011, https://hopes.stanford.edu/about-glutamate-toxicity/.

65. Annamarya Scaccia, "Serotonin: What You Need to Know," Healthline, May 18, 2017, https://www.healthline.com/health/mental-health/serotonin#functions.

66. Nancy L. Moyer, "Serotonin Deficiency: What We Do and Don't Know," Healthline, February 27, 2019, https://www.healthline.com/health/serotonin-deficiency#test.

67. Vikas Menon and Shivanand Kattimani, "Suicide and Serotonin: Making Sense of Evidence," *Indian Journal of Psychological Medicine* 37, no. 3 (2015): 377–378, https://www.ncbi.nlm.nih.gov/pmc/articles/PMC4649802/.

68. Moyer, "Serotonin Deficiency."

69. Matthew F. Muldoon et al., "The Metabolic Syndrome Is Associated With Reduced Central Serotonergic Responsivity in Healthy Community Volunteers," *Journal of Clinical Endocrinology and Metabolism* 91, no. 2 (February 1, 2006): 718–721, https://academic.oup.com/jcem/article/91/2/718/2843541.

70. James McIntosh, "What Is Serotonin and What Does It Do?," *Medical News Today*, February 2, 2018, https://www.medicalnewstoday.com/kc/serotonin-facts-232248; Colette Bouchez, "Serotonin: 9 Questions and Answers," October 12, 2011, https://www.webmd.com/depression/features/serotonin#1.

71. Bouchez, "Serotonin: 9 Questions and Answers"; "What Are MDMA's Effects on the Brain?," National Institutes of Health.

72. Jennifer Berry, "Endorphins: Effects and How to Increase Levels," *Medical News Today*, February 6, 2018, https://www.medicalnewstoday.com/articles/320839.php.

73. "Prescription Pain Medications: What You Need to Know," Scholastic, 2016, http://headsup.scholastic.com/students

/prescription-pain-medications-what-you-need-to-know; "Exercise and Opioids—What to Know Before You Go," Mayo Clinic, February 13, 2018, https://www.mayoclinic.org/healthy-lifestyle/consumer-health/in-depth/opioids-and-exercise/art-20396866.

74. David M. Lovinger, PhD, "Communication Networks in the Brain," National Institute on Alcohol Abuse and Alcoholism, National Institutes of Health, accessed July 8, 2019, http://pubs.niaaa.nih.gov/publications/arh313/196-214.htm.

75. Bouchez, "Serotonin: 9 Questions and Answers."

76. Westphalen, "What Does Gamma Aminobutyric Acid (GABA) Do?"; "Natural GABA," Integrative Psychiatry.

77. Bouchez, "Serotonin: 9 Questions and Answers."

78. Adam Hadhazy, "Think Twice: How the Gut's 'Second Brain' Influences Mood and Well-Being," *Scientific American*, February 12, 2010, https://www.scientificamerican.com/article/gut-second-brain/.

79. Bouchez, "Serotonin: 9 Questions and Answers"; Hong-Yan Qin et al., "Impact of Psychological Stress on Irritable Bowel Syndrome," *World Journal of Gastroenterology* 20, no. 39 (2014): 14126–14131, https://www.ncbi.nlm.nih.gov/pmc/articles/PMC4202343/.

80. Alan Frazer and Julie G. Hensler, "Serotonin Involvement in Physiological Function and Behavior," in G. J. Siegel et al., ed., *Basic Neurochemistry: Molecular, Cellular and Medical Aspects*, 6th edition (Philadelphia: Lippincott-Raven, 1999), https://www.ncbi.nlm.nih.gov/books/NBK27940/.

Chapter 3

1. Stacy Lu, "How Chronic Stress Is Harming Our DNA," American Psychological Association, *Monitor on Psychology* 45, no. 9 (October 2014), 28, https://www.apa.org/monitor/2014/10/chronic-stress.

2. Grant R. Jeffrey, *Creation: Remarkable Evidence of God's Design* (Colorado Springs: WaterBrook, 2003), 160–161.

3. Frederic H. Martini, Judi L. Nath, and Edwin F. Bartholomew, *Fundamentals of Anatomy and Physiology*, 11th ed. (New York: Pearson, 2018), 118, 122.

4. Jeffrey, *Creation*, 154.

5. Bing Yao et al., "DNA N6-Methyladenine Is Dynamically Regulated in the Mouse Brain Following Environmental Stress," *Nature Communications* 8, no. 1122 (October 24, 2017), https://www.nature.com/articles/s41467-017-01195-y#Sec2.

6. "How Cancer Starts, Grows, and Spreads," Canadian Cancer Society, accessed July 9, 2019, https://www.cancer.ca/en/cancer-information/cancer-101/what-is-cancer/how-cancer-starts-grows-and-spreads/?region=on.

7. Daniel Nelson, "DNA Is Called the Blueprint of Life: Here's Why," Science Trends, October 26, 2017, https://sciencetrends.com/dna-called-blueprint-life-heres/.

8. "Deoxyribonucleic Acid Fact Sheet," National Human Genome Research Institute, National Institutes of Health, June 16, 2015, https://www.genome.gov/about-genomics/fact-sheets/Deoxyribonucleic-Acid-Fact-Sheet.

9. Eberhard Fuchs and Gabriele Flügge, "Cellular Consequences of Stress and Depression," *Dialogues in Clinical Neuroscience* 6, no. 2 (2004): 171–183, https://www.ncbi.nlm.nih.gov/pmc/articles/PMC3181796/.

10. Aparna Suvrathan, Rajnish Rao, and Sumantra Chattarji, "Effects of Stress on Cognitive Versus Emotional Function: Cells, Circuits and Behavior," *Expanding Horizons of the Mind Science(s)* (2011): abstract, https://www.researchgate.net/publication/281717990_Effects_of_stress_on_cognitive_versus_emotional_function_cells_circuits_and_behavior.

11. Harvey Lodish et al., "Section 21.4: Neurotransmitters, Synapses, and Impulse Transmission," in *Molecular Cell Biology*, 4th edition (New York: W. H. Freeman, 2000), https://www.ncbi.nlm.nih.gov/books/NBK21521/.

12. Mastin, "Neurons & Synapses."

13. Patrick Toalson et al., "The Metabolic Syndrome in Patients With Severe Mental Illnesses," *Primary Care Companion to the Journal of Clinical Psychiatry* 6, no. 4 (2004): 152–158, https://www.ncbi.nlm.nih.gov/pmc/articles/PMC514841/.

14. William Rowley et al., "Diabetes 2030: Insights from Yesterday, Today, and Future Trends," *Population Health Management* 20, no. 1 (2017): 6–12, https://www.ncbi.nlm.nih.gov/pmc/articles/PMC5278808/.

Chapter 4

1. Cheryl D. Conrad, "Chronic Stress-Induced Hippocampal Vulnerability: The Glucocorticoid Vulnerability Hypothesis," *Reviews in the Neurosciences* 19, no. 6 (2008): 395–411, https://www.ncbi.nlm.nih.gov/pmc/articles/PMC2746750/.

2. Larry J. Siever, "Neurobiology of Aggression and Violence," *American Journal of Psychiatry* 165, no. 4 (2008): 429–442, https://www.ncbi.nlm.nih.gov/pmc/articles/PMC4176893/.

3. Nathalie E. Holz et al., "Role of FKBP5 in Emotion Processing: Results on Amygdala Activity, Connectivity and Volume," *Brain Structure & Function* 220, no. 3 (May 2015), 1355–1368, https://link.springer.com/article/10.1007/s00429-014-0729-5#citeas.

4. Adriana Feder, Eric J. Nestler, and Dennis S. Charney, "Psychobiology and Molecular Genetics of Resilience," *Nature Reviews: Neuroscience* 10, no. 6 (June 2009): 446–457, https://www.ncbi.nlm.nih.gov/pmc/articles/PMC2833107/.

5. "Children Reflect Parental Behavior," Urban Child Institute, October 5, 2011, http://www.urbanchildinstitute.org/articles/editorials/children-reflect-parental-behavior.

6. Jane Anderson, "The Teenage Brain: Under Construction," American College of Pediatricians, May 2016, https://www.acpeds.org/the-college-speaks/position-statements/parenting-issues/the-teenage-brain-under-construction.

7. "Children Reflect Parental Behavior," Urban Child Institute.

8. Eric Jaffe, "Mirror Neurons: How We Reflect on Behavior," Association for Psychological Science, May 1, 2007, https://www.psychologicalscience.org/observer/mirror-neurons-how-we-reflect-on-behavior.

9. Anne L. Stewart, Thomas A. Field, and Lennis G. Echterling, "Neuroscience and the Magic of Play Therapy," *International Journal of Play Therapy*

25, no. 1 (2016): 4–13, https://www.researchgate.net/publication/290175412_Neuroscience_and_the_magic_of_play_therapy.

10. Marco Iacoboni, "Imitation, Empathy, and Mirror Neurons," *Annual Reviews of Psychology* 60 (2009): 653–670, http://sites.oxy.edu/clint/physio/article/imitationempathyandmirrorneurons.pdf.

11. Laura A. Pratt, Debra J. Brody, and Qiuping Gu, "Antidepressant Use Among Persons Aged 12 and Over: United States, 2011–2014," National Center for Health Statistics, Data Brief no. 283, August 2017, https://www.cdc.gov/nchs/data/databriefs/db283.pdf.

12. Anderson, "The Teenage Brain: Under Construction"; Laurence Steinberg, "A Social Neuroscience Perspective on Adolescent Risk-Taking," *Developmental Review* 28, no. 1 (2008): 78–106, https://www.ncbi.nlm.nih.gov/pmc/articles/PMC2396566/.

13. Sonia J. Lupien et al., "Effects of Stress Throughout the Lifespan on the Brain, Behaviour, and Cognition," *Nature Reviews: Neuroscience* 10 (June 2009): 434–445, https://dublin.sciencegallery.com/memory/files/papers/Lupien_et_al_2009.pdf.

14. Kenneth H. Rubin, Robert J. Coplan, and Julie C. Bowker, "Social Withdrawal in Childhood," *Annual Review of Psychology* 60 (2009): 141–171, https://www.ncbi.nlm.nih.gov/pmc/articles/PMC3800115/.

15. "Anxiety and Physical Illness," Harvard Women's Health Watch, May 9, 2018, https://www.health.harvard.edu/staying-healthy/anxiety_and_physical_illness.

16. Sinha, "Chronic Stress, Drug Use, and Vulnerability to Addiction."

17. Sinha, "Chronic Stress, Drug Use, and Vulnerability to Addiction."

18. Ann H. Crowe and Shay Bilchik, "Consequences of Youth Substance Abuse," Drug Identification and Testing Summary, May 1998, https://www.ojjdp.gov/pubs/drugid/ration-03.html.

19. "6 Ways to Use Your Mind to Control Pain," Harvard Women's Health Watch, April 2015, https://www.health.harvard.edu/mind-and-mood/6-ways-to-use-your-mind-to-control-pain.

20. "Neurons: Reasons Why They Can Live Longer and Better," CogniFit, accessed July 10, 2019, https://www.cognifit.com/active-neurons.

21. "Marijuana," Brain Power: Grades 6–9, National Institute on Drug Abuse, June 1, 2007, https://www.drugabuse.gov/publications/brain-power/grades-6-9/weeding-out-grass-module-4/background; Rajiv Radhakrishnan, Samuel T. Wilkinson, and Deepak C. D'Souza, "Gone to Pot: A Review of the Association Between Cannabis and Psychosis," *Frontiers in Psychiatry* 5 (2014): 54, https://www.ncbi.nlm.nih.gov/pmc/articles/PMC4033190/.

22. Kirsten Schultz, "Are Childhood Trauma and Chronic Illness Connected?," Healthline, September 18, 2017, https://www.healthline.com/health/chronic-illness/childhood-trauma-connected-chronic-illness#1.

23. P. C. Konturek, T. Brzozowski, and S. J. Konturek, "Stress and the Gut: Pathophysiology, Clinical Consequences, Diagnostic Approach and Treatment Options," *Journal of Physiology and Pharmacology* 62, no. 6 (2011): 591–599, http://www.jpp.krakow.pl/journal/archive/12_11/pdf/591_12_11_article.pdf.

24. Michael Galanakis et al., "A Literature Review on the Connection between Stress and Self-Esteem," *Psychology* 7 (2016): 687–694, http://file.scirp.org/Html/5-6901721_66480.htm.

25. Anne Gold, "Why Self-Esteem Is Important for Mental Health," National Alliance on Mental Illness, July 12, 2016, https://www.nami.org/Blogs/NAMI-Blog/July-2016/Why-Self-Esteem-Is-Important-for-Mental-Health.

26. Steven Stosny, "Emotional Abuse," Compassion Power, accessed July 11, 2019, https://www.compassionpower.com/emotional-abuse/#children.

27. Anne Trafton, "How the Brain Controls Our Habits," MIT News, October 29, 2012, http://news.mit.edu/2012/understanding-how-brains-control-our-habits-1029.

28. Yi-Yuan Tang et al., "Circuitry of Self-Control and Its Role in Reducing Addiction," *Trends in Cognitive Sciences* 19, no. 8 (August 1, 2015): 439–444, https://www.cell.com/trends/cognitive-sciences/fulltext/S1364-6613(15)00144-8.

29. André Nieoullon, "Dopamine and the Regulation of Cognition and Attention," *Progress in Neurobiology* 67, no. 1 (May 2002): 53–83, https://www.sciencedirect.com/science/article/pii/S0301008202000114?via%3Dihub.

30. "How Addiction Hijacks the Brain," Harvard Mental Health Letter, July 2011, https://www.health.harvard.edu/newsletter_article/how-addiction-hijacks-the-brain.

31. "Drugs and the Brain," Drugs, Brains, and Behavior: The Science of Addiction, National Institute on Drug Abuse, July 2018, https://www.drugabuse.gov/publications/drugs-brains-behavior-science-addiction/drugs-brain.

32. Kumar et al., "Stress: Neurobiology, Consequences and Management."

33. Kate Brown, "Five Myths About Chernobyl," *Washington Post*, July 5, 2019, https://www.washingtonpost.com/outlook/five-myths/five-myths-about-chernobyl/2019/07/05/34eb2506-9214-11e9-aadb-74e6b2b46f6a_story.html?noredirect=on&utm_term=.62bed4b007ca.

34. Columbia University's Mailman School of Public Health, "Increased Risk of Thyroid Diseases Linked to Exposure at Chernobyl, Study Shows," ScienceDaily, February 22, 2008, https://www.sciencedaily.com/releases/2008/02/080219155636.htm.

35. Jenkins, Van Houten, and Bovbjerg, "Effects on DNA Damage and/or Repair Processes as Biological Mechanisms Linking Psychological Stress to Cancer Risk."

36. Serge Gauthier et al., "Mild Cognitive Impairment," *The Lancet* 367, no. 9518 (April 15–21, 2006): 1262–1270, https://www.sciencedirect.com/science/article/pii/S0140673606685425.

37. Yingxue Yang et al., "Cognitive Impairment in Generalized Anxiety Disorder Revealed by Event-Related Potential N270," *Neuropsychiatric Disease and Treatment* 11 (June 3, 2015): 1405–1411, https://www.ncbi.nlm.nih.gov/pmc/articles/PMC4461089/; Michelle A. Miller, "The Role of Sleep and Sleep Disorders in the Development, Diagnosis, and Management of Neurocognitive Disorders," *Frontiers in Neurology* 6 (October 23, 2015): 224, https://www.ncbi.nlm.nih.gov/pmc/articles/PMC4615953/.

38. Katherine Harmon, "Walking Speed Predicts Life Expectancy of Older Adults," *Scientific American*, January 4, 2011, https://www.scientificamerican.com/article/walking-speed-survival/.

39. Christopher Bergland, "Alpha Brain Waves Boost Creativity and Reduce Depression," *Psychology Today*, April 17, 2015, https://www.psychologytoday.com/us/blog/the-athletes-way/201504/alpha-brain-waves-boost-creativity-and-reduce-depression.

40. Andrew Newberg and Mark Robert Waldman, *Words Can Change Your Brain: 12 Conversation Strategies to Build Trust, Resolve Conflict, and Increase Intimacy* (New York: Plume, 2013), 24–25.

41. Shayla Love, "How Prayer and Meditation Changes Your Brain," Vice: Health, April 28, 2017, https://www.vice.com/en_us/article/nzpk9w/how-prayer-and-meditation-changes-your-brain.

42. "Neurons: Reasons Why They Can Live Longer and Better," CogniFit.

43. David Hulme, "Brain Science Has a Change of Mind," Vision, Summer 2004, https://www.vision.org/brain-science-has-change-mind-569.

44. J. P. Bounhoure, "Takotsubo or Stress Cardiomyopathy," *Cardiovascular Psychiatry and Neurology* (2012): 637672, https://www.ncbi.nlm.nih.gov/pmc/articles/PMC3465868/.

Chapter 5

1. "Prescription Opiod Data," Centers for Disease Control, accessed November 10, 2019, https://www.cdc.gov/drugoverdose/data/prescribing/prescribing-practices.html.

2. Eva Fernandez et al., "Factors and Mechanisms for Pharmacokinetic Differences Between Pediatric Population and Adults," *Pharmaceutics* 3, no. 1 (February 7, 2011): 53–72, https://www.ncbi.nlm.nih.gov/pmc/articles/PMC3857037/.

3. Berry, "Endorphins: Effects and How to Increase Levels."

4. Asma Hayati Ahmad and Rahimah Zakaria, "Pain in Times of Stress," *The Malaysian Journal of Medical Sciences* 22, special issue (2015): 52–61, https://www.ncbi.nlm.nih.gov/pmc/articles/PMC4795524/.

5. Kevin Joy, "The Cost of Chronic Pain (Infographic)," University of Michigan health blog, September 29, 2017, https://healthblog.uofmhealth.org/health-management/cost-of-chronic-pain-infographic.

6. "Module 2: Development of Children's Pain Perception," SickKids, accessed July 15, 2019, http://www.sickkids.ca/pain-centre/Health-care-Professionals/Online%20Pain%20Curriculum/Module-2/story_html5.html.

7. Harolyn M. E. Belcher and Harold E. Shinitzky, "Substance Abuse in Children: Prediction, Protection, and Prevention," *Archives of Pediatric and Adolescent Medicine* 152, no. 10 (1998), 952–960, https://jamanetwork.com/journals/jamapediatrics/fullarticle/189961.

8. Peter R. Breggin, "Psychiatric Drug-Induced Chronic Brain Impairment (CBI): Implications for Long-Term Treatment With Psychiatric Medication," *International Journal of Risk & Safety in Medicine* 23 (2011): 193–200, http://breggin.com/wp-content/uploads/2012/01/Breggin2011_ChronicBrainImpairment.pdf.

9. Ross A. Thompson, Abby Winer, and Rebecca Goodvin, "The Individual Child: Temperament, Emotion, Self, and Personality," in M. Bornstein and M. Lamb, ed., *Developmental Science: An Advanced Textbook*, 6th edition (Oxford, UK: Psychology Press/Taylor & Francis, 2010), https://www.researchgate.net/publication/232498020_The_individual_child_Temperament_emotion_self_and_personality.

10. "Children and Teens," Anxiety and Depression Association of America, accessed July 15, 2019, https://adaa.org/living-with-anxiety/children; Paul Ingraham, "Anxiety and Chronic Pain: A Self-Help Guide for People Who Worry and Hurt," PainScience.com, July 6, 2019, https://www.painscience.com/articles/anxiety.php.

11. Catherine Winters, "Painful Problem: Why Kids Face Chronic Pain," Live Science, July 1, 2013, https://www.livescience.com/37868-chronic-pain-children-teens.html.

12. "Muscle Pain: Possible Causes," Cleveland Clinic, December 3, 2017, https://my.clevelandclinic.org/health/symptoms/17669-muscle-pain/possible-causes.

13. Fernando Bessone, "Non-Steroidal Anti-Inflammatory Drugs: What Is the Actual Risk of Liver Damage?," *World Journal of Gastroenterology* 16, no. 45 (2010): 5651–5661, https://www.ncbi.nlm.nih.gov/pmc/articles/PMC2997980/; "Pain Relief: Taking NSAIDs Safely," *Harvard Women's Health Watch*, September 2013, https://www.health.harvard.edu/pain/pain-relief-taking-nsaids-safely.

14. "Harnessing the Human Body's Natural Analgesic for Pain Relief," Enzo Life Sciences, accessed July 15, 2019, http://www.enzolifesciences.com/science-center/technotes/2012/may/harnessing-the-human-bodys-natural-analgesic-for-pain-relief/.

15. Berry, "Endorphins: Effects and How to Increase Levels."

16. "Drugs and the Brain," National Institute on Drug Abuse; Emanuela Mhillaj et al., "Effects of Anabolic-Androgens on Brain Reward Function," *Frontiers in Neuroscience* 9 (August 26, 2015): 295, https://www.ncbi.nlm.nih.gov/pmc/articles/PMC4549565/.

17. Fadel Zeidan and David R. Vago, "Mindfulness Meditation-Based Pain Relief: A Mechanistic Account," *Annals of the New York Academy of Sciences* 1373, no. 1 (2016): 114–127, https://www.ncbi.nlm.nih.gov/pmc/articles/PMC4941786/.

18. Beth Moore with Dale McCleskey, *Jesus, the One and Only* (Nashville: Broadman & Holman, 2013), 97–98, 166.

19. Asmir Gračanin, Lauren M. Bylsma, and Ad J. J. M. Vingerhoets, "Is Crying a Self-Soothing Behavior?," *Frontiers in Psychology* 5 (2014): 502, https://www.ncbi.nlm.nih.gov/pmc/articles/PMC4035568/.

20. Graham, *The Journey: How to Live by Faith in an Uncertain World*, 35.

21. Larry Huch, *Free at Last: Removing the Past From Your Future* (New Kensington, PA: Whitaker House, 2004), 159.

22. Claudio Lavin et al., "The Anterior Cingulate Cortex: An Integrative Hub for Human Socially-Driven Interactions," *Frontiers in Neuroscience* 7 (May 8, 2013): 64, https://www.frontiersin.org/articles/10.3389/fnins.2013.00064/full

23. Robert D. Rogers, "The Roles of Dopamine and Serotonin in Decision Making: Evidence From Pharmacological Experiments in Humans," *Neuropsychopharmacology* 36, no. 1 (2011): 114–132, https://www.ncbi.nlm.nih.gov/pmc/articles/PMC3055502/.

24. Alice M. Isen, "Some Ways in Which Positive Affect Influences Decision Making and Problem Solving," in Michael Lewis, Jeannette M. Haviland-Jones, and Lisa F. Barrett, eds., *Handbook of Emotions*, 3rd edition (New York: Guilford Press, 2008), 568, http://dl.icdst.org/pdfs/files/4b4437cec4ba6d422c127021a46f019a.pdf.

25. Elena Răscol-Rady, *Flight to Freedom: God's Faithfulness in Communist Romania* (CreateSpace, 2015), 5.

26. John Hagee, *In Defense of Israel: The Bible's Mandate for Supporting the Jewish State* (Lake Mary, FL: FrontLine, 2007), 17–18.

Chapter 6

1. Randy L. Buckner, "Memory and Executive Function in Aging and AD: Multiple Factors That Cause Decline and Reserve Factors That Compensate," *Neuron* 44 (September 30, 2004): 195–208, https://www.cell.com/action/showPdf?pii=S0896-6273%2804%2900581-1.

2. Jingji Jin and Stephen Maren, "Prefrontal-Hippocampal Interactions in Memory and Emotion," *Frontiers in Systems Neuroscience* 9 (December 15, 2015): 170, https://www.ncbi.nlm.nih.gov/pmc/articles/PMC4678200/.

3. David J. Leeds, ed., "Earthquake in Romania: March 4, 1977," *Newsletter: Earthquake Engineering Research Institute* 11, no. 3B (May 1977): 4, https://www.eeri.org/lfe/pdf/Romania_Vrancea_PrelimReport_May77.pdf

4. Larissa Hirsch, "Abstinence," TeensHealth, May 2019, https://kidshealth.org/en/teens/abstinence.html.

5. "Takotsubo Cardiomyopathy (Broken-Heart Syndrome)," Harvard Women's Health Watch, April 2, 2018, https://www.health.harvard.edu/heart-health/takotsubo-cardiomyopathy-broken-heart-syndrome.

6. Hampton, "How Your Thoughts Change Your Brain, Cells and Genes."

7. Leah Marieann Klett, "Limbless Evangelist Nick Vujicic Announces Birth of Twin Daughters Ahead of Christmas: 'Thank You, God!,'" Gospel Herald Ministries, December 21, 2017, https://www.gospelherald.com/articles/71755/20171221/limbless-evangelist-nick-vujicic-announces-birth-twin-daughters-thank-god.htm.

8. Karen Lawson, "How Do Thoughts and Emotions Affect Health?," Taking Charge of Your Health and Wellbeing, University of Minnesota, accessed July 16, 2019, https://www.takingcharge.csh.umn.edu/how-do-thoughts-and-emotions-affect-health.

9. Riya R. Kanherkar, Naina Bhatia-Dey, and Antonei B. Csoka, "Epigenetics Across the Human Lifespan," *Frontiers in Cell and Developmental Biology* 2 (2014): 49, https://www.ncbi.nlm.nih.gov/pmc/articles/PMC4207041/.

10. James Gallagher, "'Memories' Pass Between Generations," BBC News, December 1, 2013, https://www.bbc.com/news/health-25156510.

11. T. D. Jakes, *Reposition Yourself: Living Life Without Limits* (New York: Atria Books, 2008), 172.

12. Kanherkar, Bhatia-Dey, and Csoka, "Epigenetics Across the Human Lifespan."

13. "Epigenetics: Fundamentals," What Is Epigenetics, accessed July 16, 2019, https://www.whatisepigenetics.com/fundamentals/.

14. Kanherkar, Bhatia-Dey, and Csoka, "Epigenetics Across the Human Lifespan"; "Epigenetics: Fundamentals," What Is Epigenetics.

15. Thomas Oppong, "The Neuroscience of Change: How to Train Your Brain to Create Better Habits," *Startup*, June 12, 2018, https://medium.com/swlh/to-break-bad-habits-you-really-have-to-change-your-brain-the-neuroscience-of-change-da735de9afdf.

16. Stephanie Pappas, "Divorce Plagues Kids' Social, Academic Lives for Years," Live Science, June 2, 2011, https://www.livescience.com/14402-divorce-plagues-kids-social-academic.html; Melody T. McCloud, "Borderline Personality Disorder: Who's at Risk (Part 1)," *Psychology Today*, August 8, 2011, https://www.psychologytoday.com/us/blog/black-womens-health-and-happiness/201108/borderline-personality-disorder-whos-risk-part-1.

17. *Key Substance Use and Mental Health Indicators in the United States: Results From the 2017 National Survey on Drug Use and Health*, Substance Abuse and Mental Health Services Administration (SAMHSA), September 2018, 1, https://www.samhsa.gov/data/sites/default/files/cbhsq-reports/NSDUHFFR2017/NSDUHFFR2017.pdf.

18. Eric J. Nestler, "The Neurobiology of Cocaine Addiction," *Science & Practice Perspectives* 3, no. 1 (2005): 4–10, https://www.ncbi.nlm.nih.gov/pmc/articles/PMC2851032/.

19. Committee on Child Maltreatment Research, Policy, and Practice for the Next Decade: Phase II; Board on Children, Youth, and Families; Committee on Law and Justice; Institute of Medicine; National Research Council, "4: Consequences of Child Abuse and Neglect," in Anne C. Petersen, Joshua Joseph, and Monica Feit, eds., *New Directions in Child Abuse and Neglect Research* (Washington, DC: US National Academies Press, March 25, 2014), https://www.ncbi.nlm.nih.gov/books/NBK195987/.

20. Elana Pearl Ben-Joseph, "Nightmares," KidsHealth, May 2018, https://kidshealth.org/en/parents/nightmare.html.

21. Elizabeth R. Pulgaron and Alan M. Delamater, "Obesity and Type 2 Diabetes in Children: Epidemiology and Treatment," *Current Diabetes Reports* 14, no. 8 (2014): 508, https://www.ncbi.nlm.nih.gov/pmc/articles/PMC4099943/.

22. Nestler, "The Neurobiology of Cocaine Addiction."

23. Carmine Gallo, "Brain Science Reveals the Striking Power of Optimism," *Forbes*, November 19, 2017, https://www.forbes.com/sites/carminegallo/2017/11/19/brain-science-reveals-the-striking-power-of-optimism/#55c8f5c971aa.

24. "Drug Record: Acetaminophen," National Institutes of Health, January 28, 2016, https://livertox.nih.gov/Acetaminophen.htm.

25. "Ibuprofen Dosage," Drugs.com, May 31, 2019, https://www.drugs.com/dosage/ibuprofen.html; "Nephrotoxicity (Renal Toxicity)," Chemocare, accessed July 16, 2019, http://chemocare.com/chemotherapy/side-effects/nephrotoxicity-renal-toxicity.aspx.

26. Thai Nguyen, "10 Proven Ways to Grow Your Brain: Neurogenesis and Neuroplasticity," *Huffpost*, December 7, 2017, https://www.huffpost.com/entry/10-proven-ways-to-grow-yo_b_10374730.

Chapter 7

1. Susan Reynolds, "Happy Brain, Happy Life," *Psychology Today*, August 2, 2011, https://www.psychologytoday.com/us/blog/prime-your-gray-cells/201108/happy-brain-happy-life.
2. "What's the Average Age of a Kid's First Porn Exposure?," Fight the New Drug, May 31, 2019, https://fightthenewdrug.org/real-average-age-of-first-exposure/.
3. Philippe Domenech and Etienne Koechlin, "Executive Control and Decision-Making in the Prefrontal Cortex," *Current Opinion in Behavioral Sciences* 1 (February 2015): 101–106, https://www.sciencedirect.com/science/article/pii/S2352154614000278.
4. Sam Black, "The Bible and the Brain," Covenant Eyes, March 12, 2013, http://www.covenanteyes.com/2013/03/12/biblical-neurology/.
5. Huch, *Free at Last*, 101, 268.

Chapter 8

1. William B. Strean, "Laughter Prescription," *Canadian Family Physician* 55, no. 10 (2009): 965–967, http://www.ncbi.nlm.nih.gov/pmc/articles/PMC2762283.
2. Eileen Luders et al., "The Underlying Anatomical Correlates of Long-Term Meditation: Larger Hippocampal and Frontal Volumes of Gray Matter," *NeuroImage* 45, no. 3 (2009): 672–678, https://www.ncbi.nlm.nih.gov/pmc/articles/PMC3184843/.
3. Martini, Nath, and Bartholomew, *Fundamentals of Anatomy and Physiology*, 130.
4. Phil Mason, *Quantum Glory: The Science of Heaven Invading Earth* (Maricopa, AZ: XP Publishing, 2010), 96–97.
5. Karl Deisseroth, "A Look Inside the Brain," *Scientific American* 315, no. 4 (2016): 30–37, https://www.ncbi.nlm.nih.gov/pmc/articles/PMC5846712/.
6. "Heart Murmurs Topic Review," Healio: Learn the Heart, accessed July 17, 2019, https://www.healio.com/cardiology/learn-the-heart/cardiology-review/topic-reviews/heart-murmurs.
7. Lindsey Konkel, "What Is GABA?," Everyday Health, October 17, 2015, https://www.everydayhealth.com/gaba/guide/.
8. John F. Kennedy, "Remarks of Senator John F. Kennedy," National Conference of Christians and Jews, Boston, February 16, 1956, 14, https://www.jfklibrary.org/asset-viewer/archives/JFKSEN/0895/JFKSEN-0895-002.
9. Wendy McDougal, "Macrophages: Definition, Function and Types," Armed Services Vocational Aptitude Battery (ASVAB): Practice and Study Guide, Study.com, accessed July 17, 2017, https://study.com/academy/lesson/macrophages-definition-function-types.html.
10. David L. Swanson, "Necrotizing Soft Tissue Infection," MedlinePlus, US National Library of Medicine, November 3, 2017, https://medlineplus.gov/ency/article/001443.htm.
11. LaVelle Hendricks et al., "The Effects of Anger on the Brain and Body," *National Forum Journal of Counseling and Addiction* 2, no. 1 (2013), http://www.nationalforum.com/Electronic%20Journal%20Volumes/Hendricks,%20LaVelle%20

The%20Effects%20of%20Anger%20on%20the%20Brain%20and%20Body%20 NFJCA%20V2%20N1%202013.pdf.

12. Steven Novella, "Brain Cells in the Heart?," *Neurologica* (blog), August 12, 2013, https://theness.com/neurologicablog/index.php/brain-cells-in-the-heart/.

Chapter 9

1. Rachael Link, "8 Health Benefits of Fasting, Backed by Science," Healthline, July 30, 2018, https://www.healthline.com/nutrition/fasting-benefits..

2. Everett L. Worthington Jr., "The New Science of Forgiveness," Greater Good Science Center at UC Berkeley, September 1, 2004, https://greatergood.berkeley.edu/article/item/the_new_science_of_forgiveness.

3. Christopher Bergland, "Holding a Grudge Produces Cortisol and Diminishes Oxytocin," *Psychology Today*, April 11, 2015, https://www.psychologytoday.com/us/blog/the-athletes-way/201504/holding-grudge-produces-cortisol-and-diminishes-oxytocin; McEwen, Nasca, and Gray, "Stress Effects on Neuronal Structure."

4. Scott J. Russo and Eric J. Nestler, "The Brain Reward Circuitry in Mood Disorders," *Nature Reviews: Neuroscience* 14, no. 9 (2013): 609–625, https://www.ncbi.nlm.nih.gov/pmc/articles/PMC3867253/.

5. Mason, *Quantum Glory*, 276.

6. Mason, *Quantum Glory*, 278–279.

7. Benny Hinn, *Good Morning, Holy Spirit* (Nashville: Thomas Nelson, 1997), 12–13.

8. Benedict Carey, "A Neurological Look at Speaking in Tongues," *New York Times*, November 7, 2006, https://www.nytimes.com/2006/11/07/health/07brain.html; Dirk Hanson, "Speaking in Tongues: Glossolalia and Stress Reduction," Dana Foundation, October 23, 2013, https://www.dana.org/News/Speaking_in_Tongues__Glossalalia_and_Stress_Reduction/.

9. Steve Ayan, "There Is No Such Thing as Conscious Thought," *Scientific American*, December 20, 2018, https://www.scientificamerican.com/article/there-is-no-such-thing-as-conscious-thought/.

10. Richard J. Joseph et al., "The Neurocognitive Connection Between Physical Activity and Eating Behaviour," *Obesity Reviews* 12, no. 10 (2011): 800–812, https://www.ncbi.nlm.nih.gov/pmc/articles/PMC3535467/.

11. Rodger K. Bufford, "God and Behavior Mod: Some Thoughts Concerning the Relationships Between Biblical Principles and Behavior Modification," *Journal of Psychology and Theology* 5, no. 1 (December 1977): 13–22, https://www.researchgate.net/publication/315802173.

12. "Medication," Mental Health America, accessed July 17, 2019, https://www.mentalhealthamerica.net/medication.

13. Chris Tuell, "Mental Illness, Addiction and Digital Infidelity," Lindner Center of Hope, September 30, 2016, https://lindnercenterofhope.org/blog/mental-illness-addiction-and-digital-infidelity/.

14. Joyce Meyer, *Power Thoughts: 12 Strategies to Win the Battle of the Mind* (New York: FaithWords, 2010), 116–117.

Chapter 11

1. "Female Reproductive System," Cleveland Clinic, January 19, 2019, https://my.clevelandclinic.org/health/articles/9118-female-reproductive-system.
2. Jenkins, Van Houten, and Bovbjerg, "Effects on DNA Damage and/or Repair Processes as Biological Mechanisms Linking Psychological Stress to Cancer Risk."

Chapter 12

1. Jentezen Franklin, *Right People, Right Place, Right Plan: Discerning the Voice of God* (New Kensington, PA: Whitaker House, 2007), 75.
2. Paul Ratner, "Scientists Find Out How Hope Protects the Brain," Big Think, October 20, 2017, https://bigthink.com/hope-optimism/scientists-find-out-how-hope-protects-the-brain.
3. Christopher Wanjek, "Imagination and Reality Look Different in the Brain," Live Science, December 23, 2014, https://www.livescience.com/49244-imagination-reality-brain-flow-direction.html.
4. Theresa Fisher, "43 Facts About Your Brain That Will Blow Your Mind," Mic, November 12, 2014, https://www.mic.com/articles/103518/43-facts-about-your-brain-that-will-blow-your-mind.
5. Tiz Huch, *No Limits, No Boundaries: Praying Dynamic Change Into Your Life, Family, and Finances* (New Kensington, PA: Whitaker House, 2009), 64.
6. Joseph Feher, "5.4—The Heart as a Pump," in *Quantitative Human Physiology: An Introduction* (Waltham, MA: Academic Press, 2012), 446–454, https://www.sciencedirect.com/science/article/pii/B9780123821638000475.
7. Ronan O'Rahilly, "Chapter 23: The Pericardium and Heart," Basic Human Anatomy, Dartmouth Medical School, 2008, https://www.dartmouth.edu/~humananatomy/part_4/chapter_23.html.

Chapter 13

1. Mohammad G. Saklayen, "The Global Epidemic of the Metabolic Syndrome," Current Hypertension Reports 20, no. 2 (February 26, 2018): 12, https://www.ncbi.nlm.nih.gov/pmc/articles/PMC5866840/.
2. Lea Winerman, "The Mind's Mirror," *Monitor on Psychology* 36, no. 9 (October 2005): 48, American Psychological Association, https://www.apa.org/monitor/oct05/mirror.
3. Michael Mercandetti, "Wound Healing and Repair," MedScape, April 2, 2019, https://emedicine.medscape.com/article/1298129-overview.
4. Norine Dworkin-McDaniel, "Touching Makes You Healthier," CNN Health.com, January 5, 2011, http://www.cnn.com/2011/HEALTH/01/05/touching.makes.you.healthier.health/.
5. K. Uvnas-Moberg and M. Petersson, "Oxytocin: A Mediator of Anti-Stress, Well-Being, Social Interaction, Growth and Healing," *Zeitschrift fur Psychosomatische Medizin und Psychotherapie* 51, no. 1 (2005): 57–80, https://www.ncbi.nlm.nih.gov/pubmed/15834840.

6. Andrew Newberg and Mark Robert Waldman, *How God Changes Your Brain: Breakthrough Findings From a Leading Neuroscientist* (New York: Ballantine Books, 2009), 124–125, https://books.google.com/books/about/How_God_Changes_Your_Brain.html?id=ddgo4IW1FWgC.

7. Abraham Lincoln, "Proclamation Appointing a National Fast Day," Washington, DC, March 30, 1863, http://www.abrahamlincolnonline.org/lincoln/speeches/fast.htm.

CHAPTER 14

1. "This Is What Negative Thinking Does to Your Brain and Body," Power of Positivity, accessed July 18, 2019, https://www.powerofpositivity.com/negative-thinking-affects-your-brain/.

2. "Atherosclerosis," National Heart, Lung, and Blood Institute, accessed July 18, 2019, https://www.nhlbi.nih.gov/health-topics/atherosclerosis.

3. Q. Qiao et al., "Metabolic Syndrome and Cardiovascular Disease," *Annals of Clinical Biochemistry* 44 (May 2007): 232-63, https://www.ncbi.nlm.nih.gov/pubmed/17456293, accessed August 29, 2019.

4. "Health Threats From High Blood Pressure," American Heart Association, October 31, 2016, https://www.heart.org/en/health-topics/high-blood-pressure/health-threats-from-high-blood-pressure

5. "Metabolic Syndrome," Mayo Clinic, March 14, 2019, https://www.mayoclinic.org/diseases-conditions/metabolic-syndrome/diagnosis-treatment/drc-20351921.

6. Mary Jane Brown, "Do Very Low-Carb Diets Mess Up Some Women's Hormones?," Healthline, June 4, 2016, https://www.healthline.com/nutrition/low-carb-and-womens-hormones.

7. P. Paschos and K. Paletas, "Non Alcoholic Fatty Liver Disease and Metabolic Syndrome," *Hippokratia* 13, no. 1 (2009): 9–19, https://www.ncbi.nlm.nih.gov/pmc/articles/PMC2633261/.

8. "Losing Weight," Centers for Disease Control and Prevention, February 13, 2018, https://www.cdc.gov/healthyweight/losing_weight/index.html.

9. Walter M. Bortz II, "The Disuse Syndrome," *Western Journal of Medicine* 141, no. 5 (1984): 691–694, https://www.ncbi.nlm.nih.gov/pmc/articles/PMC1011199/.

10. "Tainted Weight Loss Products," Federal Drug Administration, July 16, 2019, https://www.fda.gov/drugs/medication-health-fraud/tainted-weight-loss-products.

11. Victor Navarro et al., "Liver Injury From Herbal and Dietary Supplements," *Hepatology (Baltimore, MD)* 65, no. 1 (2017): 363–373, https://www.ncbi.nlm.nih.gov/pmc/articles/PMC5502701/.

12. Young Mi Hong, "Atherosclerotic Cardiovascular Disease Beginning in Childhood," *Korean Circulation Journal* 40, no. 1 (2010): 1–9, https://www.ncbi.nlm.nih.gov/pmc/articles/PMC2812791/.

13. Panagiota Pervanidou and George P. Chrousos, "Stress and Obesity/Metabolic Syndrome in Childhood and Adolescents," *International Journal of*

Pediatric Obesity 6 (2011): 21–28, https://www.tandfonline.com/doi/abs/10.3109/174 77166.2011.615996.

14. Dorit Koren, Magdalena Dumin, and David Gozal, "Role of Sleep Quality in the Metabolic Syndrome," *Diabetes, Metabolic Syndrome and Obesity: Targets and Therapy* 9 (2016): 281–310, https://www.ncbi.nlm.nih.gov/pmc/articles /PMC5003523/.

15. Amanda J. Kiliaan, Ilse A. C. Arnoldussen, and Deborah R. Gustafson, "Adipokines: A Link Between Obesity and Dementia?," *The Lancet: Neurology* 13, no. 9 (2014): 913–923, https://www.ncbi.nlm.nih.gov/pmc/articles/PMC4228955/.

CHAPTER 15

1. Margherita M. Lee, Andreas Reif, and Angelika Schmitt, "Major Depression: A Role for Hippocampal Neurogenesis?," *Behavioral Neurobiology of Depression and Its Treatment* 14 (2013): 153–179.

2. Princeton University, "Scientists Discover Addition of New Brain Cells in Highest Brain Area," ScienceDaily, October 15, 1999, https://www.sciencedaily.com /releases/1999/10/991015080607.htm.

3. University of Texas Medical Branch at Galveston, "Frequent Alcohol Drinking Kills New Brain Cells in Adults, Females Are More Vulnerable," Medical Xpress, November 9, 2017, https://medicalxpress.com/news/2017-11 -frequent-alcohol-brain-cells-adults.html; Wiley-Blackwell, "Smoking Linked to Brain Damage," ScienceDaily, June 23, 2009, https://www.sciencedaily.com /releases/2009/06/090623090400.htm.

4. Vishal Jinal, Sorab Gupta, and Ritwik Das, "Molecular Mechanisms of Meditation," *Molecular Neurobiology* 48, no. 3 (December 2013): 808–811, https:// link.springer.com/article/10.1007%2Fs12035-013-8468-9.

5. Jinal, Gupta, and Das, "Molecular Mechanisms of Meditation."

6. "Phytonutrients," Oral Cancer Foundation, accessed July 18, 2019, https:// oralcancerfoundation.org/nutrition/phytonutrients/.

7. "Washington Monument: History and Culture," National Park Service, April 16, 2018, https://www.nps.gov/wamo/learn/historyculture/index.htm.

8. Ravi Zacharias, "A Simple Prayer for the State of the Union," RZIM, accessed July 18, 2019, https://www.rzim.org/read/rzim-updates/a-simple-prayer-for -the-state-of-the-union.

9. Geoffrey M. Cooper, "The Development and Causes of Cancer," in *The Cell: A Molecular Approach*, 2nd edition (Sunderland, MA: Sinauer Associates, 2000), https://www.ncbi.nlm.nih.gov/books/NBK9963/.

CHAPTER 17

1. Jakes, *Reposition Yourself*, 102–103.

2. Stacy Sampson, "Serotonin Deficiency: What We Do and Don't Know," Healthline, February 27, 2019, https://www.healthline.com/health/serotonin -deficiency.

3. Anthony Wright, "Chapter 6: Limbic System: Amygdala," Neuroscience Online, McGovern Medical School at UT Health, accessed July 19, 2019, https://nba.uth.tmc.edu/neuroscience/m/s4/chapter06.html.

4. Westphalen, "What Does Gamma Aminobutyric Acid (GABA) Do?"

5. "Stress Weakens the Immune System," American Psychological Association, February 23, 2006, http://www.apa.org/research/action/immune.aspx.

6. Malcolm Pines, "Social Brain and Social Group: How Mirroring Connects People," *Group Analysis* 36, no. 4 (December 2003): 507–513, https://www.researchgate.net/publication/247735770_Social_Brain_and_Social_Group_How_Mirroring_Connects_People.

7. Kelly James Clark, ed., *Readings in the Philosophy of Religion*, 2nd ed. (New York: Broadview, 2008), 77.

8. Luke Mastin, "Memory Storage," The Human Memory, accessed July 19, 2019, http://www.human-memory.net/processes_storage.html.

9. Peg Streep, "The Enduring Pain of Childhood Verbal Abuse," *Psychology Today*, November 14, 2016, https://www.psychologytoday.com/us/blog/tech-support/201611/the-enduring-pain-childhood-verbal-abuse.

CHAPTER 18

1. Judy Squier, *His Majesty in Brokenness: Finding God's Masterpiece in Your Missing Piece* (CreateSpace, 2010), 104.

2. Gallo, "Brain Science Reveals the Striking Power of Optimism."

3. Newberg and Waldman, *How God Changes Your Brain*.

CHAPTER 19

1. Reynolds, "Happy Brain, Happy Life."

CHAPTER 20

1. "'Clueless or Clued Up: Your Right to Be Informed About Contraception' Media Report," Bayer Pharma AG, September 2011, https://www.west-info.eu/unprotected-sex-partner-contraception-drunk-your-life-uk/wcd-survey-2011-media-report-2011/.

2. "Chlamydia," Centers for Disease Control and Prevention, July 24, 2018, https://www.cdc.gov/std/stats17/chlamydia.htm.

3. "Mental Health by the Numbers," National Alliance on Mental Illness, accessed July 19, 2019, https://www.nami.org/learn-more/mental-health-by-the-numbers.

4. S. Wingate, "Cardiovascular Anatomy and Physiology in the Female," *Critical Care Nursing Clinics of North America* 9, no. 4 (December 1997): 447–452, https://www.ncbi.nlm.nih.gov/pubmed/9444167.

5. "Mental Stress, Gender, and the Heart," *Harvard Heart Letter*, March 2018, https://www.health.harvard.edu/heart-health/mental-stress-gender-and-the-heart.

6. J. C. Witteman et al., "Increased Risk of Atherosclerosis in Women after the Menopause," *BMJ (Clinical research ed.)* 298, no. 6674 (1989): 642–644, https://www.ncbi.nlm.nih.gov/pmc/articles/PMC1835855/.

7. "Males and Females Differ in Specific Brain Structures," University of Cambridge, February 11, 2014, https://www.cam.ac.uk/research/news/males-and-females-differ-in-specific-brain-structures; Theodore Rabinowicz et al., "Gender Differences in Human Cerebral Cortex: More Neurons in Males; More Processes in Females," *Journal of Child Neurology* 14, no. 2 (February 1, 1999): 98–107, https://journals.sagepub.com/doi/abs/10.1177/088307389901400207.

8. Geert J. De Vries, "Sex Differences in Neurotransmitter Systems," *Journal of Neuroendocrinology* 2, no. 1 (1990), https://onlinelibrary.wiley.com/doi/pdf/10.1111/j.1365-2826.1990.tb00385.x.

9. Caroline Leaf, *Who Switched Off Your Brain?: Solving the Mystery of He Said/She Said* (Southlake, TX: Inprov, 2011), 141.

10. Marie Ellis, "Oxytocin: The Monogamy Hormone?," Medical News Today, November 26, 2013, https://www.medicalnewstoday.com/articles/269365.php.

11. Markus MacGill, "Oxytocin: What Is the Link Between Love and Oxytocin?," Medical News Today, September 4, 2017, http://www.medicalnewstoday.com/articles/275795.php.

12. Luciana Gravotta, "Be Mine Forever: Oxytocin May Help Build Long-Lasting Love," *Scientific American*, February 12, 2013, http://www.scientificamerican.com/article/be-mine-forever-oxytocin/.

13. Ellis, "Oxytocin: The Monogamy Hormone?"; Gravotta, "Be Mine Forever."

14. Susan Weiss, "The Power of Touch: Stimulate Oxytocin, Stimulate Love," FOR A.tv, YouTube, June 25, 2013, https://www.youtube.com/watch?v=8gMA7XLoYJA.

15. M. Galbally et al., "The Role of Oxytocin in Mother-Infant Relations: A Systematic Review of Human Studies," *Harvard Review of Psychiatry* 19, no. 1 (January–February 2011): 1–14, https://www.ncbi.nlm.nih.gov/pubmed/21250892.

16. Ana Sandoiu, "Low Oxytocin May Lead to Low Empathy, Study Finds," Medical News Today, November 7, 2016, https://www.medicalnewstoday.com/articles/313911.php.

17. Universität Bonn, "Oxytocin Helps to Better Overcome Fear," ScienceDaily, November 13, 2014, https://www.sciencedaily.com/releases/2014/11/141113110014.htm.

18. Loretta Breuning, "The Neurochemistry of Love," *Psychology Today*, February 13, 2018, https://www.psychologytoday.com/us/blog/your-neurochemical-self/201802/the-neurochemistry-love.

19. Breuning, "The Neurochemistry of Love."

20. Beni Johnson, *The Happy Intercessor* (Shippensburg, PA: Destiny Image, 2009), 131.

Chapter 21

1. "Queen's Christmas Message—Full Text," *Guardian*, December 25, 2013, https://www.theguardian.com/uk-news/2013/dec/25/queen-christmas-message-time-to-reflect.

2. Joel Osteen, "Focus on His Freedom," Today's Word With Joel and Victoria, November 18, 2015, https://www.joelosteen.com/Pages/MessageViewer.aspx?date=2015-11-18.

3. Divya Krishnakumar, Michael R. Hamblin, and Shanmugamurthy Lakshmanan, "Meditation and Yoga Can Modulate Brain Mechanisms That Affect Behavior and Anxiety: A Modern Scientific Perspective," *Ancient Science* 2, no. 1 (2015): 13–19, https://www.ncbi.nlm.nih.gov/pmc/articles/PMC4769029/.

Chapter 22

1. Joanna Weaver, *Having a Mary Heart in a Martha World: Finding Intimacy With God in the Busyness of Life* (Colorado Springs: WaterBrook, 2002), 197.
2. Joel Osteen, *Your Best Life Now: 7 Steps to Living at Your Full Potential*, rev. ed. (New York: FaithWords, 2014), 241.
3. Winerman, "The Mind's Mirror,"
4. Moore, *Jesus, the One and Only*, 328.
5. "How the Growth and Evolution of the Over-the-Air TV Home Fits into Today's Viewing Landscape," Nielsen, January 31, 2019, https://www.nielsen.com/us/en/insights/article/2019/how-the-growth-and-evolution-of-the-over-the-air-tv-home-fits-into-media-landscape/.
6. John Bevere, *Honor's Reward: How to Attract God's Favor and Blessing* (New York: FaithWords, 2007), 209.
7. Dodie Osteen, *Healed of Cancer* (Houston: Lakewood Church, 1986), https://www.hopefaithprayer.com/books/Healed%20of%20Cancer%20-%20Osteen.pdf.
8. Patricia L. Lockwood, "The Anatomy of Empathy: Vicarious Experience and Disorders of Social Cognition," *Behavioural Brain Research* 311 (2016): 255–266, https://www.ncbi.nlm.nih.gov/pmc/articles/PMC4942880/.
9. Newberg and Waldman, *How God Changes Your Brain*, 43.
10. John M. Allman et al., "The von Economo Neurons in the Frontoinsular and Anterior Cingulate Cortex," *Annals of the New York Academy of Sciences* 1225 (2011): 59–71, https://www.ncbi.nlm.nih.gov/pmc/articles/PMC3140770/.

Chapter 23

1. "Strengthen Your Brain Through the Power of Prayer," interview with Dr. Andrew Newberg, *Mind Health Report*, 2017, http://fgbt.org/Health-Tips/strengthen-your-brain-through-the-power-of-prayer.html.
2. "Strengthen Your Brain Through the Power of Prayer," *Mind Health Report*.
3. Jessie Dezutter, Amy Wachholtz, and Jozef Corveleyn, "Prayer and Pain: The Mediating Role of Positive Re-appraisal," *Journal of Behavioral Medicine* 34, no. 6 (December 2011): 542–549, https://link.springer.com/article/10.1007%2Fs10865-011-9348-2.
4. Dezutter, Wachholtz, and Corveleyn, "Prayer and Pain"; Leeds Beckett University, "Meditation Could Be a Cheapter Alternative to Traditional Pain Medication, Study Suggests," ScienceDaily, June 12, 2017, https://www.sciencedaily.com/releases/2017/06/170612094633.htm.
5. Jessica Tartaro, Linda J. Luecken, and Heather E. Gunn, "Exploring Heart and Soul: Effects of Religiosity/Spirituality and Gender on Blood Pressure

and Cortisol Stress Responses," *Journal of Health Psychology* 10, no. 6 (December 1, 2005): 753–766, https://journals.sagepub.com/doi/abs/10.1177/1359105305057311.

6. Lynn Rew, Y. Joel Wong, and R. Weylin Sternglanz, "The Relationship Between Prayer, Health Behaviors, and Protective Resources in School-Age Children," *Issues in Comprehensive Pediatric Nursing* 27, no. 4 (October–December 2004): 245–255, https://www.tandfonline.com/doi/abs/10.1080/01460860490884156?needAccess=true.

7. Gail Ironson et al., "The Ironson-Woods Spirituality/Religiousness Index Is Associated With Long Survival, Health Behaviors, Less Distress, and Low Cortisol in People With HIV/AIDS," *Annals of Behavioral Medicine* 24, no. 1 (February 2002): abstract, https://academic.oup.com/abm/article-abstract/24/1/34/4631542?redirectedFrom=fulltext.

8. J. A. Ciesla et al., "Dispositional Mindfulness Moderates the Effects of Stress Among Adolescents: Rumination as a Mediator," *Journal of Clinical Child and Adolescent Psychology* 41, no. 6 (2012): 760–770, https://www.ncbi.nlm.nih.gov/pubmed/22775559.

9. Shaowei Xue, Yi-Yuan Tang, and Michael I. Posner, "Short-Term Meditation Increases Network Efficiency of the Anterior Cingulate Cortex," *NeuroReport* 22, no. 12 (August 24, 2011): 570–574, https://journals.lww.com/neuroreport/Abstract/2011/08240/Short_term_meditation_increases_network_efficiency.2.aspx.

10. Helming, "Healing Through Prayer."

11. David I. Levy with Joel Kilpatrick, *Gray Matter: A Neurosurgeon Discovers the Power of Prayer...One Patient at a Time* (Carol Stream, IL: Tyndale House, 2011), 11.

12. Charles Stanley, *Handle With Prayer: Discovering God's Strength for Living* (Colorado Springs, CO: Cook Communications, 2004), 118.

Chapter 24

1. Priscilla Shirer, "The Armor of God: Prayer Strategies," Friday Feature, LifeWay Groups Ministry, August 7, 2015, https://groupministry.lifeway.com/2015/08/07/the-armor-of-god-prayer-strategies/. Excerpt from Priscilla Shirer, *The Armor of God* (Nashville: LifeWay Press, 2015).

2. Carrie Murphy, "This Is How Joy Affects Your Body," Healthline, June 27, 2018, https://www.healthline.com/health/affects-of-joy#7.

3. "Study: Gratitude Is a Healthy Attitude," American Heart Association, November 21, 2016, https://news.heart.org/study-gratitude-is-a-healthy-attitude/.

4. Gloria Copeland, *Blessed Beyond Measure: Experience the Extraordinary Goodness of God* (Tulsa, OK: Harrison House, 2004), 185.

Chapter 25

1. A. V. Rzheshevsky, "Fatal 'Triad': Lipotoxicity, Oxidative Stress, and Phenoptosis," *Biochemistry (Moscow)* 78, no. 9 (2013): abstract, http://www.protein.bio.msu.ru/biokhimiya/contents/v78/pdf/bcm_0991.pdf.

2. Scott M. Grundy et al., "Diagnosis and Management of the Metabolic Syndrome: An American Heart Association/National Heart, Lung, and Blood Institute Scientific Statement," *Circulation* 112 (2005): 2735–2752, https://www.ahajournals.org/doi/10.1161/circulationaha.105.169404.

3. G. V. Ramesh Prasad, "Metabolic Syndrome and Chronic Kidney Disease: Current Status and Future Directions," *World Journal of Nephrology* 3, no. 4 (2014): 210–219, https://www.ncbi.nlm.nih.gov/pmc/articles/PMC4220353/.

4. Grundy et al., "Diagnosis and Management of the Metabolic Syndrome."

5. Grundy et al., "Diagnosis and Management of the Metabolic Syndrome"; Scott M. Grundy, "A Changing Paradigm for Prevention of Cardiovascular Disease: Emergence of the Metabolic Syndrome as a Multiplex Risk Factor," *European Heart Journal Supplements* 10, suppl. B (March 2008): B16–B23, https://academic.oup.com/eurheartjsupp/article/10/suppl_B/B16/415890.

6. Grundy et al., "Diagnosis and Management of the Metabolic Syndrome."

7. Grundy et al., "Diagnosis and Management of the Metabolic Syndrome."

8. Trevor Orchard et al., "The Effect of Metformin and Intensive Lifestyle Intervention on the Metabolic Syndrome: The Diabetes Prevention Program Randomized Trial," *Annals of Internal Medicine* 142, no. 8 (2005): 611–619, https://www.ncbi.nlm.nih.gov/pmc/articles/PMC2505046/.

9. Evaggelia Fappa et al., "Lifestyle Intervention in the Management of Metabolic Syndrome: Could We Improve Adherence Issues?," *Nutrition* 24, no. 3 (March 2008): abstract, https://www.sciencedirect.com/science/article/abs/pii/S0899900707003541?via%3Dihub.

10. Rodica Malos, "Independent Case Report," Doctor of Nursing Practice Portfolio, *OHSU Digital Collections* (2009): 10, https://doi.org/10.6083/M4ZP443X.

11. Johannes Bohacek and Isabelle M. Mansuy, "Epigenetic Inheritance of Disease and Disease Risk," *Neuropsychopharmacology* 38, no. 1 (2013): 220–236, https://www.ncbi.nlm.nih.gov/pmc/articles/PMC3521963/.

12. Allison Stevens, "Methyl Diet," LiveStrong, accessed July 23, 2019. https://www.livestrong.com/article/387247-methyl-diet/.

13. Rick Nauert, "Dehydration Influences Mood, Cognition," Psychology Central, August 8, 2018, https://psychcentral.com/news/2012/02/20/dehydration-influences-mood-cognition/35037.html.

14. "Depression on Melatonin: Can the Supplement Make Your Depression Worse?," Family Service Foundation, June 29, 2018, https://www.fsfinc.org/mental-health/depression-melatonin-can-supplement-make-depression-worse/; Therapeutic Research Faculty, "Melatonin," WebMD, accessed July 26, 2019, https://www.webmd.com/vitamins/ai/ingredientmono-940/melatonin.

15. Thomas Unbehaun, Andreas Jähne, and Dieter Riemann, "The Relationship Between Addiction and Sleep: Basic Information on Sleep Regulation," *Sucht: Zeitschrift fur Wissenschaft und Praxis* 59, no. 1 (February 2013): 17–23, https://econtent.hogrefe.com/doi/abs/10.1024/0939-5911.a000226.

16. Zhi-Li Huang, Yoshihiro Urade, and Osamu Hayaishi, "The Role of Adenosine in the Regulation of Sleep," *Current Topics in Medicinal Chemistry* 11 (2011): 1047–1057, https://www.researchgate.net/profile/Zhi_Li_Huang

/publication/50393713_The_Role_of_Adenosine_in_the_Regulation_of_Sleep/links/551d4de80cf2a15336261c59.pdf.

17. Italo Biaggioni, "Contrasting Excitatory and Inhibitory Effects of Adenosine in Blood Pressure Regulation," *Hypertension* 20, no. 4 (October 1992): 457–465, https://www.ahajournals.org/doi/pdf/10.1161/01.HYP.20.4.457.

18. "Sleep and Mental Health," *Harvard Mental Health Letter*, March 18, 2019, https://www.health.harvard.edu/newsletter_article/sleep-and-mental-health; Rosie Osmun, "Oversleeping: The Effects and Health Risks of Sleeping Too Much," Amerisleep, *Early Bird* (blog), July 10, 2019, https://www.amerisleep.com/blog/oversleeping-the-health-effects/.

19. Colin Gerber, "These Neurotransmitters Are Probably Keeping You Up at Night," *Forbes*, October 5, 2016, https://www.forbes.com/sites/quora/2016/10/05/these-neurotransmitters-are-probably-keeping-you-up-at-night/#499cf9bc1228.

20. "What Happens When You Sleep?," National Sleep Foundation, accessed July 24, 2019, https://www.sleepfoundation.org/articles/what-happens-when-you-sleep; "Nocturnal Asthma (Nighttime Asthma)," WebMD, May 15, 2018, https://www.webmd.com/asthma/guide/nocturnal-asthma-nighttime-asthma#1.

21. "How Sleep Affects Your Blood Sugar," WebMD, May 4, 2019, https://www.webmd.com/diabetes/sleep-affects-blood-sugar#1.

22. Zane Bartlett, "Apoptosis in Embryonic Development," *Embryo Project Encyclopedia*, June 8, 2017, https://embryo.asu.edu/pages/apoptosis-embryonic-development.

23. *Merriam-Webster*, s.v. "apoptosis," accessed July 24, 2019, https://www.merriam-webster.com/dictionary/apoptosis.

24. Elizabeth George, *A Woman After God's Own Heart*, updated and expanded edition (Eugene, OR: Harvest House, 2006), 186.

25. "Transcript for VitalSigns Teleconference: Preventing 1 Million Heart Attacks and Strokes," Centers for Disease Control and Prevention, September 7, 2018, https://www.cdc.gov/media/releases/2018/t0906-vital-signs-preventing-heart-attacks-strokes.html; "Cardiovascular Disease: Prevention and Reversal," Cleveland Clinic, December 20, 2018, https://my.clevelandclinic.org/health/articles/17385-cardiovascular-disease-prevention--reversal.

26. Emelia J. Benjamin et al., "Heart Disease and Stroke Statistics 2018: At-a-Glance," American Heart Association/American Stroke Association, January 31, 2018, https://www.heart.org/-/media/data-import/downloadables/heart-disease-and-stroke-statistics-2018---at-a-glance-ucm_498848.pdf.

27. "Ischemic Heart Disease: Risk Factors," National Heart, Lung, and Blood Institute, accessed July 24, 2019, https://www.nhlbi.nih.gov/health-topics/ischemic-heart-disease.

28. Hans Diehl and Aileen Ludington, *Dynamic Health* (Lake Mary, FL: Siloam, 2003), 33.

29. Cleveland Clinic, "Cardiovascular Disease: Prevention and Reversal."

30. "High Blood Pressure Fact Sheet," Centers for Disease Control and Prevention, accessed September 6, 2019, https://www.cdc.gov/dhdsp/data_statistics/fact_sheets/fs_bloodpressure.htm.

31. Mary E. Cogswell et al., "Dietary Sodium and Cardiovascular Disease Risk—Measurement Matters," *The New England Journal of Medicine* 375, no. 6 (2016): 580–586, https://www.ncbi.nlm.nih.gov/pmc/articles/PMC5381724/.

32. "Estrogen & Hormones," Cleveland Clinic, April 29, 2019, https://my.clevelandclinic.org/health/articles/16979-estrogen--hormones.

33. Annadora J. Bruce-Keller, Jeffrey N. Keller, and Christopher D. Morrison, "Obesity and Vulnerability of the CNS," *Biochimica et Biophysica Acta—Molecular Basis of Disease* 1792, no. 5 (May 2009): 395–400, https://www.sciencedirect.com/science/article/pii/S0925443908001968.

34. "Stroke," National Heart, Lung, and Blood Institute, accessed July 24, 2019, https://www.nhlbi.nih.gov/health-topics/stroke.

35. Preetha Anand et al., "Cancer Is a Preventable Disease That Requires Major Lifestyle Changes," *Pharmaceutical Research* 25, no. 9 (2008): 2097–2116, https://www.ncbi.nlm.nih.gov/pmc/articles/PMC2515569/.

36. Anand et al., "Cancer Is a Preventable Disease That Requires Major Lifestyle Changes"; Sarah Lie, Chikezie O. Madu, and Yi Lu, "The Role of Melatonin in Cancer Development," *Oncomedicine* 3 (2018): 37–47, http://www.oncm.org/v03p0037.htm.

CHAPTER 26

1. Heidi Baker, *Birthing the Miraculous: The Power of Personal Encounters With God to Change Your Life and the World* (Lake Mary, FL: Charisma House, 2014), 108.

2. David Stoop, *You Are What You Think* (Grand Rapids: Revell, 1996), 136.

3. "Strengthen Your Brain Through the Power of Prayer," *Mind Health Report*.

4. "Strengthen Your Brain Through the Power of Prayer," *Mind Health Report*; Richard Schiffman, "Why People Who Pray Are Healthier Than Those Who Don't," *HuffPost*, March 19, 2012, https://www.huffpost.com/entry/why-people-who-pray-are-heathier_b_1197313.

5. "Strengthen Your Brain Through the Power of Prayer," *Mind Health Report*.

6. Larry Dossey, *Healing Words: The Power of Prayer and the Practice of Medicine* (New York: HarperCollins. 1994), 70.

7. Lee Strobel, *The Case for Christ: A Journalist's Personal Investigation of the Evidence for Jesus* (Grand Rapids: Zondervan, 1998), 268.

8. Don Colbert, *Toxic Relief: Restore Health and Energy Through Fasting and Detoxification*, rev. and expanded edition (Lake Mary, FL: Siloam, 2012), 147–149.

9. Jentezen Franklin, *Fasting: Opening the Door to a Deeper, More Intimate, More Powerful Relationship With God* (Lake Mary, FL: Charisma House, 2011), 135–136.

10. Intermountain Medical Center, "Fasting Reduces Cholesterol Levels in Prediabetic People Over Extended Period of Time, New Research Finds," Newswise, June 10, 2014, https://www.newswise.com/articles/fasting-reduces-cholesterol-levels-in-prediabetic-people-over-extended-period-of-time-new-research-finds

11. Barbara Ormond et al., "Potential National and State Medical Care Savings From Primary Disease Prevention," *American Journal of Public Health* 101, no. 1 (2011): 157–164, https://www.ncbi.nlm.nih.gov/pmc/articles/PMC3000727/.

Chapter 27

1. Louis Cozolino, *The Neuroscience of Human Relationships: Attachment and the Developing Social Brain*, 2nd ed. (New York: W. W. Norton, 2014), xi–xii.
2. Book description for Cozolino, *The Neuroscience of Human Relationships*, accessed July 25, 2019, https://books.google.com/books?id=dYUYAwAAQBAJ.
3. "Peer Support Key to Sustaining Recovery," Behavioral Health Evolution, Hazelden Publishing, 2016, http://www.bhevolution.org/public/peer_support_research.page.
4. "Want to Stay Sharp? Maintain Your Social Brain," UNC Health Talk, July 23, 2018, https://healthtalk.unchealthcare.org/want-to-stay-sharp-maintain-your-social-brain/.
5. Yuan Bo Peng et al., "GABAA and 5-HT3 Receptors Are Involved in Dorsal Root Reflexes: Possible Role in Periaqueductal Gray Descending Inhibition," *Journal of Neurophysiology* 86, no. 1 (July 2001): 49–58, https://www.physiology.org/doi/full/10.1152/jn.2001.86.1.49?url_ver=Z39.88-2003
6. Leif Hetland, *Seeing Through Heaven's Eyes: A Worldview That Will Transform Your Life* (Shippensburg, PA: Destiny Image, 2011), 192.

Chapter 28

1. Felix Just, "Have No Fear! Do Not Be Afraid!," Catholic Resources for Bible, Liturgy, Art, and Theology, April 6, 2012, https://catholic-resources.org/Bible/HaveNoFear.htm.
2. Randy Alcorn, *Heaven* (Carol Stream, IL: Tyndale, 2004), 440–441.
3. Paul Manwaring, *What on Earth Is Glory?: A Practical Approach to a Glory-Filled Life* (Shippensburg, PA: Destiny Image, 2011), 222–223.
4. Irvin D. Yalom, *Staring at the Sun: Overcoming the Terror of Death* (San Francisco: Jossey-Bass, 2009), 5.

Conclusion

1. Jeffrey Barsch, *Praying for the Brain: Rewiring the Brain Through Prayer* (Ventura, CA: Beneath His Wings Publishing Company, 2013), 56.
2. Lucinda Bassett, *From Panic to Power: Proven Techniques to Calm Your Anxiety, Conquer Your Fears, and Put You in Control of Your Life* (New York: HarperCollins, 1995), 246.
3. Carol Kinsey Goman, "Why We Resist Change and What Leaders Can Do About It," *Forbes*, December 19, 2011, https://www.forbes.com/sites/carolkinseygoman/2011/12/19/why-we-resist-change-and-what-leaders-can-do-about-it/#3eb9de77e0f2.
4. Brian King, "The Habits of Happy People: A Seminar for Health Professionals," Institute for Brain Potential (seminar, Portland, OR, October 23, 2015).
5. Bill Johnson, *The Power That Changes the World: Creating Eternal Impact in the Here and Now* (Grand Rapids: Chosen Books, 2015), 14.

INDEX

A

abstinence 80, 82, 186–187, 247
Academy of Economic Studies 67, 229
acetylcholine xviii, 6, 16–17, 21, 226–227
acute stress syndrome 41
addiction 3, 21, 35–37, 40, 46, 55–56, 62, 65–66, 72, 82, 91, 119, 165, 170–171, 178, 196, 241, 250–251
adenosine 226–227
adolescents 35–38, 56, 192, 211.
See also teenagers
adrenal glands xvii, 17, 21
adrenaline xviii, 52, 226
adrenocorticotropic hormone axis 17
AIDS 37, 186, 211
Alcorn, Randy 258
aldosterone 17
Alzheimer's disease xviii, 6, 21, 42, 60, 77, 154, 194, 210, 212, 232, 236–237, 250
amino acids 12, 97
amotivational syndrome 13, 20, 37
amygdala 13, 18–19, 27, 32–33, 57, 79, 82–83, 87, 168, 191, 207

analgesics 56–57
anandamide 56
anhedonia 55, 154
anterior cingulate 40, 65–66, 145, 206–208, 210
antiaging xix, 13, 20, 78, 155, 194, 210, 212, 233, 235, 237
antidepressants 10, 23, 35, 165, 190, 218, 232
antioxidants 155, 230, 246
anxiety xvii–xix, xxiii–xxv, 3–9, 13, 17–18, 20–21, 23, 25–28, 31–33, 35–37, 39, 41–45, 47–48, 50, 53, 55–56, 60, 63–64, 66–67, 69, 77–78, 82–83, 87–92, 97, 106, 108, 112, 119–122, 131, 137, 143–145, 154–155, 157, 166, 169, 176–178, 180–181, 185, 188, 190–191, 210–211, 218–220, 225–227, 236, 238–239, 245, 249, 261–262, 266, 270–272
apoptosis 15, 227, 252
arthritis 6, 233
asthma 5, 224, 233, 242
atheists 43, 51–52, 67, 95, 160, 245
atherosclerosis 150, 188, 223–224, 230–231, 242–243
attitude xvii, 12, 17, 28, 42–43, 59–60, 68, 77,

79–81, 84, 89–90, 93–94, 98, 100, 105–106, 109, 134–135, 138, 153, 155, 159, 164–175, 177–178, 181, 187–189, 199–200, 204, 208–211, 216–220, 222, 229, 234, 236, 242, 244
autoimmune diseases xxv, 6, 155
axons 12–13, 19–20, 43

B

Baker, Heidi 236
Barsch, Jeffrey 271
basal ganglia 39
Bassett, Lucinda 271
Bevere, John 203
bitterness 3, 13, 32, 47–50, 56, 62–64, 67, 69–73, 81, 87, 94, 105, 111–112, 128, 169, 177, 182–183, 188, 190, 219, 235, 256, 261
blood pressure xvii, 5, 13, 18, 22, 47, 112, 123, 210–211, 219, 224–225, 227, 230–233, 236, 247.
See also hypertension
breathing xxv, 5, 11, 13, 22, 36, 42, 56, 70, 90, 103, 111, 123, 125, 128, 135–136, 138, 176, 191, 213, 220–221, 239, 252, 256
shortness of breath 5–6, 232

303

broken heart syndrome 52, 60, 69, 80, 186
burnout 42, 62

C

cancer xxv, 3, 6–7, 15, 18–19, 26, 34, 37, 51–52, 56, 82, 104, 110, 119, 131, 158, 160, 191, 205, 207, 211, 224, 230, 233, 242, 246, 267
cannabinoids 20, 56
carbohydrates 6, 21–22, 25, 152, 231–232
cardiovascular system 5, 18, 112, 143, 150, 155, 225
carotenoids 155
catecholamines 16, 19, 52
Ceausescu, Nicolae 43
cerebellum 9
cerebral cortex 17, 124, 155, 172, 191
Chernobyl 41
children 32–39, 41, 45–46, 51–52, 55, 58–59, 63, 66–68, 73, 79–85, 88, 92, 99–100, 110–111, 113–114, 117–118, 120, 125, 131–132, 136, 140–141, 148, 151–152, 159–160, 162–163, 167, 172–173, 180, 182, 190, 200–201, 203, 211, 216–217, 223–225, 234, 238–239, 247, 253, 259–260, 266
cholesterol 22, 83, 112, 150, 224, 230–233, 243, 247
chromosomes 25–26, 97
chronic pain 54–57, 211, 242
cingulate gyrus 13, 40, 65–66, 145, 155, 206–208, 210–211
circulatory system xviii, 5, 7, 14, 16, 80, 106, 187, 191, 231–232, 247
cirrhosis 150
Clarke, Shaneen 4, 61
cognition 5, 9, 14–15, 21, 27, 41–42, 151, 154–155, 194, 211–212, 225
    cognitive impairment 6, 18, 20–22, 42, 77, 92, 152, 154
Colbert, Don 242
comorbidities 8, 150
compassion xix, 52, 58–59, 62, 70, 78, 88, 111, 119, 128, 143, 145, 159, 171, 177, 190–191, 198–201, 206–208, 210, 215–216, 227, 239, 244, 247, 254, 271
compromise 16, 68–69, 100, 157
constipation 6, 16, 18, 242
Copeland, Gloria 221
coronary artery disease. *See* atherosclerosis
cortisol xviii, 6–7, 17–19, 31, 35, 62, 64, 106, 111, 140, 154–155, 169, 211, 220, 226
Cozolino, Louis 248

D

decision making xix, xxiii, xxv, 16–17, 20, 36, 40, 46, 58, 64–68, 84–87, 90, 92, 106, 110, 135, 139, 149, 156, 159–160, 168, 171, 177, 204, 211, 219, 246, 262, 267, 269–270
degenerative diseases xxv, 6, 15
dementia 6, 60, 62, 77, 150, 152, 154, 178, 194, 225, 231–232, 250
dendrites 12, 17, 19, 106, 117, 212
depression xvii–xix, xxiii–xxv, 3–6, 8–9, 13, 22–23, 28, 32–33, 35–37, 39, 41–43, 45, 47–50, 53, 55, 60, 62, 68–69, 78, 82–83, 87–89, 91, 96–97, 105, 112, 119–121, 143–144, 150, 152, 154, 157, 166, 168–169, 172, 176–178, 180–181, 196–197, 210, 219–220, 225–227, 232–233, 236, 239, 242–243, 245, 247, 249, 267, 270–272
diabetes xviii, 6, 22, 28, 39, 83, 112, 143, 152, 211, 224–225, 230, 232–233, 242–243, 247
diarrhea 5–6, 18, 23, 242
diet xviii–xix, 13, 149–152, 224–225, 230–233, 245–247

discouragement 32, 34, 42, 47–49, 62–64, 68, 71, 81, 105, 122, 125, 132–134, 140–141, 146, 156, 173, 175, 177, 182, 192, 197, 201, 216, 237–238, 241, 250, 267–268

DNA 15, 18–19, 24–26, 33, 41, 47, 87, 91, 97–98, 111–112, 118, 128, 131, 133–134, 144, 161, 166, 168, 177, 179, 204, 225, 227–228, 243, 263–264

dopamine 13, 17, 21, 36, 40, 64, 66, 78, 82–84, 170, 176, 188, 191, 207, 218, 226–227

Dossey, Larry 237

dreams 26, 39, 49, 62–63, 81, 85, 94, 104, 122, 133–137–140, 157, 169, 195, 237, 241, 272

dyslipidemia 28, 39, 143, 224

E

eczema 6, 242

embryology 129, 262

emotions xvii–xviii, xxiii–xxiv, 8–9, 12–13, 17, 19–22, 26–28, 32–34, 36–40, 42–43, 47, 49–50, 52, 55, 59, 62–63, 65, 69, 79–83, 87, 89–90, 93, 111, 115, 118, 121, 134, 138–140, 146, 152, 154–155, 164, 168–169, 172, 178, 185–186, 189, 191, 196, 199, 201, 206–207, 210, 212–213, 223–226, 236, 244, 249, 257, 261–262, 271–272
    emotional healing 72, 87, 121, 145
    emotional health 89, 99, 112, 210, 213, 219, 232, 236
    emotional pain 8, 10, 12, 34, 42, 49–50, 54, 56–57, 59, 63, 65, 69–73, 80, 96, 141, 143–144, 146, 157, 180, 186, 202, 210–211, 221, 230, 237, 249, 256, 260
    emotional stress 8–9, 82
    emotional support 36, 82, 200, 214

endocrine system 6, 13–14, 16–18, 20, 224

endorphins 21–22, 55–57, 64, 66, 78, 145, 155, 165, 168, 176, 188, 190, 218, 232

epigenetics xvii, 41, 67, 81–83, 88, 159, 170, 225, 247

epinephrine 5, 16–17, 21, 66, 188, 245

Eternal Perspective Ministries 258

euphoria 40, 55

evolution 16, 95, 160

exercise xviii–xix, 13, 20, 39, 42, 84, 149–151, 154, 215, 224, 226, 229–232, 247

F

faith xvii, 4, 9, 35, 39, 42–43, 49–50, 57, 61–62, 64–68, 70, 73, 78, 87, 89–90, 95, 101, 118, 120, 123–124, 127–132, 136–139, 143–145, 164–165, 167, 170–173, 176–180, 182, 184, 186, 188, 190, 196, 204, 206, 215, 218–220, 222, 234–236, 238, 241–242, 249, 260, 262–263, 265–268

fasting xix, 13, 49, 61, 84, 87, 94, 104, 111, 135–136, 142, 146–147, 149, 159, 165, 171, 180, 188, 192, 206, 215, 217, 220, 224, 230, 233–235, 237–238, 240, 242–247, 249–250, 269, 271
    Daniel Fast 217, 230, 242, 245–246

fatigue 5–6, 41, 50, 242

fatty liver 150, 224

favor 68, 84, 127, 130, 133, 136–138, 156, 159–160, 162–163, 168, 192, 199, 203, 205, 219, 234, 241, 245, 249, 265

fear xvii–xix, xxiii–xxv, 3, 5, 7–9, 13, 17–18, 20–21, 23–25, 27–28, 31–32, 36–37, 42–47, 53, 55–56, 61–64, 66, 69, 72, 78, 81, 83, 86, 88–90, 92–93, 97, 102, 108–109, 111–113, 119–123, 125, 130–132, 137–140, 144, 146, 154–155, 157, 166,

168–169, 176–177, 181, 185, 188, 190–191, 193, 220, 225, 227, 236–241, 243, 245, 249, 251, 253, 256, 258–263, 265, 269–272
    fear of death 61, 236, 253, 255–256, 258, 260, 262, 268
    spirit of fear 62, 125, 260–261
fear of the Lord 43, 45, 65–67, 79, 123, 130–132, 159–161, 171, 188, 195
fibromyalgia 6, 242
fibrosis 150
finances 7–8, 31, 34, 45–46, 56, 63–66, 81, 92–93, 122, 137, 151, 203, 205, 208, 247
flavonoids 155
forgiveness 7, 31, 39, 46–47, 49–51, 68, 70, 72, 81, 85, 87, 92, 94, 99–100, 105–109, 111–113, 120–121, 128–130, 138, 140–143, 147, 162, 164–165, 169–170, 180, 183, 187, 190, 203, 205, 211, 217, 241, 244, 251, 258, 267
Franklin, Jentezen 133, 243
frontal lobe xviii, 40, 65–66, 91, 210, 237

G

GABA 21, 23, 44, 101, 168, 195, 226–227, 250
gambling 5, 21, 40, 187, 247
gamma-aminobutyric acid. *See* GABA
gastrointestinal system xxv, 6, 14, 18, 23
gender 185, 188–189
generational curses xvii, 67–68, 225
genetic mutations 7, 19, 26, 82, 138, 160, 228
genitourinary system 14
George, Elizabeth 229
Global Mission Awareness 251
gluconeogenesis 18
glucose xviii, 28, 224, 227
glutamate 21
glycogen 18
gratitude xix, 67, 183, 217, 219–220, 271–272. *See also* Thanksgiving
guilt xxiii, 32, 50, 55, 103, 255–256

H

headaches 5–6, 56, 242
heart disease xxv, 22, 86, 150–151, 169, 187, 225, 230–233, 247
heaven 12, 15, 33, 35, 46, 53, 58–59, 61, 68, 90, 93–94, 99, 104–105, 107, 113, 115–118, 120–121, 125, 127–128, 130–131, 136, 138–139, 146–147, 159, 162, 169, 178, 180, 191, 199, 203, 214, 220–221, 236, 238, 249, 251–268, 272
Helming, Mary Blaszko xxiv, 213
heroin 20, 22, 38, 57
Hetland, Leif 251
Hinn, Benny 116
hippocampus xvii–xviii, 6, 13, 18–20, 27, 31–33, 79, 82–83, 106, 111, 154–155, 168, 226
HIV 158, 186
hormones 5–6, 14, 16–18, 31, 55, 62, 111, 150, 154–155, 165, 169, 188–190, 211, 224, 232
Horne, Benjamin 243
Huch, Larry 62, 93
Huch, Tiz 137
hypertension xviii, 28, 39, 83, 143, 150, 223, 230–231, 242. *See also* blood pressure
hypoglycemia 102
hypothalamic-pituitary-adrenal axis xviii
hypothalamus 6, 9, 13, 17, 19, 23, 111, 168, 189

I

identity 23, 73, 98, 100, 124, 126, 173, 181, 224, 264

Index

imagination 56–57, 87, 98, 102, 111, 115, 119–121, 125, 134–135, 140, 147, 165, 191, 193, 203, 214, 216, 259

immune system xviii, 6–7, 15–16, 18, 23, 82, 105, 169, 180, 191, 211, 219, 230, 246

inflammation xviii, 5–7, 18, 56, 86, 224, 227, 232, 246

insomnia 226–227, 242

integumentary system 6, 14

irritable bowel syndrome 6, 23, 242

J

Jakes, T. D. 81, 165
Jeffrey, Grant R. 24
Jesus movement 116
joy xvii–xviii, 42, 45, 47, 50, 55, 57–58, 62, 64–65, 69–71, 78, 82, 84, 88, 90–91, 93, 96, 101, 103, 108–109, 111–112, 114–117, 121, 123, 134, 137–140, 146, 153–154, 156, 160, 162, 165, 168–169, 175–178, 180–183, 186, 188–189, 191–192, 199–201, 203–205, 208, 212, 215, 218–219, 221, 237, 256–257, 260–261, 263, 267, 272

K

King, Brian 272

L

Lakewood Church 198
laminin 15
Leaf, Caroline 14, 17, 188–189
Levy, David 213
lifestyle xvii–xviii, 28, 39–40, 79, 81–84, 90, 95, 112, 143, 149–152, 158, 170, 183–184, 186, 205, 210, 223–225, 228, 230–233, 242–244, 247–248, 271
limbic system 9, 13, 20, 32, 47, 57, 82–83, 138, 155, 249
lipids 25, 56, 143, 225
lipoprotein 224, 230
loneliness 5, 31, 48, 50, 55, 58, 68, 71–73, 88, 91–92, 104–105, 177, 192, 221, 239, 251, 256
lymphatic system 6–7
lymphocytes 7

M

macrophages 7, 105
Manwaring, Paul 261
marijuana 13, 20, 22, 36–38, 56, 82
marriage 3, 66, 80, 93, 170, 180, 185–190, 207
Mason, Phil 98, 114
meditation xvii–xix, 13, 20, 39, 41–42, 47, 51, 57, 62, 68, 77–79, 82, 87, 91, 96–97, 101, 110, 134, 145–146, 151, 154–156, 165, 167, 174, 178, 188, 194–196, 210–212, 219, 227, 237–238, 243, 271–272

medulla xvii
melatonin 6, 17, 23, 226, 233
memory xviii, 9, 12–14, 17–21, 26–27, 32, 34, 36, 39–40, 44, 49, 57, 79, 81–83, 87, 89–90, 120–121, 134–135, 138, 140, 154–155, 162, 168, 172, 174, 181, 212, 219, 250, 258
  memory loss xix, 13, 20, 42, 242
metabolic syndrome xviii, 22–23, 28, 39–40, 83, 143, 150–152, 224–225, 230
Midwest Center for Stress and Anxiety 271
migraines 22
money. *See* finances
mood 5, 9, 22, 27, 37, 57, 138, 154–155, 162, 211, 225
Moore, Beth 57, 200
morphine 22, 55–57
motivation 13, 20, 40, 56, 83–84, 93, 122, 225, 264, 266
musculoskeletal system xxv, 6, 14

N

narcotics 36, 55–56, 226
necrosis 106
nervous system 12, 14, 17, 36, 55, 130
   autonomic nervous system 13, 16, 20–21, 155
   parasympathetic nervous system 16
   sympathetic nervous system xvii, 16
   central nervous system 14, 17, 227
   peripheral nervous system 14
neurocognitive disorders xix, 6, 20, 42, 60, 62, 77, 89, 120, 152, 202, 212, 236, 249
neurological system xxv, 6, 18, 155, 211, 248
neurons xvii–xviii, 6, 8–9, 12–14, 17–22, 27, 31, 33–35, 37, 40–41, 43, 55–58, 62, 77–78, 87, 89, 91, 97–98, 102, 105–106, 110, 116, 118, 124, 134, 138, 143, 145, 154–155, 171–172, 178, 188–189, 191, 194–195, 198–201, 206–208, 210–212, 219, 227, 237, 248–249, 271–272
   neurochemicals xvii–xviii, 3, 5, 9, 12, 16–22, 27, 31, 40–41, 43, 47, 49, 62, 80, 91, 93, 96, 106, 109, 123, 130, 140, 145, 151, 165, 168, 176, 188, 207, 218, 220, 237, 250, 271–272
neurogenesis xvii, 41, 77, 97, 154–155, 194, 211–212, 272
neuroplasticity xvii–xviii, 53, 64, 271
neurotransmitters xvii–xviii, 3, 5–6, 8–9, 12–14, 16–22, 27, 31, 36, 41, 44, 49, 57, 63–64, 78, 83, 87, 90, 92, 96–97, 101, 106, 108, 111, 116, 123, 150, 155, 162, 165, 168–169, 176, 181, 188–192, 195, 206–207, 211–212, 218, 226–227, 232–233, 239, 250, 271
New Beginnings Christian Center 202
nicotine 22, 154
non-pharmacological interventions 120, 179
norepinephrine xvii, 5, 16–17, 21, 57, 188, 226–227
nucleus accumbens 21, 27, 79

O

obesity 6, 28, 39, 143, 152, 224–225, 231–232, 242
occipital lobe 134
opioids 22, 36, 54–55
orbitofrontal cortex 33
Oregon Health & Science University xv, 4, 205, 224
orexin 226–227
Osteen, Dodie 205
Osteen, Joel 195, 198, 205
osteoporosis xviii, 6
overeating 39–40, 224, 233, 243, 247
oxygenation 5–6, 141, 152, 191, 230–231
oxytocin 21, 64, 78, 145, 168, 176, 188–190, 207, 218, 262

P

pandemic xxiv, 28, 92
panic attacks xxiv, 4–5, 18, 23, 39, 55, 210, 219, 236, 272
parents 7, 32–37, 44, 46, 48, 51, 56, 59, 66, 70, 81–82, 84, 111, 113, 118, 120–121, 125, 135, 141, 180, 203, 208, 216–217, 228, 239, 259, 262
parietal lobe 206, 210
pharmacological interventions 120, 179
pituitary gland xviii, 6, 16–17, 21, 189
pornography 32, 40, 80, 91, 120, 170, 186–187
Portland Adventist Community Services Health Clinic 37

Index

praise 8, 24, 27, 53, 61, 90, 92, 121, 131, 143, 157, 172, 175, 180, 182, 203, 216–221, 243, 250. *See also* worship

prayer xix, xxiv, 43–44, 47–50, 61, 63–64, 66–67, 72, 77–78, 85, 87, 91, 104–107, 110, 113–114, 118, 120–121, 131, 135–139, 142–143, 145–147, 156–157, 163, 165–166, 169–171, 173, 178, 180–183, 188, 192, 194, 200, 206, 210–211, 213–221, 227, 230, 234–242, 244, 249–250, 265–268, 271

prefrontal cortex 36, 39–40, 79, 82, 91, 117, 168

premarital sex 79–80, 229

prescriptions xvii–xix, xxv, 3, 8–11, 16, 18, 22–23, 25, 28, 32, 35–36, 38, 41–42, 50–51, 54–56, 58, 63–66, 69, 72, 77–80, 82–86, 90–92, 94–100, 104, 106, 108, 117–118, 121, 123–124, 127–128, 132, 141, 145–147, 151–154, 157, 163–164, 166, 170, 172–173, 175, 178, 180, 184–186, 188–191, 197, 199–200, 204, 208, 211–212, 215, 218, 220, 223–226, 232–233, 240, 243–244, 249, 255–256, 260, 265, 267, 270–272

priorities 62, 87–88

proteins xvii–xviii, 6, 15, 18, 25–26, 33, 56, 97–98,

150, 152, 223, 225, 246, 272

psychological stress xxv, 3, 8–9, 19, 36, 38, 42, 52, 80, 111, 121, 151, 188, 211

R

Răscol-Rady, Elena 70
Răscol-Rady, Vasile 70
rejection 31–32, 35–37, 46, 60, 83, 87, 92, 136, 251
relationships 42, 47, 50, 61–62, 64, 67, 80, 82–83, 91, 93, 99–100, 103, 105, 109, 114, 118, 120, 128, 140, 145, 162, 165, 170, 172, 180, 182, 185–186, 188–191, 194, 208, 212, 215, 235–236, 240, 243, 248–250, 252, 256

relaxation 13, 16, 92, 123, 130, 191, 258
    relaxation techniques 36, 42

repentance 48–51, 68, 93, 99, 103–106, 111, 146–147, 162, 183, 187, 241, 245

respiratory system 5, 16, 20, 22. *See also* breathing

RNA 25, 97

Rzheshevsky, A. V. 223

S

self-control 7, 21, 80, 117, 135, 149, 165, 169, 176–177, 186, 189

self-discipline 165, 170, 237, 261

self-esteem 23, 32, 35–38, 45–46, 82, 87, 90, 93–94, 113

sensory receptors 12, 19

serotonin xviii, 6, 17, 21–23, 35, 64, 66, 78, 168, 176, 188, 218, 220, 226, 227

shame 5, 50, 73, 134, 175, 251

Shirer, Priscilla 217

sin 47, 49–51, 58–59, 68–69, 81, 85, 88, 94, 98–100, 103–109, 111–113, 124–125, 128–130, 132, 138, 140–141, 143, 146–148, 154, 158–160, 162–164, 175, 187, 192, 194, 198–199, 203, 213, 226, 244, 250, 255–256, 266–268

sleep xviii, 6, 13, 21–23, 26, 42, 66, 80, 94, 102, 122, 138, 156, 225–227, 229, 233, 237, 239, 245, 257, 259
    REM sleep 21, 226
    sleep apnea 83, 152
    sleep disturbances xviii, 6, 36, 41, 56, 169, 224, 226

spiritual health xvii, xxiii–xxv, 4, 9–10, 22, 32, 39, 47, 50, 52–54, 59, 69, 85–86, 89, 92, 95, 97–101, 103–105, 108–109, 111, 115, 118, 126, 128–131, 143–144, 146, 152–153, 158–159, 164, 194, 198, 205–206,

212–213, 215, 224–225, 233, 243–244, 249, 266–267
Squier, Judy 175
Stanley, Charles 214
Star of Hope 66
stenosis 101, 231
Stoop, David 236
stress management xvii, xix, xxiv, 4, 6, 8, 13, 20, 28, 37, 41, 56, 90, 103, 149–150, 152, 177, 179, 187–188, 197, 204, 211, 216, 224, 229, 232, 242, 248, 250, 259, 270–271
Strobel, Lee 241
stroke 18, 22, 143, 150, 224–225, 230–233, 236
substance abuse 21–22, 32, 36, 38–39, 55, 62, 80, 82, 187, 249
suicide 3, 5, 22, 32, 37, 39, 46, 63, 176, 187, 260
symptoms xvii, xxiv, 5–9, 17–18, 21, 23, 27, 38, 40–41, 50, 52, 55, 60, 62, 78, 102, 116, 120–121, 165, 170, 187, 220, 231, 237, 239, 241, 258, 263
synapses 12–13, 19–21, 27, 43, 116

T

Tabor Crest 258
teenagers 32, 44, 46, 55–56, 69, 79, 82, 118, 159, 187, 200, 211, 234–235, 240, 247, 256. *See also* adolescents
ten Boom, Corrie 272
thalamus 9, 17, 19, 168
thanksgiving 77, 91, 106, 142, 216–222, 237, 244. *See also* gratitude
thyroid 6, 17, 41
thyroxine axis 17
toxicity xviii, 8, 20–21, 25, 41, 80, 86–87, 89, 131, 155, 158, 166, 189, 226, 228, 230, 242–243, 246–247, 252

V

vasopressin axis 17
Vujicic, Nick 80–81

W

Weaver, Joanna 197
will of God 31, 39, 47, 51–52, 64, 66–67, 78, 87, 92, 102, 128, 131, 136, 140, 143, 166, 177, 179–183, 188, 192, 214, 216–219, 232, 236–237, 246, 265
worry xix, xxiii–xxv, 3–5, 7–9, 13, 17–18, 21, 23–28, 31–32, 36, 38–42, 44–45, 47–48, 53, 56, 63–64, 69, 72, 77–78, 82–83, 88–93, 97, 104, 106, 108, 111–112, 120–122, 125, 127, 130–132, 137–138, 141, 144, 154–155, 163, 166, 177–178, 185, 188, 195, 197, 199, 210, 219–221, 225, 227, 230, 236, 238–239, 243, 246, 258, 262, 270–272
worship xix, 31, 59, 68, 78, 90, 113, 131, 139, 143, 147, 173, 204, 214, 220–221, 242, 250–251, 258, 266, 271. *See also* praise

Z

Zacharias, Ravi 157